T0263218

Liver Pathology

Editor

JAY H. LEFKOWITCH

GASTROENTEROLOGY
CLINICS OF NORTH AMERICA

www.gastro.theclinics.com

June 2017 • Volume 46 • Number 2

ELSEVIER

1600 John F. Kennedy Boulevard • Suite 1800 • Philadelphia, Pennsylvania, 19103-2899
http://www.theclinics.com

GASTROENTEROLOGY CLINICS OF NORTH AMERICA Volume 46, Number 2
June 2017 ISSN 0889-8553, ISBN-13: 978-0-323-53009-5

Editor: Kerry Holland
Developmental Editor: Alison Swety

Gastroenterology Clinics of North America (ISSN 0889-8553) is published quarterly by Elsevier Inc., 360 Park Avenue South, New York, NY 10010-1710. Months of issue are March, June, September, and December. Business and Editorial Offices: 1600 John F. Kennedy Blvd., Suite 1800, Philadelphia, PA 19103-2899. Customer Service Office: 6277 Sea Harbor Drive, Orlando, FL 32887-4800. Periodicals postage paid at New York, NY and additional mailing offices. Subscription prices are $330.00 per year (US individuals), $100.00 per year (US students), $616.00 per year (US institutions), $361.00 per year (Canadian individuals), $220.00 per year (Canadian students), $756.00 per year (Canadian institutions), $458.00 per year (international individuals), $220.00 per year (international students), and $756.00 per year (international institutions). Foreign air speed delivery is included in all *Clinics* subscription prices. All prices are subject to change without notice. **POSTMASTER**: Send address changes to *Gastroenterology Clinics of North America*, Elsevier Health Sciences Division, Subscription Customer Service, 3251 Riverport Lane, Maryland Heights, MO 63043. **Telephone: 1-800-654-2452 (U.S. and Canada); 314-447-8871 (outside U.S. and Canada). Fax: 314-447-8029. E-mail: journalscustomerservice-usa@elsevier.com (for print support); journalsonlinesupport-usa@elsevier.com (for online support)**.

Reprints. For copies of 100 or more, of articles in this publication, please contact the Commercial Reprints Department, Elsevier Inc., 360 Part Avenue South, New York, New York 10010-1710. Tel. 212-633-3874, Fax: 212-633-3820, E-mail: reprints@elsevier.com.

Gastroenterology Clinics of North America is also published in Italian by Il Pensiero Scientifico Editore, Rome, Italy; and in Portuguese by Interlivros Edicoes Ltda., Rua Commandante Coelho 1085, 21250 Cordovil, Rio de Janeiro, Brazil.

Gastroenterology Clinics of North America is covered in *MEDLINE/PubMed (Index Medicus)*, *Excerpta Medica*, *Current Contents/Clinical Medicine*, *Science Citation Index*, *ISI/BIOMED*, and *BIOSIS*.

Contributors

EDITOR

JAY H. LEFKOWITCH, MD
Professor, Department of Pathology and Cell Biology, Columbia University Medical Center, College of Physicians and Surgeons, Columbia University, New York, New York

AUTHORS

CHARLES BALABAUD, MD
Inserm U 1053, Université Bordeaux, Bordeaux, France

PAULETTE BIOULAC-SAGE, MD
Inserm U 1053, Université Bordeaux, Bordeaux, France

HERSCHEL A. CARPENTER, MD
Professor Emerita of Pathology, Department of Laboratory Medicine and Pathology, Mayo Clinic College of Medicine, Rochester, Minnesota

JONATHAN H. CHEN, MD, PhD
Department of Pathology, Massachusetts General Hospital, Harvard Medical School, Boston, Massachusetts

WON-TAK CHOI, MD, PhD
Assistant Professor, Department of Pathology, University of California at San Francisco, San Francisco, California

ALBERT J. CZAJA, MD
Professor Emeritus of Medicine, Division of Gastroenterology and Hepatology, Mayo Clinic College of Medicine, Rochester, Minnesota

VIKRAM DESHPANDE, MD
Department of Pathology, Massachusetts General Hospital, Harvard Medical School, Boston, Massachusetts

MILTON J. FINEGOLD, MD
Professor, Department of Pathology and Immunology, Texas Children's Hospital, Baylor College of Medicine, Houston, Texas

SARAH E. FLEET, MD
Clinical Fellow, Division of Pediatric Gastroenterology, Hepatology and Nutrition, Columbia University Medical Center, New York, New York

SANJAY KAKAR, MD
Professor, Department of Pathology, University of California at San Francisco, San Francisco, California

DAVID E. KLEINER, MD, PhD
Senior Research Physician, Chief Post-Mortem Section, Laboratory of Pathology, National Cancer Institute, Bethesda, Maryland

ANNE KNOLL KOEHNE DE GONZALEZ, MD
Gastrointestinal and Liver Pathology Fellow, Professor, Department of Pathology and Cell Biology, Columbia University, New York, New York

JOEL E. LAVINE, MD, PhD
Professor and Vice Chairman of Pediatrics, Columbia College of Physicians and Surgeons, Division of Pediatric Gastroenterology, Hepatology and Nutrition, Columbia University Medical Center, New York, New York

MICHAEL LEE, MD
Assistant Professor of Pathology and Cell Biology, Columbia University, New York, New York

JAY H. LEFKOWITCH, MD
Professor, Department of Pathology and Cell Biology, Columbia University Medical Center, College of Physicians and Surgeons, Columbia University, New York, New York

DANIELA LENGGENHAGER, MD
Department of Pathology and Molecular Pathology, University Hospital Zurich, Zurich, Switzerland

TANIA ROSKAMS, MD, PhD
Head, Liver Research Unit, Department of Imaging and Pathology, KU Leuven and University Hospitals Leuven, Leuven, Belgium

DEBORAH A. SCHADY, MD
Assistant Professor, Department of Pathology and Immunology, Texas Children's Hospital, Baylor College of Medicine, Houston, Texas

CHRISTINE SEMPOUX, MD, PhD
Service of Clinical Pathology, Lausanne University Hospital, Institute of Pathology, Lausanne, Switzerland

MARK W. SONDERUP, MBChB, FCP (SA), MMED (MED)
Associate Professor, Division of Hepatology, Department of Medicine, Groote Schuur Hospital and Faculty of Health Sciences, University of Cape Town, Observatory, Cape Town, South Africa

MICHAEL S. TORBENSON, MD
Professor of Pathology, Department of Laboratory Medicine and Pathology, Mayo Clinic Rochester, Rochester, Minnesota

MATTHIAS VAN HAELE, MD
Liver Research Unit, Department of Imaging and Pathology, KU Leuven and University Hospitals Leuven, Leuven, Belgium

HELEN CECILIA WAINWRIGHT, MBChB, FFPath
Associate Professor and Principle Pathologist, Department of Anatomical Pathology,
National Health Laboratory Services and Faculty of Health Sciences, D7 Groote Schuur
Hospital, University of Cape Town, Observatory, Cape Town, South Africa

ACHIM WEBER, MD
Department of Pathology and Molecular Pathology, University Hospital Zurich, Zurich,
Switzerland

Contents

> Pathologists are likely to encounter IgG4-related disease in several organ systems. This article focuses on helping pathologists diagnose IgG4-related disease in the hepatobiliary system. Missing the diagnosis can result in unnecessary organ damage and/or unnecessary surgical and cancer therapy. In the liver, tumefactive lesion(s) involving the bile ducts with storiform fibrosis and an IgG4-enriched lymphoplasmacytic infiltrate are highly concerning for IgG4-related disease. The recent identification of oligoclonal populations of T cells and B cells in IgG4-related disease may lead to molecular tests, new therapeutics, and a greater mechanistic understanding of the disease.

> Nonalcoholic fatty liver disease (NAFLD) represents a spectrum of disease. Its increasing prevalence is a direct result of historically high rates of obesity. Hepatocyte lipid accumulation is the first step in a cascade of metabolic and inflammatory events thought to precipitate NAFLD. Histologic findings provide insight into these events. Lifestyle modification remains the primary therapy in children. Current recommendations include vitamin E treatment in those with biopsy-proven NASH. Trials of novel drugs are ongoing in adults. As efficacy/safety are established, these therapies may be tenable for use in children. At the current time, biopsy-driven histology endpoints are necessary to establish whether future therapies can improve pediatric or adult-type NASH in children.

> Liver disease in the neonate, infant, child, and adolescent may manifest differently depending on the type of disorder. These disorders show marked overlap clinically and on light microscopy. Histology and ultrastructural examination are used in tandem for the diagnosis of most disorders. A final diagnosis or interpretation of the pediatric liver biopsy depends on appropriate and adequate clinical history, laboratory test results, biochemical assays, and molecular analyses, as indicated by the light microscopic and ultrastructural examination.

Mark W. Sonderup and Helen Cecilia Wainwright

The improvement in antiretroviral therapy has significantly impacted the lives of people living with human immunodeficiency virus (HIV). In high-income countries, HIV deaths are predominated by liver disease consequent to viral hepatitis coinfection, alcohol, and nonalcoholic fatty liver disease. Published liver pathology findings have shifted from being predominated by opportunistic infections to the metabolic effects of HIV and antiretroviral therapy as well as drug-induced liver injuries. Differences remain between high-income and low-income countries, where opportunistic infections and immune reconstitution syndromes, dominate findings.

Albert J. Czaja and Herschel A. Carpenter

Autoimmune hepatitis (AIH) may have an atypical serum alkaline phosphatase elevation, antimitochondrial antibodies, histologic features of bile duct injury/loss, or cholangiographic findings of focal biliary strictures and dilations. These manifestations characterize the overlap syndromes. Patients can be classified as having AIH with features of primary biliary cholangitis, primary sclerosing cholangitis, or a cholestatic syndrome. The gold standard of diagnosis is clinical judgment. Histologic evaluation is a major diagnostic component. Treatment is based on algorithms; outcomes vary depending on the predominant disease component. Combination therapy has been the principal recommendation.

Michael S. Torbenson

Hepatocellular carcinomas can be further divided into distinct subtypes that provide important clinical information and biological insights. These subtypes are distinct from growth patterns and are on based on morphologic and molecular findings. There are 12 reasonably well-defined subtypes as well as 6 provisional subtypes, together making up 35% of all hepatocellular carcinomas. These subtypes are discussed, with an emphasis on their definitions and the key morphologic findings.

Daniela Lenggenhager and Achim Weber

Infection with hepatitis E virus (HEV) is a leading cause of acute hepatitis worldwide, now increasingly recognized also in nonendemic regions. Clinical manifestation of hepatitis E includes mostly asymptomatic/subclinical presentations or acute, self-limiting hepatitis, but also potentially fatal liver failure or chronic hepatitis in immunocompromised individuals. Accordingly, hepatitis E histolpathologic patterns range from an unremarkable histology over acute (cholestatic) hepatitis with variable degree of necrosis to chronic hepatitis with fibrosis. Awareness of hepatitis E and its differential diagnoses, knowledge of its clinico-pathologic manifestations and familiarity with its diagnostic tools will enable clinicians and pathologists to competently make this diagnosis.

> Liver regeneration is a fascinating and complex process with many medical implications. An important component of this regenerative process is the hepatic progenitor cell (HPC). These appealing cells are able to participate in the renewal of hepatocytes and cholangiocytes when the normal homeostatic regeneration is exhausted. Moreover, the HPC niche is of vital importance toward the activation, differentiation, and proliferation of the HPC. This niche provides a rich microenvironment for the regulation of the HPC, thanks to the intercellular secretion of molecules. New findings indicate that the regenerative possibilities in the liver could provide a diverse basis for therapeutic targets.

> Liver injury due to acute and chronic heart failure has long been recognized. This article discusses the concepts of acute cardiogenic liver injury (ACLI) and cardiac or congestive hepatopathy (CH) along with their clinical manifestations and sequelae. Histologically, ACLI manifests as centrilobular hepatocellular necrosis, whereas CH is associated with centrilobular hepatocyte atrophy, dilated sinusoids, and perisinusoidal fibrosis, progressing to bridging fibrosis and ultimately cirrhosis. ACLI is associated with marked increases in aminotransferase levels, whereas CH is associated with a cholestatic pattern of laboratory tests. Certain cardiac medications have also been implicated as a cause of liver fibrosis.

GASTROENTEROLOGY
CLINICS OF NORTH AMERICA

RELATED INTEREST

Surgical Pathology Clinics
June 2013 (Vol. 6, Issue 2)
Liver Pathology
Sanjay Kakar and Dhanpat Jain, *Editors*
Available at: http://www.surgpath.theclinics.com

THE CLINICS ARE AVAILABLE ONLINE!
Access your subscription at:
www.theclinics.com

Preface

Liver Pathology

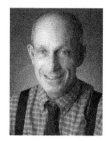

Jay H. Lefkowitch, MD
Editor

This issue of *Gastroenterology Clinics of North America* is devoted to liver pathology. It has been a pleasure to serve as guest editor and to assemble an esteemed roster of experts from the United States, Europe, and South Africa to provide their insights (and striking photomicrographs) on a spectrum of "of the moment" topics in hepatology. Over the past decade, IgG4-related disease (IgG4-RD) has entered the differential diagnostic lists of many organ systems. For the liver, the major representation of IgG4-RD is either as a biliary tract disease resembling primary sclerosing cholangitis (IgG4-sclerosing cholangitis or IgG4-SC) or as a mass obstructing the large bile ducts, resembling cholangiocarcinoma. Drs Chen and Deshpande make an important point about IgG4-RD involving the hepatobiliary system: although it may be an isolated condition, it is usually associated with other organ manifestations (eg, pancreatitis, tubulointerstitial nephritis). The useful photomicrographs and rich characterization of the pathogenesis and epidemiology of this unusual disorder are a helpful diagnostic resource.

Pediatric liver disease is represented by articles on nonalcoholic fatty liver disease and interpretation of the pediatric liver biopsy. Dr Fleet, Dr Lavine, and I cover the breadth of current knowledge on the demographics, histopathologic correlates (including the lesion referred to as type 2 nonalcoholic steatohepatitis [type 2 NASH], which involves portal and periportal regions, in contrast to the centrilobular involvement seen in adults with type 1 NASH). The pathogenesis of pediatric NASH is related to multiple hits, and the authors discuss roles for reactive oxygen species, overexpression of cytochrome p450 2E1, activation of hepatic stellate cells, and the adiponectin-leptin axis.

Interpretation of pediatric liver biopsies is a unique subspecialty within liver pathology that requires a different set of eyes from adult liver biopsies. As Drs Schady and Finegold concisely describe in their article, the diseases of neonates and children differ from adult conditions and include extrahepatic biliary atresia, metabolic disorders, mutations of bile salt transporter proteins, and others that may require different diagnostic techniques (transmission electron microscopy, genomic analysis, immunohistochemistry)

Gastroenterol Clin N Am 46 (2017) xiii–xv
http://dx.doi.org/10.1016/j.gtc.2017.03.001
0889-8553/17/© 2017 Published by Elsevier Inc.

to reach the correct diagnosis. They provide updates on the pathogenesis of biliary atresia (eg, maternal chimeric CD8+ T cells as the initial "hit") and two additional forms of progressive familial intrahepatic cholestasis: types 4 and 5. Their article serves as an excellent "primer" on the spectrum of pediatric liver disease.

The issue includes several articles on liver tumors, including hepatocellular adenomas (HCAs) and hepatocellular carcinoma (HCC). The astounding progress made during the last two decades in understanding the pathogenesis of HCAs is highlighted by Drs Bioulac-Sage, Sempoux, and Balabaud. The four recognized types of HCAs are now genomically correlated with their primary pathologic features and include steatotic, atypical, inflammatory, and unclassified types. The subtleties required for the pathologist handling these neoplasms are fully discussed and illustrated in their update. Practitioners who enjoy and/or want to learn more about the morphologic aspects of the liver will appreciate the comprehensive coverage of HCC in all its subtypes in Dr Torbenson's article. Dr Torbenson subdivides each of the subtypes into categories regarding morphology, clinical findings, molecular correlates, and prognostic elements. Twelve major subtypes, including steatohepatitic, clear cell, cirrhotomimetic, fibrolamellar, and others (including several proposed new candidate subtypes), are discussed at length and are accompanied by outstanding photomicrographs. Further amplification on the immunohistochemical menu available for confirming the presence of HCC (or differentiating it from metastatic neoplasms) is presented in the article by Drs Choi and Kakar.

There are multiple articles on medical liver diseases (including posttransplantation issues such as antibody-mediated rejection, or AMR). Dr Kleiner carefully outlines a pathway for the pathologist to pursue in order to optimize recognition of drug-induced liver injury (DILI). DILI may have a varied histologic spectrum, including cholestatic hepatitis, acute hepatitis, chronic hepatitis, chronic cholestasis, and acute cholestasis. Key images help distinguish among these and other lesions such as eosinophilia and/or granulomas. The clinical and (sometimes) pathologic conundrum of so-called overlap syndromes (autoimmune hepatitis-primary biliary cholangitis and autoimmune hepatitis-primary sclerosing cholangitis) reflects a mismatch of serologic test results and morphologic findings that do not sit happily together. This contentious topic is covered by longtime experts, Drs Czaja and Carpenter, with superb tables that provide enormous clarification. Drs Czaja and Carpenter provide very specific details on approaches to medication that should be most helpful for guiding therapy in these atypical cases.

Drs Sonderup and Wainwright provide a masterful and global look at how HIV and its treatment with antiretroviral medications impact the liver. The statistic that 37 million people worldwide are currently living with HIV is astonishing, and for those with concomitant chronic hepatitis B or C, there has been a well-recognized negative prognostic impact. Questions regarding potential DILI from antiretrovirals come up frequently in clinical practice, and their article is extremely helpful in distilling the liver pathology according to each of six classes of antiretroviral drugs (nucleoside reverse transcriptase inhibitors; nonnucleoside reverse transcriptase inhibitors; protease inhibitors; integrase inhibitors; fusion inhibitors; and chemokine receptor antagonists). This is a "must-read" article for pathologists, gastroenterologists, and hepatologists who take care of individuals with HIV.

The liver pathology associated with hepatitis E virus (HEV) has for many years been terra incognita. In this issue, Drs Lenggenhager and Weber bring many fascinating insights regarding HEV, including discussion of its structure, diagnostic testing (serum tests vs. molecular analysis), and the pathologic features of acute and chronic HEV infection. Their article is handsomely illustrated with pertinent examples of HEV infection in different clinical settings.

Individuals with acute or chronic heart failure may have serious hepatic complications that come to be further evaluated by liver biopsy, particularly if a heart transplant is contemplated and a possible heart-liver transplantation is on the horizon. In an article from my own medical center with Dr Koehne de Gonzalez, we discuss and illustrate the spectrum of morphologic changes in cardiac hepatopathy, from centrilobular congestion to cirrhosis, and rarely, to HCC. Cardiologists increasingly call on the pathologist to stage the degree of fibrosis in order to evaluate the need for combined heart-liver transplantation.

In their update on hepatic progenitor cells (HPCs), Drs Van Haele and Roskams review the role of these fascinating cells in liver disease, their prime location (the canal of Hering between the terminal segment of the bile duct epithelium and hepatocytes), and several of the immunohistochemical stains that are used in their identification, including EpCAM, NCAM, SOX9, CK7, and CK19, among others (Epithelial Cell Adhesion Molecule, Neural Cell Adhesion Molecule/CD56, sex-determining region Y-box 9, cytokeratin 7, and cytokeratin 19, respectively). The authors cite the multiple studies that corroborate that the ductular reaction is derived from activated HPCs, including their own work, which clarified that 50% of liver parenchyma must be lost before HPCs become activated. Senescence of hepatocytes as a driving factor is emphasized. There remains controversy on how regenerative activity and replacement of effete hepatocytes are accomplished, with the authors pointing out that the Zajicek concept of the "streaming liver" (the proceeding of new progeny hepatocytes in a "streaming" gradient from periportal HPCs downward toward the central veins) is at odds with other studies showing the possibility of more local replacement at lobular sites of cell loss, such as a self-renewing centrilobular population of hepatocytes.

Although the histopathology of acute cellular rejection following liver transplantation is widely known, the topic of AMR is currently a contentious one, with many unanswered questions (particularly for the hepatic pathologist). What is the best method for demonstrating C4d: immunofluorescence or immunohistochemistry? Dr Lee's pragmatic approach is to review the described light microscopic features and anticipated C4d staining (all well illustrated) in the context of other diagnostic criteria, including the presence of donor-specific antibodies.

I am indebted to all of the contributors to this issue who provided such superbly detailed articles and helpful illustrations. I greatly appreciate the invitation to serve as guest editor from Kerry Holland, editor of Gastroenterology Clinics of North America. I am also grateful to my longtime colleague in hepatology, Dr Norman Gitlin, who several decades ago first entrusted me with writing and guest editing for the Clinics in Liver Disease series. This issue points up the inextricable interrelationship between clinical hepatology and liver pathology, a link that has existed since the founding days of modern hepatology in the 1950s and continues unchanged into the future.

Jay H. Lefkowitch, MD
Department of Pathology and Cell Biology
Columbia University Medical Center
630 West 168th Street
PH 15 West, Room 1574
New York, NY, 10032, USA

E-mail address:
JHL3@columbia.edu

Erratum

Errors were made in the December 2016 issue of *Gastroenterology Clinics* (Volume 45, Issue 4) on pages 683–684 of the article, "Endoscopic Management," by Michael C. Bennett, Ricardo Badillo, and Shelby Sullivan. The "Mucosal resurfacing" section on page 683 incorrectly states that the Revita duodenal mucosal resurfacing procedure involves "the use of radiofrequency ablation." The correct procedure involves "the use of hydrothermal ablation." In the "Mucosal resurfacing" section on page 683, and in the Figure 12 caption on page 684, the location for Fractyl Laboratories was incorrectly listed as "Cambridge, Massachusetts." The correct location is "Lexington, Massachusetts."

http://dx.doi.org/10.1016/j.gtc.2017.05.001
0889-8553/17/© 2016 Elsevier Inc. All rights reserved.

gastro.theclinics.com

IgG4-related Disease and the Liver

Jonathan H. Chen, MD, PhD, Vikram Deshpande, MD*

KEYWORDS

- IgG4-related disease • IgG4 • IgG4-related sclerosing cholangitis
- Primary sclerosing cholangitis • Autoimmune pancreatitis

KEY POINTS

- IgG4-related disease (IgG4-RD) can present in the liver as cholangitis with or without tumefactive lesions. IgG4-RD affects a wide range of ages and both genders, but most commonly middle-aged to elderly men.
- Although imperfect, histology currently represents the single best gold standard for diagnosis of IgG4-RD. Classic histologic appearance is storiform fibrosis, obliterative phlebitis, and an IgG4-enriched lymphoplasmacytic infiltrate.
- An enriched IgG4+ lymphoplasmacytic infiltrate (IgG4:IgG ratio >0.4) supports, but is not sufficient for, a diagnosis. An interdisciplinary approach integrating pathologic features, imaging, and clinical history is necessary for diagnosis.
- IgG4-related sclerosing cholangitis (IgG4-SC) is an uncommon disease and a wide differential diagnosis should be considered, one that includes primary sclerosing cholangitis (PSC), bile duct carcinoma, intrahepatic cholangiocarcinoma, inflammatory myofibroblastic tumor (IMT), and lymphoproliferative disorders.
- Recent evidence suggests that IgG4-RD is associated with unique T-cell and B-cell oligoclonal populations that may help with diagnosis of IgG4-RD and uncover unique therapeutic targets.

INTRODUCTION

IgG4-RD is a recently described entity that generally presents with multifocal mass-forming lesions that are frequently concerning for cancer.[1,2] Like sarcoidosis and granulomatosis with polyangiitis (GPA) (formerly Wegener granulomatosis), this protean disease can affect 1 or more organs, synchronously or metachronously, and may present differently from patient to patient. Previously, the manifestations in each organ system were classified as unrelated diseases (eg, type 1 autoimmune

Disclosure Statement: The authors have nothing to disclose.
Department of Pathology, Massachusetts General Hospital, Harvard Medical School, 55 Fruit Street, Boston, MA 01224, USA
* Corresponding author.
E-mail address: vikramdirdeshpande@gmail.com

Gastroenterol Clin N Am 46 (2017) 195–216
http://dx.doi.org/10.1016/j.gtc.2017.01.001
0889-8553/17/© 2017 Elsevier Inc. All rights reserved.

gastro.theclinics.com

pancreatitis, Riedel thyroiditis, Küttner tumor [submandibular gland], and Mikulicz disease [salivary and lacrimal glands]).

The realization that patients often had lesions in multiple organs and expressed high levels of IgG4,[3] however, led to unification of these diseases under the IgG4-RD umbrella.[4,5] Currently, IgG4-RD is primarily diagnosed based on its characteristic histologic appearance notable for storiform fibrosis, obliterative phlebitis, and a lymphoplasmacytic infiltrate.[6] This lymphocytic infiltrate contains predominantly CD4[+] T cells but is especially remarkable for an increased number of plasma cells class-switched to express the IgG4 antibody isotype, with a high ratio of IgG4[+] to IgG[+] plasma cells. Most patients respond to steroids or rituximab in the short term.[7,8] Relapse is common, however, and better therapies are needed.

This review focuses on the diagnosis of IgG4-RD in the hepatobiliary system — commonly termed, *IgG4-SC*.[9–11] Diagnosing IgG4-SC can be especially challenging for the practicing pathologist because its lesions can mimic bile duct carcinoma, PSC, and other entities. Prior to the recognition of IgG4-SC, a majority of these cases were labeled as PSC. For example, retrospective review of a case published as PSC in the "Case Records of the Massachusetts General Hospital" series in *The New England Journal of Medicine* in 1982 reveals that the overall findings are more in keeping with IgG4-SC (**Fig. 1**).[12]

Further adding to the diagnostic difficulty is that bile duct biopsies are often small and may contain crush artifact, and needle biopsies from the liver may not show classic histologic features. Because biopsies may miss areas with neoplastic cells, the absence of malignant cells on a slide does not rule out cancer in a fibrotic specimen. Additionally, demographic features of age and gender provide little assistance in diagnosis. IgG4-RD generally presents in middle-aged to elderly men, which is a common presentation for bile duct carcinoma. Importantly, although IgG4-RD isolated to the hepatobiliary system occurs, it usually presents with other organ manifestations. A history of IgG4-RD, pancreatitis, sialadenitis, tubulointerstitial nephritis, dacryoadenitis, or retroperitoneal fibrosis should raise the possibility of IgG4-RD. Given that it generally portends a good prognosis with immunosuppressive therapy and can spare

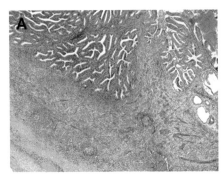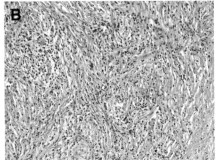

Fig. 1. The gallbladder (*A*, hematoxylin-eosin, original magnification ×40) shows an extramural fibroinflammatory infiltrate with storiform pattern of fibrosis (*B*, hematoxylin-eosin, original magnification ×100). Obliterative phlebitis was observed (not shown). An immunohistochemical stain for IgG4 performed retrospectively showed greater than 100 IgG4[+] plasma cells per HPF and an IgG4:IgG ratio greater than 40%. Collectively, the evidence supports a diagnosis of IgG4-SC. In the past, most examples of IgG4-SC were diagnosed PSC, as in this example.

patients surgery, radiation, and chemotherapy, astute pathologists can benefit patients with a timely diagnosis of IgG4-RD.

EPIDEMIOLOGY

The prevalence of IgG4-RD in North America is currently unknown. In the largest study to date in the United States,[13] IgG4-RD was found to affect both men and women, although a slight male predominance was identified. The mean age at presentation was 55 years. The disease was found in all ethnicities, although whites constituted a majority of cases. The most commonly involved sites were submandibular gland (28%), lymph node (27%), orbit (22%), pancreas (19%), retroperitoneal fibrosis (18%), lung (18%), and parotid gland (17%).[13] With the obvious exception of ethnicity, these data are fairly consistent with several recent large studies of patients in China and Japan.[14–17]

IgG4-RD commonly involves the hepatobiliary system. In the United States cohort, 10% presented with bile duct lesions.[13] In a Japanese study of 235 consecutive IgG4-RD patients, 13 (6%) presented with bile duct lesions.[14] Smaller Italian and Spanish studies each found 4% of IgG4-RD patients presented with bile duct lesions.[18,19] In Japan, it has been estimated that the annual incidence of autoimmune pancreatitis is 1.44 per 100,000, with a prevalence of 4.6 per 100,000.[20,21] Among patients with autoimmune pancreatitis, 10.3% have disease at the hepatic hilum and 24% had disease involving the intrahepatic tree.[20,21]

In 1 of the largest single institutional series of IgG4-SC, the Mayo Clinic reported 53 patients with IgG4-RD involving the liver, bile duct, or pancreas. This study refers to the hepatobiliary manifestations of IgG4-RD as IgG4-associated cholangitis (IAC), although IgG4-SC now represents the more widely used term.[22] This population had a mean age of 62 years and 85% of patients were male. Intrapancreatic bile duct lesions were found in 70% and were an isolated finding in 51% of patients. Proximal extrahepatic biliary strictures were found in 34% and were an isolated finding in 9% of patients. Intrahepatic strictures were found in 36% and were an isolated finding in 8% of patients. Thus, within this cohort of IgG4-SC patients, fully 17% had isolated lesions in the hepatobiliary system outside of the pancreas. Similarly, a more recent British study of patients with autoimmune pancreatitis/IgG4-SC found that 8% of IgG4-SC cases lacked involvement of the pancreas.[23] Nevertheless, any pathologist considering a diagnosis of IgG4-RD of the hepatobiliary system should look for a history of lesions in the pancreas and other organs. For example, within the 235-patient Japanese IgG4-RD cohort, 95% of patients had at least one of the 5 most common manifestations: pancreatitis (60%), sialadenitis (34%), tubulointerstitial nephritis (23%), dacryoadenitis (23%), and periaortitis (20%).[14]

Additional epidemiologic work indicates that approximately 6% to 10% of IgG4-SC patients also have inflammatory bowel disease (IBD), predominantly ulcerative colitis, with a minority having Crohn disease.[22,23] Also intriguingly, Dutch and UK cohorts revealed that 61% to 88% of patients with IgG4-SC or type 1 autoimmune pancreatitis were from the blue collar workforce, compared with 14% of patients with PSC, suggesting that chronic chemical exposure might play a role in this disease.[24] Additional studies are needed to clarify whether these detected associations occurred by chance alone or are truly associated with IgG4-RD.

PATHOPHYSIOLOGY

Recent works highlighting aberrant oligoclonal B-cell and cytotoxic CD4+ T-cell populations as well as increased plasmablasts constitute important new discoveries, improving understanding of IgG4-RD pathophysiology.[25,26] Next-generation sequencing of the B-cell repertoire revealed multiple dominant IgG4 clones among the IgG clones in IgG4-SC patients but not those with PSC or pancreatobiliary carcinoma.[25] These B-cell clones were greatly reduced by steroid therapy.

Although plasma cells are expanded in IgG4-RD, T cells are actually the dominant mononuclear cell infiltrate. Recent characterization of the T-cell infiltrate in patients with IgG4-RD has revealed aberrant clonal populations of cytotoxic CD4$^+$ T cells expressing the marker SLAMF7[26] (**Fig. 2**). These aberrant CD4$^+$ T cells expressed the cytotoxic molecule granzyme A as well as the profibrotic molecules interleukin (IL)-1β and transforming growth factor (TGF)-β1, suggesting that these T cells promote fibrosis in IgG4-RD.[26] The mechanism behind obliterative phlebitis, a highly characteristic finding, remains unresolved.

Next-generation sequencing of these CD4$^+$SLAMF7$^+$ T cells showed them to be oligoclonal, suggesting an antigen-driven phenomenon. Interestingly, rituximab therapy induced loss of the CD4$^+$SLAMF7$^+$ population, indicating that maintenance of the CD4$^+$SLAMF7$^+$ T-cell population likely depends on B cells in IgG4-RD. The identification of oligoclonal plasmablast and CD4$^+$SLAMF7$^+$ T-cell populations may lead to a better understanding of IgG4-RD pathophysiology. Further validation may also lead to acceptance of molecular diagnostics for IgG4-RD and possibly therapeutic targeting of this T-cell population.

Epithelial organs are the primary targets of IgG4-RD, supporting the hypothesis that epithelial proteins are antigenic targets. The antigens that drive disease, however, remain elusive. IgG4 antibodies from the serum of IgG4-RD patients bind to the

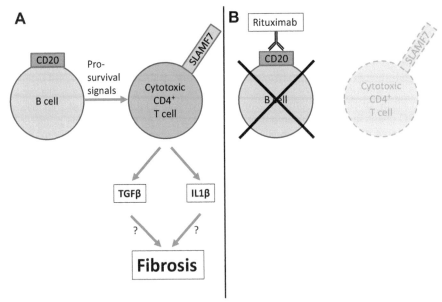

Fig. 2. (*A*) IgG4-RD is associated with oligoclonal populations of aberrant cytotoxic CD4$^+$ T cells characterized by SLAMF7 expression. These cytotoxic CD4$^+$ T cells express IL-1β and TGF-β1, which may promote the characteristic fibrosis observed in IgG4-RD. (*B*) It is hypothesized that these cytotoxic CD4$^+$ T cells depend on B cells for their survival. Therapeutic depletion of B cells with the anti-CD20 antibody rituximab may lead to a decrease of this aberrant cytotoxic CD4$^+$ T-cell population.

epithelium lining the pancreatic ducts, salivary gland ducts, intrahepatic and extrahepatic ducts, and gallbladder.[27] Some studies indicate that the antigens recognized are carbonic anhydrases II and IV as well as secretory products of these epithelia, such as lactoferrin, amylase α-2A, pancreatic trypsinogens, and pancreatic secretory trypsin inhibitor.[2,28–32] These antibodies, however, are neither specific nor sensitive for IgG4-RD, and the presence of these antibodies may simply be indicative of epitope spreading.

While some research suggests that IgG4-RD is a Type 2 T helper (T_H2)-mediated disease, other research calls this into question. There are a few features of IgG4-RD that argue for a T_H2-type disease.[33] First, the IgG4 and IgE isotypes, which are enriched in IgG4-RD, are generally induced in diseases with a prominent T_H2 skew. IgG4 selection in particular has been shown to be driven by the presence of T_H2 cytokines in conjunction with IL-10.[34,35] Second, T_H2 conditions have been shown to promote fibrosis in other disease models, whereas T_H1 conditions are thought to inhibit fibrosis. These findings have led researchers to search for a link between IgG4-RD and T_H2 factors. A recent study found that T_H2 CD4$^+$ T cells isolated from the blood of IgG4-RD patients more potently induced naïve B cell differentiation into plasmablasts than T_H1 and T_H17 T cells from these same patients.[36] However, it should be noted that this same study found relatively similar T_H1 and T_H2 CD4$^+$ T cell upregulation in the blood of IgG4-RD patients, each correlating with disease activity. Other studies have found that a substantial percentage of IgG4-RD patients report a history of allergy. For example, a Mayo Clinic study found that 15% of autoimmune pancreatitis patients reported allergic symptoms, such as hay fever, allergic rhinitis, or asthma, whereas only 4% of the healthy control group did.[37] However, this cohort group seems to under-represent the actual combined prevalence of hay fever, allergic rhinitis, and asthma. The prevalence of allergic rhinitis alone likely exceeds 15% in the United States.[38] Thus, it is not clear that the IgG4-RD population is enriched for patients with atopy. Furthermore, calling a T_H2-type immune response into question, the study that found oligoclonal expansion of CD4$^+$SLAMF7$^+$ cells failed to find any clonal expansion of T_H2-skewed CD4$^+$ T cells in the same patient cohort.[26] Another study from the same group found that T cells from patients with IgG4-related dacryoadenitis and sialoadenitis expressed a predominantly cytolytic CD4$^+$ T-cell infiltration but not a T_H2 gene profile compared with chronic sialoadenitis patients and healthy controls.[39,40] Taken together, although the extensive fibrosis and predominance of IgG4 and IgE isotypes are certainly suggestive, characterization of IgG4-RD patients has not yet yielded definitive evidence that IgG4-RD is a T_H2-type disease.

The mechanistic role of IgG4 antibodies in IgG4-RD is unclear, in large part because the function of IgG4 antibodies is not well understood in general. In comparison to other IgG subtypes, the constant (Fc) portion of the IgG4 antibody seems to be relatively immunologically inert. It binds poorly to the C1q complex and does not activate the classic complement pathway.[41,42] Additionally, the Fc region of IgG4 antibody binds poorly to Fc receptors.[41,42] Intriguingly, the IgG4 molecules possess the unique ability to undergo half-antibody exchange, a process whereby a given IgG4 antibody can split in 2 and recombine with a different IgG4 antibody, such that the recombined antibody has 2 different Fab fragments, each specific for a different epitope. This half-antibody exchange is thought to occur in approximately half of IgG4 molecules and may limit the ability of IgG4 to cross-link antigen, possibly further limiting the biologic reactivity of the IgG4 antibody.[41,43] The lack of clear immune function of IgG4 antibodies has led some to speculate that the antibody is either noninflammatory or anti-inflammatory.[41,44] In sum, knowledge of the function of the IgG4 antibody provides no solid explanation why this isotype is enriched in IgG4-RD. It can be speculated that the IgG4 antibodies may actually be part of a counter-regulatory process that develops to inhibit progression of IgG4-RD. Alternatively, the IgG4$^+$ plasmablasts play a role in promoting IgG4-RD outside of their secretion of antibodies, perhaps serving as antigen presenting cells for the CD4$^+$ cytotoxic T cells.

CLINICAL PRESENTATION

As discussed previously, either gender can be affected across a wide age range, but patients are generally middle-aged to elderly and predominantly male. The clinical presentation of IgG4-RD patients usually correlates with the location of disease. The typical presentation of IgG4-SC is obstructive jaundice, often in the setting of abnormal liver function tests.[22,23] In addition to these, IgG4-RD involving the pancreas (type 1 autoimmune pancreatitis) can also present with weight loss, steatorrhea, mild abdominal pain, and new-onset diabetes mellitus.[22]

RADIOLOGIC PRESENTATION

Cross-sectional imaging detects either a hilar or perihilar mass. Biliary strictures and thickening of bile duct walls may be the only radiologic signs, although these lesions may also be associated with a mass. Long and multifocal strictures with mild upstream dilatation are features supportive of a diagnosis of IgG4-SC. Even in expert hands, however, the sensitivity of ERCP findings is low (45%), highlighting the challenge of distinguishing IgG4-SC from PSC and bile duct carcinoma.[45] Involvement of the gallbladder and pancreas also be may observed. The imaging findings of the pancreas are generally highly characteristic — a "sausage-shaped" swollen pancreas.

A cholangiogram-based classification of IgG4-SC highlights the diverse patterns of biliary involvement in IgG4-RD.[10] Among these patterns, isolated involvement of the common bile duct (type I) and isolated hilar stricture (type IV) are most likely to be confused with bile duct and hilar carcinoma, respectively.[10]

SEROLOGY

Among IgG isotype antibodies, IgG1, IgG2, IgG3, and IgG4 are named in approximately descending order of serum levels. IgG4 has a wide range of expression among healthy individuals but is fairly constant over time in any individual.[41,46]

Serum IgG4 concentrations are normal in approximately 10% to 40% patients with IgG4-RD.[47–50] Thus, a normal serum IgG4 does not exclude the diagnosis of IgG4-RD.

Despite this limitation, serum IgG4 is perhaps the most important component of the diagnostic algorithm.[50] In a European cohort, serum IgG4 greater than 1.4 g/L had a 90% sensitivity, 85% specificity, and 59% positive predictive value (PPV) in diagnosing IgG4-SC over PSC. For serum IgG4 greater than 2.8 g/L, there was a 70% sensitivity, 98% specificity, and 88% PPV for IgG4-SC over PSC. Finally, for IgG4 greater than 5.6 g/L, there was a 42% sensitivity, 100% specificity, and 100% PPV for IgG4-SC over PSC.

Given the importance of serum IgG4, the most problematic patients are those with normal serum IgG4 concentrations, constituting approximately 10% to 20% of cases of IgG4-SC.[48,50] It has been suggested that this group might be clinically distinct, with limited sites of involvement and reduced risk of relapse. It has been shown that serum IgG4 concentrations are frequently not elevated in patients with isolated organ involvement.[47] A serum-based quantitative polymerase chain reaction test that analyzes the IgG4:IgG mRNA ratio may assist in evaluating patients with normal serum

IgG4 levels: a ratio of greater than 0.05 was 94% sensitive and 99% specific for IgG4-RD over PSC and biliary/pancreatic malignancy.[25]

A peripheral blood test that may have diagnostic implications is the presence of elevated numbers of plasmablasts in IgG4-RD.[51,52] Plasmablasts, however, are also identified in a variety of other immunologically mediated diseases, such as rheumatoid arthritis and systemic lupus erythematosus. Increased plasmablasts in blood may be an early indicator of relapse in patients with IgG4-RD.[51,52] Additionally, elevated rheumatoid factor, antinuclear antibodies (ANAs), and hypergammaglobulinemia are common in IgG4-RD.[11]

GENERAL PATHOLOGIC FEATURES OF IgG4-RELATED DISEASE

The combination of the characteristic histologic features and increased numbers of IgG4+ plasma cells are currently central to diagnosis of IgG4-RD.[6] Although the same characteristic histologic features identified in other organs are also present in IgG4-RD of the hepatobiliary system, the small and often fragmented biopsy specimens, a wide differential diagnosis and numerous histologic mimics mandate extraordinary caution on the part of pathologists.

The so-called Boston consensus criteria describe 3 principal histologic and a couple of additional minor criteria for the diagnosis of IgG4-RD.[6] Generally, a diagnosis requires at least 2 of the 3 major criteria:

- Dense lymphoplasmacytic infiltrate (**Fig. 3**)
- Fibrosis, arranged at least focally in a storiform pattern (see **Fig. 3**)
- Obliterative phlebitis (**Fig. 4**)

Additional findings that are neither sensitive nor specific are

- Phlebitis that does not obliterate the lumen
- Increased eosinophil numbers

In addition to the histologic findings, 2 principal supporting immunohistochemistry findings are described (**Fig. 5**):

- Elevated IgG4+ cells
- IgG4:IgG ratio greater than 40%

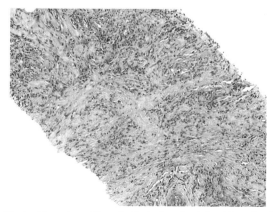

Fig. 3. IgG4-RD with storiform-type fibrosis. Note the short fascicles of spindle-shaped cells, accompanied by a lymphoplasmacytic infiltrate, seem to emanate from the central portion of the image (hematoxylin-eosin, original magnification ×100).

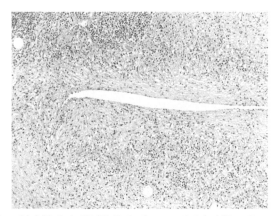

Fig. 4. Obliterative phlebitis in IgG4-SC. Note the near total obliteration of the vein (hematoxylin-eosin, original magnification ×40).

Storiform fibrosis refers to cartwheel patterns with spokes of fibroblasts radiating outward from a central nidus. The spindle cells comprise either myofibroblasts or fibroblasts and contain a lymphoplasmacytic infiltrate. Some cases may lack storiform-type fibrosis and instead show a cellular form of fibrosis. Biopsy samples may not capture either form of fibrosis. Nevertheless, deposition of collagen seems to be a cardinal feature of IgG4-RD, and its absence is exceptionally uncommon. Keloid-type collagen is, however, an uncommon finding in IgG4-RD.

Obliterative phlebitis is characterized by a dense lymphoplasmacytic infiltrate that destroys the vein. Lymphocytes and plasma cells expand the wall and occupy the lumen of the vein. This infiltrate is similar to that noted in the adjacent involved parenchyma and is accompanied by fibroblasts. Fibrinoid necrosis is not a feature of IgG4-RD. The biopsy may capture veins at varying phases of obliteration. Although mural and perivenular inflammation with only limited obliteration (<50%) supports a diagnosis, it is not considered specific for IgG4-RD. Alternatively, in more advanced cases of phlebitis, an elastic stain may be required to identify the obliterated vein. Obliterative arteritis is occasionally observed, with histologic features similar to those

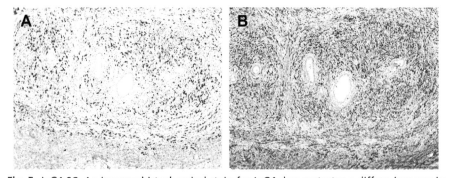

Fig. 5. IgG4-SC. An immunohistochemical stain for IgG4 demonstrates a diffuse increase in IgG4+ plasma cells (IgG4 immunohistochemistry) (A). The diffuse increase in IgG4+ plasma cells (as opposed to patchy and focal) is suggestive of IgG4-RD. An IgG stain was also performed (IgG immunohistochemistry) (B). The IgG4:IgG ratio was greater than 40%.

observed in an obliterated vein. Obliterative arteritis is typically confined to the pancreas, lung, and occasionally the retroperitoneum.

Histologic features that are generally considered to be atypical for IgG4-RD include the presence of necrosis, large numbers of giant cells, a predominantly histiocytic infiltrate, and necrotizing arteritis. Special stains for histiocytes, however, such as CD163, invariably reveal a substantial number of tissue macrophages.

The number of IgG4+ plasma cells per high-power field (HPF) (400-fold magnification) and the IgG4+:IgG+ plasma cell ratio are key diagnostic elements that can support a diagnosis of IgG4-RD. For a diagnosis of IgG4-RD, it is thought that the minimum number of IgG4 cells per HPF ranges from 10 to 100, depending on the organ involved.[6] For the liver or bile ducts, the cutpoints suggested are greater than 50 IgG4+ cells/HPF for surgical resection specimens and greater than 10 IgG4+ cells/HPF for biopsies.[6] An IgG4:IgG ratio of greater than 0.4 on immunohistochemistry is a commonly cited cutoff in the diagnosis of IgG4-RD.[6,53–56] The IgG4:IgG ratio is often the single most useful parameter on biopsy specimens. Pathologists should be aware that quantification of IgG and IgG4 on immunohistochemical staining can be problematic. IgG staining in particular must be evaluated with caution because it may have high background. The authors recommend counting the 3 HPFs with the highest density of IgG4+ plasma cells and using these same 3 fields for IgG+ counts to generate the IgG4:IgG ratio. In the authors' experience, this is also the case in hepatobiliary IgG4-RD. The ratio should be interpreted, however, with care when few plasma cells are present (eg, 10 plasma cells/HPF). In this situation, the small population of positive cells may not be representative, resulting in an incorrect IgG4:IgG ratio. Pathologists must keep in mind that bile duct carcinomas can also show elevated numbers of IgG4+ cells. In studies of extrahepatic cholangiocarcinoma (bile duct carcinoma), greater than 10 IgG4+ plasma cells per HPF were identified in 37% to 43% of cases, and greater than 50 IgG4+ cells per HPF were counted in 6% of cases.[57,58] Thus, an undersampled bile duct carcinoma may be misdiagnosed as IgG4-SC if a pathologist is overly reliant on the IgG4+ cell count. PSC may also be misdiagnosed as IgG4-SC in a similar manner. For example, a study of PSC liver explants found that 23% of livers showed greater than 10 IgG4+ cells per HPF.[59] Additionally, 22% of cases showed increased IgG4 serum levels. Characteristic histologic features, however, of IgG4-RD were not identified.[59]

PATHOLOGIC FEATURES SPECIFIC TO IgG4-RELATED SCLEROSING CHOLANGITIS
Hepatic and Perihilar Lesions

Grossly, the disease may mimic bile duct carcinoma, with thickening of the bile duct as well as expansion and fibrosis at the porta hepatis. Less commonly, a well-circumscribed intrahepatic mass may be identified (**Fig. 6**). The characteristic histologic features of IgG4-RD are generally identified in the hilar region, adjacent to large-caliber bile ducts. The tissue between vascular and biliary structures is expanded by a fibroinflammatory infiltrate and storiform-type fibrosis is virtually always seen (**Figs. 7** and **8**). Obliterated large and small caliber venous channels are easily identified. The linings of large caliber bile ducts, although surrounded by a dense inflammatory infiltrate, are intact (**Fig. 9**). In more peripheral portions of the liver, the portal tracts are expanded and typically infiltrated by a mixed inflammatory infiltrate composed of lymphocytes, plasma cells, and eosinophils (**Fig. 10**). A majority of portal tracts lack fibrosis. In a minority of cases, however, a portal-based expansile inflammatory nodule is identified, one composed of fibrosis and inflammation, and this

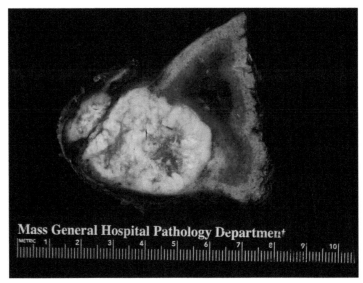

Fig. 6. On histologic evaluation, this 6-cm mass lesion showed pathologic features of IgG4-SC. The disease was confined to the liver, and hepatic hilar involvement was not identified.

appearance is characteristic for IgG4-RD (see **Fig. 7**).[60] These fibroinflammatory nodules are generally not captured on a needle biopsy.

Involvement of the Bile Duct

The involvement of the bile duct creates a highly characteristic histologic appearance (**Fig. 11**). The most reliable feature is the presence of a full-thickness, uniformly dense inflammatory infiltrate. The involvement of the outer half of the biliary wall is particularly characteristic, and obliterative phlebitis and storiform-type fibrosis are typically observed in this region. The lining epithelium is generally intact, although the presence of a stent could precipitate extensive loss of epithelium.

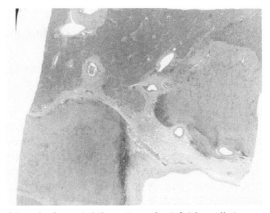

Fig. 7. IgG4-SC involving the hepatic hilum. Note the 2 fairly well circumscribed fibroinflammatory lesions. Similar nodules, albeit somewhat smaller, may also be detected in the peripheral portions of the liver (hematoxylin-eosin, original magnification ×20).

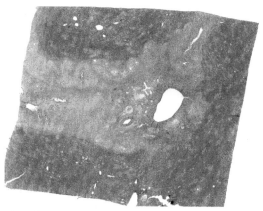

Fig. 8. Low-power view showing an expansile fibroinflammatory lesion involving the secondary branches of the biliary tree. In addition, note the portal tracts seem expanded (hematoxylin-eosin, original magnification ×20).

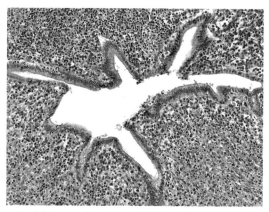

Fig. 9. The bile duct in this image is surrounded by a dense lymphoplasmacytic infiltrate. This stellate-shaped narrowing of the bile duct — a feature also seen in type 1 autoimmune pancreatitis — is a common feature noted in IgG4-SC. Also note that the biliary epithelium appears preserved (hematoxylin-eosin, original magnification ×100).

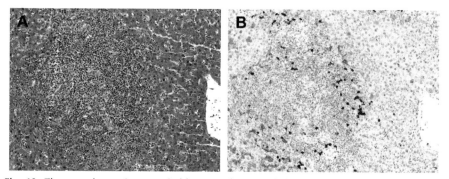

Fig. 10. The portal tract is expanded by a predominantly lymphocytic infiltrate with interface activity. Apoptotic hepatocytes are conspicuously absent (A) (hematoxylin-eosin, original magnification ×200). The increased numbers of IgG4$^+$ plasma cells (B) (Immunohistochemistry for IgG4), although suggestive of IgG4-RD, in and of themselves are not diagnostic, and would not definitively distinguish IgG4-RD from PSC.

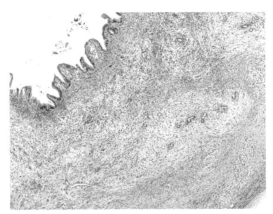

Fig. 11. A section from the common bile duct showing full-thickness inflammation, a characteristic histologic appearance of IgG4-RD involving the bile duct (hematoxylin-eosin, original magnification ×20).

BIOPSY DIAGNOSIS

Because the diagnostic areas are localized to the outer portion of the bile duct, biopsies are often non-diagnostic. The diagnosis is consequently greatly reliant on documentation of elevated numbers of IgG4+plasma cells and an elevated IgG4:IgG ratio. Compounding the difficulties described previously, immunohistochemical stains for IgG4 and IgG on small biopsies typically show strong background signal. Histologic mimics of IgG4-SC in the hepatobiliary system, in particular bile duct carcinoma and pancreatic adenocarcinoma, warrant careful consideration and are discussed later. As a general rule, a definitive diagnosis of IgG4-RD is seldom possible on a bile duct biopsy, although the histologic findings may provide supportive information. The primary role of such biopsies is generally to rule out malignancy.

AMPULLARY BIOPSIES FOR THE DIAGNOSIS OF IgG4-RELATED SCLEROSING CHOLANGITIS

Biopsies from the pancreas, bile duct, and liver are technically challenging, and these limited samples may not provide the necessary diagnostic information. Ampullary biopsies are often used as a surrogate test for IgG4-RD. Ampullary disease, when present, is generally clinically asymptomatic. The histologic features of IgG4-RD are virtually absent on ampullary biopsies. The diagnosis thus relies entirely on the presence of greater than 10 IgG4+ plasma cells per HPF.[61] Although an elevated IgG4:IgG ratio adds an additional layer of security, a diagnosis that relies solely on enumeration of these cells is fraught with danger. In the authors' experience, ampullary biopsies show a low sensitivity and are also reported to show low specificity.[62] Nevertheless, they can be of some assistance but only when viewed in the broader clinical context.

DIAGNOSTIC ALGORITHM

In most instances, diagnosis of IgG4-SC is made in conjunction with clinical and radiologic appearance. The acronym, HISORt, initially created for autoimmune pancreatitis and subsequently applied to IgG4-SC, highlights the 5 cardinal diagnostic features of

IgG4-RD: (1) histology, (2) imaging, (3) serology — specifically elevated serum IgG4, (4) other organ involvement, and (5) response to immunosuppressive therapy.[22,63] Two or more of these parameters are generally required before a diagnosis of IgG4-RD is considered. Clinical, biochemical, and/or cholangiographic improvement is generally seen within 4 to 6 weeks after starting steroids. In instances where there is uncertainty about the diagnosis, clinicians may resort to a trial of steroids. A swift response may provide an additional layer of reassurance but is not in and of itself diagnostic. Bile duct carcinomas and pancreatic ductal adenocarcinomas may show limited but not sustained response to steroids.

DIFFERENTIAL DIAGNOSIS
Primary Sclerosing Cholangitis

The many overlapping features between PSC and IgG4-SC make this distinction a difficult problem, and occasionally an insurmountable challenge (**Box 1**). Distinguishing IgG4-SC from PSC is important, given that IgG4-RD lesions resolve with immunosuppressive therapy. PSC is associated with a much poorer prognosis and a substantially increased risk of bile duct carcinoma. The American College of Gastroenterology recommends the measurement of serum IgG4 levels in all patients with possible PSC to exclude IgG4-SC.[64]

The average age at presentation in PSC (44 years old) is younger than IgG4-SC (63 years old)[60] (**Table 1**). A majority of cases of PSC come to light at laboratory evaluation for liver function tests, whereas most cases of IgG4-SC present with clinical and enzymatic changes of cholestasis. An overwhelming majority of patients with PSC have evidence of inflammatory bowel disease. There seems a small but significant association, however, of IgG4-RD with inflammatory bowel disease.[22,23] A careful evaluation of the HISORt criteria is helpful in many instances.

Histologic features may assist in the distinction of IgG4-SC from PSC but are seldom pathognomonic in isolation. Inflammatory nodules, alluded to previously, are not seen in PSC. It is suggested that the loss of bile ducts may assist in the distinction, with a paucity of bile ducts uncommon in IgG4-SC. Onion skin–type periductal fibrosis, although a characteristic finding of PSC, has also been observed in IgG4-SC (**Fig. 12**). Elevated numbers of IgG4+ plasma cells, although more common in IgG4-RD, are observed in a small proportion of cases of PSC. Increased numbers of IgG4+ cells or serum IgG4 concentrations must be interpreted in the context of clinical and histologic features to differentiate PSC from IgG4-RD (**Fig. 13**).

Box 1
Differential diagnosis of IgG4-related sclerosing cholangitis

- PSC
- Bile duct carcinoma and intrahepatic cholangiocarcinoma
- Lymphoproliferative disorder
- Follicular cholangitis
- Sclerosing cholangitis with granulocytic epithelial lesions
- IMT
- Fibrohistiocytic variant of inflammatory pseudotumor

Table 1
Contrasting IgG4-related sclerosing cholangitis and primary sclerosing cholangitis

	IgG4-related Sclerosing Cholangitis	Primary Sclerosing Cholangitis
Age	50–70 years old	30–50 years old
Gender	M > F	M > F
Cholangiographic appearance	Thickening of bile duct walls; long strictures with upstream dilatation	Bile duct with short segment strictures and interspersed normal caliber or dilated segments (beads-on-a-string appearance)
Other organ involvement	IgG4-RD frequently involves pancreas, salivary glands, kidneys, periorbital tissues, aorta, lymph nodes, lungs, meninges, etc.	Inflammatory bowel disease
Serum IgG4 >140 mg/dL	90%	15%
Histology	Dense lymphoplasmacytic infiltrate; storiform fibrosis; obliterative phlebitis; onion skin–type periductal fibrosis (rare)	Loss of bile ducts; onion skin–type periductal fibrosis
Immunohistochemistry: > 10 IgG4+ cells/HPF or IgG4:IgG ratio >0.4	Usually	Occasionally
Response to immunosuppressive therapy	Swift	Minimal

The presence of characteristic radiologic or histologic features of IgG4-RD in other organs is greatly reassuring and in many instances sufficient evidence to render a categorical diagnosis of IgG4-RD, sparing patients an invasive procedure and a potentially nondiagnostic biopsy. Prior biopsies are often available in these patients, most

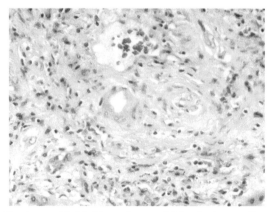

Fig. 12. IgG4-SC. The image highlights a damaged bile duct as well as subtle periductal fibrosis (hematoxylin-eosin, original magnification ×400).

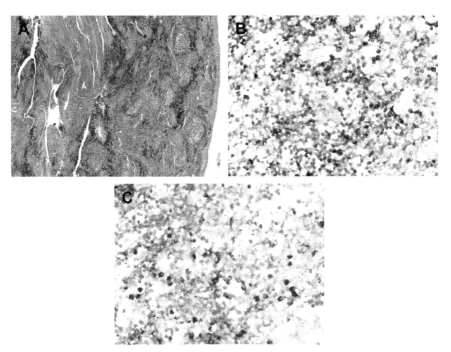

Fig. 13. A subcapsular liver biopsy was performed during a cholecystectomy procedure (*A*) (hematoxylin-eosin, original magnification ×20). This 64-year-old woman carried a diagnosis of ulcerative colitis and PSC. Multiple lymphoid aggregates are identified, and the inflammatory infiltrate appears to spare the bile duct (*A*). Note the lack of the characteristic histologic features of IgG4-RD. Immunohistochemical stains for IgG4 and IgG showed strong background signal and could not be interpreted. An *in situ* hybridization stain for IgG4 (*B*) and IgG (*C*) shows greater than 50 IgG4⁺ plasma cells per HPF in an IgG4:IgG ratio greater than 40%. The serum IgG4 was 850 mg/dL (greater than 6 times normal). There was no evidence, however, of systemic disease. The patient was not placed on immunosuppressive therapy. The case highlights the general reluctance of hepatologist to treat isolated IgG4-SC (B and C, *in situ* hybridization stain for IgG4 and IgG).

commonly from the salivary gland and gallbladder. The pathologic changes of IgG4-related gallbladder disease are highly characteristic: a fibroinflammatory infiltrate on the serosal aspect, often in the form of a well-circumscribed nodule[65] (see **Fig. 1**).

Many cases misdiagnosed as PSC prior to widespread recognition of IgG4-RD would now be classified as IgG4-SC.[66] Conversely, with increasing awareness of IgG4-SC, cases of PSC are now occasionally misclassified as IgG4-SC — often based primarily on serologic features or elevated numbers of IgG4⁺ plasma cells. Thus, the pendulum may be shifting from under-recognition to overdiagnosis.

Follicular Cholangitis

Like IgG4-SC, the recently described entity, follicular cholangitis, typically affects elderly individuals and presents with obstructive jaundice.[67] On histology, the large bile ducts are surrounded by a dense lymphoid infiltrate and germinal centers are prominent. Unlike IgG4-RD, IgG4⁺ plasma cells are either absent or sparse. The characteristic histopathologic features of IgG4-RD are not identified. A disease similar to follicular cholangitis has also been recognized in the pancreas.[68]

Sclerosing Cholangitis with Granulocytic Epithelial Lesions

Sclerosing cholangitis with granulocytic epithelial lesions is an uncommon form of sclerosing cholangitis that typically affects individuals in the first two decades of life. It is characterized by the presence of neutrophilic aggregates within bile ducts, the so-called granulocytic epithelial lesions[69] (**Fig. 14**). IgG4+ cells are not elevated and serum IgG4 levels are normal. The histologic appearance is remarkably similar to the type 2 variant of autoimmune pancreatitis.[70] Patients go into remission with prednisolone and/or ursodeoxycholic acid and do not seem to relapse.

Bile Duct Carcinoma

The distinction between bile duct carcinoma and IgG4-SC, although not as challenging as for PSC, is perhaps more critical, given the narrow window of opportunity for surgical resection in these patients.[71] On imaging there can be significant overlap between the 2 entities, and the characteristic histologic changes of IgG4-RD may not be evident on a limited biopsy from the bile duct. In the absence of overt malignancy on a biopsy, cytologic examination and next-generation sequencing analyses that identify common genetic alterations in bile duct carcinoma may be of great value.[72] Additionally, next-generation sequencing of the B-cell repertoire shows the existence of dominant IgG4 subclones in IgG4-SC that do not exist in PSC or biliary/pancreatic malignancies.[25] Genetic analyses, such as fluorescence *in situ* hybridization assays, may be falsely positive in IgG4-SC. Aneuploidy in bile duct brushing specimens, a feature of malignancy, may also be detected in patients with IgG4-RD.[71]

Hepatic Inflammatory Pseudotumor and Inflammatory Myofibroblastic Tumor

Prior to the recognition of IgG4-RD and IMTs, inflammatory mass-forming lesions were referred to as hepatic inflammatory pseudotumors. A significant proportion of these would currently be reclassified as IgG4-RD and a smaller proportion recategorized as IMTs. IMTs are mesenchymal neoplasms that are frequently accompanied by a dense inflammatory infiltrate composed of lymphocytes and plasma cells.[73] Although higher-grade IMTs are readily distinguished from IgG4-RD, the hypocellular examples may be indistinguishable from this entity, particularly on needle biopsy

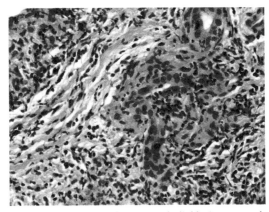

Fig. 14. Sclerosing cholangitis with granulocytic epithelial lesion. Note the neutrophilic infiltrate involving the bile duct (hematoxylin-eosin, original magnification ×200).

samples. Both lesions show spindle-shaped cells in an inflammatory background with little to no atypia. Although obliterative phlebitis and storiform-type fibrosis are uncommon in IMTs, the authors' group has encountered both features. While IgG4-RD is usually associated with significantly higher numbers of IgG4[+] plasma cells, some IMTs also show elevations at levels comparable with IgG4-RD.[74] The 2 most common genetic alterations in IMTs are *ALK* and *ROS1* translocations, and immunohistochemical assays serve as fairly robust surrogates for the translocation.[75] Pathologists must be aware that rare alternate translocations have been identified in IMTs that cannot be detected on immunohistochemical stains for ALK-1 and ROS1 (**Fig. 15**).

Other mesenchymal tumors also may be associated with elevated numbers of IgG4[+] plasma cells. The inflammatory variant of liposarcoma — a lesion that preferentially involves the retroperitoneum and abdomen — is a particularly close mimic of IgG4-RD. Both lesions are associated with a dense lymphoplasmacytic infiltrate and show elevated numbers of IgG4[+] plasma cells.

In addition to IgG4-RD and IMTs, a third category teased out from the inflammatory pseudotumor cohort is the so-called fibrohistiocytic-type inflammatory pseudotumor.[76] This lesion affects men and women equally, is mass forming, is usually found in the peripheral portion of the liver rather than hilar bile ducts, and is associated with abundant histiocytes and giant cells — a xanthogranulomatous inflammatory response. It seems unrelated to IgG4-RD.[76]

Granulomatosis with Polyangiitis (Formerly Wegener)

GPA is yet another disease that shows considerable clinical and pathologic overlap with IgG4-RD.[17,77] Involvement of the biliary tract or pancreas, however, is uncommon. More significantly, patients seldom present with hepatic manifestations. Nevertheless, pathologists need to be cognizant of the histologic overlap between the 2 diseases. Storiform-type fibrosis and elevated numbers of IgG4[+] plasma cells are also seen in GPA. The presence, however, of poorly formed granulomas, large numbers of giant cells, and necrosis — classic features of GPA — are virtually never seen in IgG4-RD. A positive antineutrophil cytoplasmic autoantibody test, found in greater than 90% of cases of GPA, argues strongly against the diagnosis of IgG4-RD.

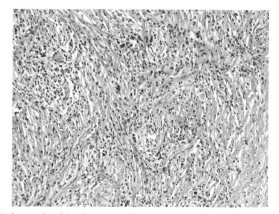

Fig. 15. This IMT showed a histologic and immunohistochemical appearance compatible with IgG4-RD. Immunohistochemistry for ALK and ROS1 were negative. On a next-generation sequencing platform, however, an ETV6-NTRK3 translocation was identified. This genetic abnormality has been noted in rare cases of IMT (hematoxylin-eosin, original magnification ×100).

Multicentric Castleman Disease

The human herpesvirus (HHV)-negative plasma cell variant of Castleman disease, although widely reported in the Japanese literature, is seldom diagnosed in North America or Europe.[78] The HHV-negative plasma cell variant of Castleman disease is reported to show remarkable overlap with IgG4-RD, clinically, radiologically, and pathologically. Multiorgan involvement is often seen. Storiform-type fibrosis and elevated numbers of IgG4+ plasma cells are widely prevalent. The distinction of MCD from IgG4-RD requires careful correlation with clinical and serologic features. MCD typically shows elevations in erythrocyte sedimentation rate, C-reactive protein, and interleukin (IL)-6 — features uncommon in IgG4-RD.[6,79] IL-6 inhibitors are the front-line therapy for MCD.[78]

TREATMENT

IgG4-RD responds rapidly to immunosuppressive therapy.[80] The absence of a quick response should prompt a thorough evaluation to exclude an alternative diagnosis, the most serious concern being malignancy. Unfortunately, a majority of patients relapse after withdrawal of immunosuppression. In an attempt to prevent flares, patients are placed on low-dose corticosteroid therapy. Maintenance therapy is often used in Asia, whereas in North America steroids are withdrawn after slow steroid taper. Several steroid-sparing agents have been investigated, most prominently rituximab, an anti-CD20 antibody. IgG4-RD responds swiftly to rituximab therapy, although relapses are common, typically at approximately the 6-month mark, a time at which the B cells reappear.[7,81] Although the disease is responsive to immunosuppressive therapy, there seems to be a risk of progressive fibrosis, and cases of cirrhosis have also been recognized.

REFERENCES

1. Stone JH, Zen Y, Deshpande V. IgG4-related disease. N Engl J Med 2012;366: 539–51.
2. Mahajan VS, Mattoo H, Deshpande V, et al. IgG4-related disease. Annu Rev Pathol 2014;9:315–47.
3. Hamano H, Kawa S, Horiuchi A, et al. High serum IgG4 concentrations in patients with sclerosing pancreatitis. N Engl J Med 2001;344:732–8.
4. Kamisawa T, Egawa N, Nakajima H. Autoimmune pancreatitis is a systemic autoimmune disease. Am J Gastroenterol 2003;98(12):2811–2.
5. Deshpande V, Mino-Kenudson M, Brugge W, et al. Autoimmune pancreatitis: more than just a pancreatic disease? A contemporary review of its pathology. Arch Pathol Lab Med 2005;129(9):1148–54.
6. Deshpande V, Zen Y, Chan JK, et al. Consensus statement on the pathology of IgG4-related disease. Modern Pathology 2012;25:1181–92.
7. Khosroshahi A, Carruthers MN, Deshpande V, et al. Rituximab for the treatment of IgG4-related disease: lessons from 10 consecutive patients. Medicine (Baltimore) 2012;91(1):57–66.
8. Carruthers MN, Topazian MD, Khosroshahi A, et al. Rituximab for IgG4-related disease: a prospective, open-label trial. Ann Rheum Dis 2015;74(6):1171–7.
9. Stone JH. IgG4-related disease: nomenclature, clinical features, and treatment. Semin Diagn Pathol 2012;29(4):177–90.
10. Culver EL, Chapman RW. IgG4-related hepatobiliary disease: an overview. Nat Rev Gastroenterol Hepatol 2016;13(10):601–12.

11. Zen Y, Kawakami H, Kim JH. IgG4-related sclerosing cholangitis: all we need to know. J Gastroenterol 2016;51:295–312.

12. Case records of the Massachusetts General Hospital. Weekly clinicopathological exercises. Case 6-1982. A 55-year-old man with eight months of obstructive jaundice. N Engl J Med 1982;306(6):349–58.

13. Wallace ZS, Deshpande V, Mattoo H, et al. IgG4-related disease: clinical and laboratory features in one hundred twenty-five patients. Arthritis Rheumatol 2015;67:2466–75.

14. Inoue D, Yoshida K, Yoneda N, et al. IgG4-related disease: dataset of 235 consecutive patients. Medicine 2015;94:e680.

15. Lin W, Lu S, Chen H, et al. Clinical characteristics of immunoglobulin G4-related disease: a prospective study of 118 Chinese patients. Rheumatology (Oxford) 2015;54(11):1982–90.

16. Chen Y, Zhao JZ, Feng RE, et al. Types of organ involvement in patients with immunoglobulin G4-related disease. Chin Med J (Engl) 2016;129(13):1525–32.

17. Zen Y, Nakanuma Y. IgG4-related disease: a cross-sectional study of 114 cases. Am J Surg Pathol 2010;34(12):1812–9.

18. Campochiaro C, Ramirez GA, Bozzolo EP, et al. IgG4-related disease in Italy: clinical features and outcomes of a large cohort of patients. Scand J Rheumatol 2016;45(2):135–45.

19. Fernandez-Codina A, Martinez-Valle F, Pinilla B, et al. IgG4-related disease: results from a multicenter spanish registry. Medicine (Baltimore) 2015;94(32):e1275.

20. Kanno A, Masamune A, Okazaki K, et al. Nationwide epidemiological survey of autoimmune pancreatitis in Japan in 2011. Pancreas 2015;44(4):535–9.

21. Kanno A, Nishimori I, Masamune A, et al. Nationwide epidemiological survey of autoimmune pancreatitis in Japan. Pancreas 2012;41(6):835–9.

22. Ghazale A, Chari ST, Zhang L, et al. Immunoglobulin G4-associated cholangitis: clinical profile and response to therapy. Gastroenterology 2008;134:706–15.

23. Huggett MT, Culver EL, Kumar M, et al. Type 1 autoimmune pancreatitis and IgG4-related sclerosing cholangitis is associated with extrapancreatic organ failure, malignancy, and mortality in a prospective UK cohort. Am J Gastroenterol 2014;109(10):1675–83.

24. de Buy Wenniger LJ, Culver EL, Beuers U. Exposure to occupational antigens might predispose to IgG4-related disease. Hepatology 2014;60(4):1453–4.

25. Doorenspleet ME, Hubers LM, Culver EL, et al. Immunoglobulin G4(+) B-cell receptor clones distinguish immunoglobulin G 4-related disease from primary sclerosing cholangitis and biliary/pancreatic malignancies. Hepatology 2016;64(2):501–7.

26. Mattoo H, Mahajan VS, Maehara T, et al. Clonal expansion of CD4(+) cytotoxic T lymphocytes in patients with IgG4-related disease. J Allergy Clin Immunol 2016;138(3):825–38.

27. Aoki S, Nakazawa T, Ohara H, et al. Immunohistochemical study of autoimmune pancreatitis using anti-IgG4 antibody and patients' sera. Histopathology 2005;47(2):147–58.

28. Okazaki K, Uchida K, Ohana M, et al. Autoimmune-related pancreatitis is associated with autoantibodies and a Th1/Th2-type cellular immune response. Gastroenterology 2000;118(3):573–81.

29. Nishimori I, Miyaji E, Morimoto K, et al. Serum antibodies to carbonic anhydrase IV in patients with autoimmune pancreatitis. Gut 2005;54(2):274–81.

30. Lohr JM, Faissner R, Koczan D, et al. Autoantibodies against the exocrine pancreas in autoimmune pancreatitis: gene and protein expression profiling and immunoassays identify pancreatic enzymes as a major target of the inflammatory process. Am J Gastroenterol 2010;105(9):2060–71.

31. Endo T, Takizawa S, Tanaka S, et al. Amylase alpha-2A autoantibodies: novel marker of autoimmune pancreatitis and fulminant type 1 diabetes. Diabetes 2009;58(3):732–7.

32. Asada M, Nishio A, Uchida K, et al. Identification of a novel autoantibody against pancreatic secretory trypsin inhibitor in patients with autoimmune pancreatitis. Pancreas 2006;33(1):20–6.

33. Zen Y, Fujii T, Harada K, et al. Th2 and regulatory immune reactions are increased in immunoglobin G4-related sclerosing pancreatitis and cholangitis. Hepatology 2007;45(6):1538–46.

34. Akdis CA, Blesken T, Akdis M, et al. Role of interleukin 10 in specific immunotherapy. J Clin Invest 1998;102(1):98–106.

35. Jeannin P, Lecoanet S, Delneste Y, et al. IgE versus IgG4 production can be differentially regulated by IL-10. J Immunol 1998;160(7):3555–61.

36. Akiyama M, Yasuoka H, Yamaoka K, et al. Enhanced IgG4 production by follicular helper 2 T cells and the involvement of follicular helper 1 T cells in the pathogenesis of IgG4-related disease. Arthritis Res Ther 2016;18:167.

37. Sah RP, Pannala R, Zhang L, et al. Eosinophilia and allergic disorders in autoimmune pancreatitis. Am J Gastroenterol 2010;105:2485–91.

38. Wheatley LM, Togias A. Clinical practice. Allergic rhinitis. N Engl J Med 2015; 372(5):456–63.

39. Maehara T, Mattoo H, Ohta M, et al. Lesional CD4+ IFN-gamma+ cytotoxic T lymphocytes in IgG4-related dacryoadenitis and sialoadenitis. Ann Rheum Dis 2016;76:377–85.

40. Mattoo H, Stone JH, Pillai S. Clonally expanded cytotoxic CD4+ T cells and the pathogenesis of IgG4-related disease. Autoimmunity 2017;50:19–24.

41. Nirula A, Glaser SM, Kalled SL, et al. What is IgG4? A review of the biology of a unique immunoglobulin subtype. Curr Opin Rheumatol 2011;23:119–24.

42. Aalberse RC, Schuurman J. IgG4 breaking the rules. Immunology 2002;105(1): 9–19.

43. van der Neut Kolfschoten M, Schuurman J, Losen M, et al. Anti-inflammatory activity of human IgG4 antibodies by dynamic Fab arm exchange. Science 2007; 317:1554–7.

44. van de Veen W, Stanic B, Yaman G, et al. IgG4 production is confined to human IL-10-producing regulatory B cells that suppress antigen-specific immune responses. J Allergy Clin Immunol 2013;131:1204–12.

45. Kalaitzakis E, Levy M, Kamisawa T, et al. Endoscopic retrograde cholangiography does not reliably distinguish IgG4-associated cholangitis from primary sclerosing cholangitis or cholangiocarcinoma. Clin Gastroenterol Hepatol 2011; 9(9):800–3.e2.

46. Aucouturier P, Danon FO, Daveau M, et al. Measurement of serum IgG4 levels by a competitive immunoenzymatic assay with monoclonal antibodies. J Immunol Methods 1984;74:151–62.

47. Culver EL, Sadler R, Simpson D, et al. Elevated Serum IgG4 levels in diagnosis, treatment response, organ involvement, and relapse in a prospective igg4-related disease UK cohort. Am J Gastroenterol 2016;111(5):733–43.

48. Oseini AM, Chaiteerakij R, Shire AM, et al. Utility of serum immunoglobulin G4 in distinguishing immunoglobulin G4-associated cholangitis from cholangiocarcinoma. Hepatology 2011;54:940–8.

49. Carruthers MN, Khosroshahi A, Augustin T, et al. The diagnostic utility of serum IgG4 concentrations in IgG4-related disease. Ann Rheum Dis 2015;74:14–8.

50. Boonstra K, Culver EL, de Buy Wenniger LM, et al. Serum immunoglobulin G4 and immunoglobulin G1 for distinguishing immunoglobulin G4-associated cholangitis from primary sclerosing cholangitis. Hepatology 2014;59:1954–63.

51. Wallace ZS, Mattoo H, Carruthers M, et al. Plasmablasts as a biomarker for IgG4-related disease, independent of serum IgG4 concentrations. Ann Rheum Dis 2015;74:190–5.

52. Mattoo H, Mahajan VS, Della-Torre E, et al. De novo oligoclonal expansions of circulating plasmablasts in active and relapsing IgG4-related disease. J Allergy Clin Immunol 2014;134(3):679–87.

53. Umehara H, Okazaki K, Masaki Y, et al. Comprehensive diagnostic criteria for IgG4-related disease (IgG4-RD), 2011. Mod Rheumatol 2012;22(1):21–30.

54. Sato Y, Kojima M, Takata K, et al. Systemic IgG4-related lymphadenopathy: a clinical and pathologic comparison to multicentric Castleman's disease. Mod Pathol 2009;22(4):589–99.

55. Cheuk W, Chan JK. IgG4-related sclerosing disease: a critical appraisal of an evolving clinicopathologic entity. Adv Anat Pathol 2010;17(5):303–32.

56. Cheuk W, Yuen HK, Chu SY, et al. Lymphadenopathy of IgG4-related sclerosing disease. Am J Surg Pathol 2008;32(5):671–81.

57. Harada K, Shimoda S, Kimura Y, et al. Significance of immunoglobulin G4 (IgG4)-positive cells in extrahepatic cholangiocarcinoma: molecular mechanism of IgG4 reaction in cancer tissue. Hepatology 2012;56(1):157–64.

58. Kimura Y, Harada K, Nakanuma Y. Pathologic significance of immunoglobulin G4-positive plasma cells in extrahepatic cholangiocarcinoma. Hum Pathol 2012; 43(12):2149–56.

59. Zhang L, Lewis JT, Abraham SC, et al. IgG4+ plasma cell infiltrates in liver explants with primary sclerosing cholangitis. Am J Surg Pathol 2010;34:88–94.

60. Deshpande V, Sainani NI, Chung RT, et al. IgG4-associated cholangitis: a comparative histological and immunophenotypic study with primary sclerosing cholangitis on liver biopsy material. Mod Pathol 2009;22(10):1287–95.

61. Moon SH, Kim MH, Park DH, et al. IgG4 immunostaining of duodenal papillary biopsy specimens may be useful for supporting a diagnosis of autoimmune pancreatitis. Gastrointest Endosc 2010;71(6):960–6.

62. Cebe KM, Swanson PE, Upton MP, et al. Increased IgG4+ cells in duodenal biopsies are not specific for autoimmune pancreatitis. Am J Clin Pathol 2013; 139(3):323–9.

63. Chari ST, Smyrk TC, Levy MJ, et al. Diagnosis of autoimmune pancreatitis: the Mayo Clinic experience. Clin Gastroenterol Hepatol 2006;4(8):1010–6 [quiz: 1934].

64. Lindor KD, Kowdley KV, Harrison ME, American College of Group. ACG Clinical Guideline: Primary Sclerosing Cholangitis. Am J Gastroenterol 2015;110(5): 646–59 [quiz: 660].

65. Wang WL, Farris AB, Lauwers GY, et al. Autoimmune pancreatitis-related cholecystitis: a morphologically and immunologically distinctive form of lymphoplasmacytic sclerosing cholecystitis. Histopathology 2009;54(7):829–36.

66. Portmann B, Zen Y. Inflammatory disease of the bile ducts-cholangiopathies: liver biopsy challenge and clinicopathological correlation. Histopathology 2012;60: 236–48.
67. Zen Y, Ishikawa A, Ogiso S, et al. Follicular cholangitis and pancreatitis - clinicopathological features and differential diagnosis of an under-recognized entity. Histopathology 2012;60(2):261–9.
68. Gupta RK, Xie BH, Patton KT, et al. Follicular pancreatitis: a distinct form of chronic pancreatitis-an additional mimic of pancreatic neoplasms. Hum Pathol 2016;48:154–62.
69. Zen Y, Grammatikopoulos T, Heneghan MA, et al. Sclerosing cholangitis with granulocytic epithelial lesion: a benign form of sclerosing cholangiopathy. Am J Surg Pathol 2012;36(10):1555–61.
70. Shinagare S, Shinagare AB, Deshpande V. Autoimmune pancreatitis: a guide for the histopathologist. Semin Diagn Pathol 2012;29(4):197–204.
71. Graham RPD, Smyrk TC, Chari ST, et al. Isolated IgG4-related sclerosing cholangitis: a report of 9 cases. Hum Pathol 2014;45:1722–9.
72. Dudley JC, Zheng Z, McDonald T, et al. Next-generation sequencing and fluorescence in situ hybridization have comparable performance characteristics in the analysis of pancreaticobiliary brushings for malignancy. J Mol Diagn 2016; 18(1):124–30.
73. Coffin CM, Watterson J, Priest JR, et al. Extrapulmonary inflammatory myofibroblastic tumor (inflammatory pseudotumor). A clinicopathologic and immunohistochemical study of 84 cases. Am J Surg Pathol 1995;19(8):859–72.
74. Saab ST, Hornick JL, Fletcher CD, et al. IgG4 plasma cells in inflammatory myofibroblastic tumor: inflammatory marker or pathogenic link? Mod Pathol 2011; 24(4):606–12.
75. Lovly CM, Gupta A, Lipson D, et al. Inflammatory myofibroblastic tumors harbor multiple potentially actionable kinase fusions. Cancer Discov 2014;4(8):889–95.
76. Zen Y, Fujii T, Sato Y, et al. Pathological classification of hepatic inflammatory pseudotumor with respect to IgG4-related disease. Mod Pathol 2007;20:884–94.
77. Chang SY, Keogh KA, Lewis JE, et al. IgG4-positive plasma cells in granulomatosis with polyangiitis (Wegener's): a clinicopathologic and immunohistochemical study on 43 granulomatosis with polyangiitis and 20 control cases. Hum Pathol 2013;44(11):2432–7.
78. Liu AY, Nabel CS, Finkelman BS, et al. Idiopathic multicentric Castleman's disease: a systematic literature review. Lancet Haematol 2016;3(4):e163–75.
79. Sato Y, Notohara K, Kojima M, et al. IgG4-related disease: historical overview and pathology of hematological disorders. Pathol Int 2010;60(4):247–58.
80. Khosroshahi A, Wallace ZS, Crowe JL, et al. International consensus guidance statement on the management and treatment of IgG4-related disease. Arthritis Rheumatol 2015;67(7):1688–99.
81. Pa Hart, Topazian MD, Witzig TE, et al. Treatment of relapsing autoimmune pancreatitis with immunomodulators and rituximab: the Mayo Clinic experience. Gut 2013;62:1607–15.

Current Concepts in Pediatric Nonalcoholic Fatty Liver Disease

Sarah E. Fleet, MD[a], Jay H. Lefkowitch, MD[b], Joel E. Lavine, MD, PhD[c],*

KEYWORDS

- Steatohepatitis • NASH • Obesity • Metabolic syndrome • Histopathology

KEY POINTS

- Nonalcoholic fatty liver disease (NAFLD) manifests as a spectrum of disease (steatosis to steatohepatitis to cirrhosis) and its increasing prevalence is a direct result of rapidly rising obesity rates.
- Pediatric NAFLD may be distinctly different from that found in adults by histologic evaluation; however, the cause of these differences is unknown.
- The exact pathophysiology of NAFLD is largely unknown, but histologic findings provide insight into possible mechanisms and targets for therapy.
- Few effective therapies are successful in treating NAFLD, and lifestyle modification remains the first-line of therapy in children.
- Randomized, controlled trials demonstrate resolution of NASH with vitamin E therapy, which is the current recommended treatment in pediatrics by expert guidelines.

PEDIATRIC EPIDEMIOLOGY AND RISK FACTORS

Nonalcoholic fatty liver disease (NAFLD) is the most common cause of liver disease in children and its increasing prevalence is associated with the concomitant rise in obesity.[1] Features of the metabolic syndrome criteria are each associated with NAFLD, including obesity, insulin resistance, and hypertriglyceridemia, and children with the metabolic syndrome have 5 times the odds of having NAFLD as overweight and obese children without metabolic syndrome.[2] Although the prevalence rates of pediatric obesity have remained stable over the past decade,[1] estimates on the prevalence of NAFLD in pediatrics vary widely.

[a] Division of Pediatric Gastroenterology, Hepatology and Nutrition, Columbia University Medical Center, 622 West 168th Street, PH17-119, New York, NY 10032, USA; [b] Department of Pathology, Columbia University Medical Center, 630 West 168th Street, PH 15W 1574, New York, NY 10032, USA; [c] Division of Pediatric Gastroenterology, Hepatology and Nutrition, Columbia University Medical Center, 622 West 168th Street, PH17-105F, New York, NY 10032, USA
* Corresponding author.
E-mail address: jl3553@cumc.columbia.edu

Gastroenterol Clin N Am 46 (2017) 217–231
http://dx.doi.org/10.1016/j.gtc.2017.01.002
0889-8553/17/© 2017 Elsevier Inc. All rights reserved.

The variability in prevalence estimates is in part owing to a relative lack of sensitive screening methods. Alanine transaminase (ALT) is a marker of hepatic injury and when combined with imaging that has sensitivity to fat infiltration, and when combined with other laboratory tests to eliminate other causes of fatty liver clinical suspicion, can be used to diagnose NAFLD. However, ALT is not sensitive, and normal cutoff values are based on adult values; appropriate cutoffs have not yet been defined in children, and are likely lower than current cutoffs, because "normal" ranges have shifted upward with the trend in higher body mass index z-scores.[3] More work is needed to determine appropriate cutoffs in children, and to determine other more sensitive markers of disease.

Despite this challenge, attempts have been made to get accurate prevalence rates in children. The SCALE study conducted a retrospective review of 742 children from the San Diego, California area, between the ages of 2 and 19 years, who had an autopsy performed by a county medical examiner for reasons related to unnatural rapid death. In this study, 9.6% of all children and 38% of obese children were found to have NAFLD.[4] In contrast, in a large European cohort of children, the prevalence of elevated ALT was 11% of the study population, and 17% in the extremely obese children.[5] Finally, in an National Health and Nutrition Examination Survey cohort of children, 8% of the population had an elevated ALT.[6] Across all 3 studies, however, older, male, Hispanic children were found to be at greatest risk.[4–6]

NONALCOHOLIC FATTY LIVER DISEASE AS A SPECTRUM OF DISEASE

NAFLD results from an accumulation of excess free fatty acids and triglycerides, demonstrated by hepatocellular macrovesicular steatosis.[7] NAFLD is an all-encompassing term that refers to a spectrum of disease. Although nonalcoholic fatty liver refers to steatosis without inflammation or necrosis and is considered relatively benign, this condition may progress or present with inflammation, hepatocyte injury and cell death, called nonalcoholic steatohepatitis (NASH).[8] NASH may be present with or without fibrosis, with potential progression to cirrhosis and increasing the risk of hepatocellular carcinoma.[9]

THE ROLE OF LIVER BIOPSY

Liver biopsy is required for definitive diagnosis and staging of NAFLD owing to insufficiently validated or developed biomarkers or imaging techniques.[10] For example, pediatric ultrasound imaging has shown good correlation with steatosis but not with fibrosis or liver injury.[11] Liver biopsy is also required to rule out comorbid disease as cause of elevated ALT. Skelly and colleagues[12] found that one-third of patients with suspected NAFLD were diagnosed with a condition other than NAFLD by biopsy, reinforcing the role of biopsy and the lack of specificity of ALT. Furthermore, biopsy is required for determination of nonprogressive (NAFL) versus progressive (NASH) disease.[8]

Unfortunately, liver biopsy carries significant risks of morbidity and mortality, rendering it an unacceptable screening tool.[13] Therefore, guidelines have been developed to help clinicians balance possible risk with the need for accurate diagnosis. The American Association for the Study of Liver Disease published guidelines in 2012 that recommend clinicians reserve liver biopsy for only subjects who will benefit and for children with unclear diagnosis or consideration for medication.[14] Its European counterpart, the European for the Study of Liver Disease, released a position statement that acknowledged liver biopsy provides both diagnostic and prognostic information on fibrosis, and potential for progression if fibrosis is suspected by noninvasive methods. No specific pediatric recommendations were made.[15]

PEDIATRIC DISEASE PROGRESSION

Although biopsy is desirable for the evaluation of fibrosis, only a minority of children will progress to it. Published data on the natural history in children is minimal. In a single retrospective longitudinal study, 66 children with NAFLD were followed for 20 years. In this group, 2 children died and 2 underwent liver transplantation owing to decompensated cirrhosis. Of 5 children with diagnostic biopsy at the start of the study, 2 developed fibrosis and 2 developed fibrosis with cirrhosis.[16] Most of the other literature available is adult focused. In adult studies, one-third of patients with NASH progress to cirrhosis, and NASH was identified as the leading risk factor for hepatocellular carcinoma.[17–19] Hepatocellular carcinoma is very rarely seen in children with NASH; however, those patients who acquire NAFLD earlier in life are likely have increased vulnerability to further liver disease in the future, and longer exposure to disease-related provocation.

HISTOLOGIC FEATURES OF PEDIATRIC FATTY LIVER DISEASE

Liver biopsies for NAFLD demonstrate a wide range of histologic findings. Simple steatosis, or nonalcoholic fatty liver, has the same threshold in children and adults, which is lipid accumulation evident in greater than 5% of hepatocytes.[7] Steatosis must be primarily macrovesicular, indicating there is a single large fat droplet with or without multiple smaller intracytoplasmic droplets, accompanied by nuclear displacement to the cellular periphery (**Fig. 1**A). A smaller proportion of patients

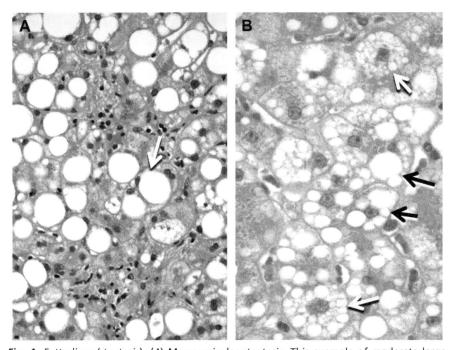

Fig. 1. Fatty liver (steatosis). (*A*) Macrovesicular steatosis. This example of moderate large droplet steatosis, the hepatocyte nuclei are pushed to the periphery of the cell by large vacuoles of triglyceride (*yellow arrow*). (*B*) Microvesicular steatosis. The majority of lipid vacuoles in this case are small (*yellow arrows*), with the hepatocyte nuclei remaining central in the hepatocyte cytoplasm. Note that in some hepatocytes the small vacuoles are coalescing into large droplets (*black arrows*). (Hematoxylin and eosin stain; original magnification: *A*, ×200, *B*, ×400).

may have a mix of small and large droplet accumulation.[20] There is an even smaller subset of patients who may have microvesicular steatosis, where there are many tiny lipid droplets with preservation of a centrally located nucleus (**Fig. 1**B).[20] In adults, steatosis severity is positively associated with a progression to NASH. Chalasani and colleagues[21] found that levels of steatosis severity positively correlated with lobular inflammation, zone 3 fibrosis, and definite steatohepatitis.

Although steatosis is consistent between adults and children, steatohepatitis often differs significantly. Children can have the same features as adult-type NASH (type 1), but a subset of children have different histologic features known as type 2 NASH. These children are younger, male, Asian, Hispanic, and Native American.[22] Pediatric NASH may also have features of both types.[23] In a study of 100 pediatric patients with NAFLD, Schwimmer and colleagues[22] found type 1 (adult type) NASH in 17% of subjects, and type 2 (pediatric type) NASH in 51%. It has been proposed that the switch from pediatric to adult type NASH, which is more common in older children, is related to the hormonal changes of puberty or possibly to nutritional factors.[24]

Type 1 NASH is defined by a set of minimal criteria. These criteria include steatosis, hepatocellular ballooning, and perivenular (zone 3) lobular inflammation (**Figs. 2** and **3**).[25] Hepatocellular ballooning is marked by enlarged hepatocytes with rarefied

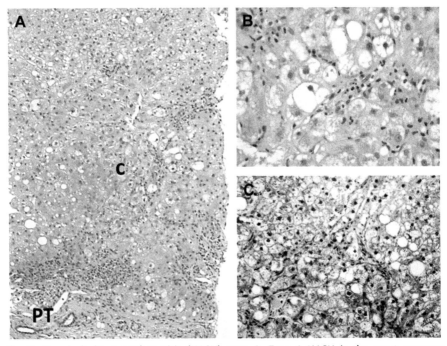

Fig. 2. Nonalcoholic steatohepatitis (NASH) type 1. Type 1 NASH is the most common pattern seen in adults and at its onset involves centrilobular regions (acinar zones 3). (*A*) At low magnification there is centrilobular (c) large droplet fat, hepatocyte ballooning, and inflammation (the minimal criteria for NASH). Note that the portal tract (PT) is also mildly inflamed. (*B*) Centrilobular steatosis, ballooned hepatocytes and inflammation are evident. (*C*) The typical "chicken-wire" perisinusoidal and pericellular pattern of fibrosis is evident on this trichrome stain (*A*, stain: hematoxylin and eosin stain; original magnification, ×100; *B*, ×400; *C*, stain: Masson trichrome; original magnification, ×200).

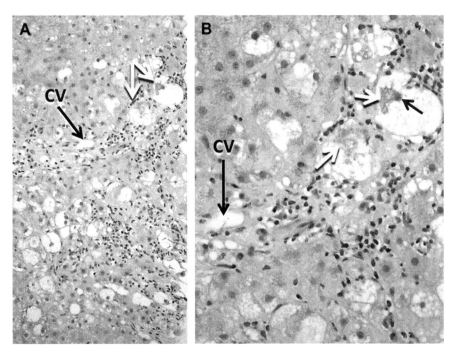

Fig. 3. Type 1 nonalcoholic steatohepatitis (NASH). (A) The hepatocytes in the centrilobular region show ballooning and considerable nearby inflammation. Mallory-Denk bodies are present in several ballooned hepatocytes (*yellow arrows*) (seen to better advantage in B). (B) At the upper right, several ballooned hepatocytes with wispy, rarefied cytoplasm contain Mallory-Denk bodies (*yellow arrows*). The blue arrow indicates the hepatocyte nucleus. The surrounding inflammatory infiltrate is mixed, predominantly lymphocytes with a few neutrophils (A, stain: hematoxylin and eosin; original magnification, ×200; B, ×400). CV, central vein.

reticular cytoplasm indicating cell injuries that are the result of alterations in intermediate filament cytoskeleton.[26] Owing to this change, loss of keratin 8/18 immunostaining may serve as marker for recognition of hepatocyte ballooning.[26] Apoptotic bodies and lytic necrosis also may be present.[20] Lobular inflammation in type 1 NASH is, by definition, in zone 3 or perivenular. This lobular inflammation seen in type 1 NASH is often mild with a mixed inflammatory cell infiltrate. Polymorphs sometimes surround ballooned hepatocytes (which usually also show intracytoplasmic Mallory-Denk bodies), a phenomenon referred to as "satellitosis" (**Fig. 4**). Scattered lobular microgranulomas and lipogranulomas are common. It is possible to have mild chronic lobular and portal lymphocytic inflammation that can indicate resolution in treated NAFLD. It should be noted that fibrosis is not required for the diagnosis of steatohepatitis but, when present, is usually perisinusoidal (**Fig. 2C; Table 1**).[27]

In contrast, however, borderline zone 1 or type 2 NASH is quite different histologically, and is more common than type 1 in children, and relatively unique to the pediatric population.[25] The distinctive features of type 2, or pediatric type NASH, are portal-based (zone 1) chronic inflammation and fibrosis, moderate to severe steatosis, and absence of zone 3 lesions (**Figs. 5 and 6**).[22] It is less common to find hepatocellular ballooning, or Mallory-Denk bodies (see **Fig. 3B**), as found in type 1.

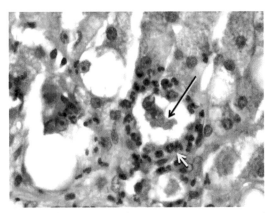

Fig. 4. Satellitosis. The swollen, steatotic hepatocyte at center contains an eosinophilic Mallory-Denk body (*black arrow*). The *yellow arrow* denotes the neutrophil infiltrate surrounding the affected hepatocyte ("satellitosis") (stain: hematoxylin and eosin; original magnification, ×400).

Finally, both types 1 and 2 can progress to fibrosis. Noncirrhotic, NASH-related fibrosis has a characteristic perisinusoidal and pericellular (chicken wire) pattern in zone 3, but generally shows portal tract predominance in type 2 NASH. This fibrosis is associated frequently with active lesions of NASH, but also may be seen in their absence, possibly indicating prior episodes of steatohepatitis.[27] In the progression of NASH, portal and periportal fibrosis may be observed leading to bridging fibrosis. Although steatosis is the first step in the progression of NAFLD, in advanced fibrosis and cirrhosis, steatosis can be absent (**Fig. 7**). Once NASH has become true cirrhosis, it is most commonly macronodular or mixed.[7]

SYSTEMS PROPOSED FOR HISTOLOGIC EVALUATION

Because NAFLD is a spectrum of disease from steatosis to cirrhosis, and histologic appearance has direct implications for prognosis, attempts have been made to standardize histologic evaluation of NAFLD liver biopsies. Two main scoring systems have been used, the NAFLD Activity Score and the Brunt scoring system.[28]

The NAFLD Activity Score was developed by the NASH Clinical Research Network and was designed as a quantitative tool for evaluation of NASH. This score uses degree of steatosis, lobular inflammation, and ballooning with a separate grade for fibrosis.[29] The Brunt scoring system is a semiquantitative assessment by using

Table 1
Histologic differences in adult and pediatric types of nonalcoholic steatohepatitis

	Type 1 (Adult)	Type 2 (Pediatric)
Steatosis	+	++
Hepatocellular ballooning	+	−
Mallory-Denk bodies	+	−
Inflammation	+ (Lobular)	++ (Portal)
Fibrosis	−/+ (Perisinusoidal)	−/+ (Portal)

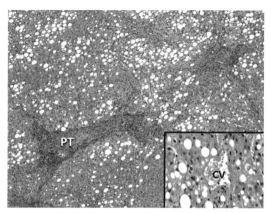

Fig. 5. Type 2 nonalcoholic steatohepatitis (NASH). This common pediatric type of NASH is centered on the portal tracts (PT), which show chronic inflammation and periportal fibrosis reminiscent of chronic hepatitis. The centrilobular hepatocyte ballooning and inflammation are absent. *Inset,* A central vein (CV) is shown, further emphasizing the absence of hepatocyte ballooning and inflammation from this region (stain: hematoxylin and eosin; original magnification, ×100; inset: stain: hematoxylin and eosin; original magnification, ×200).

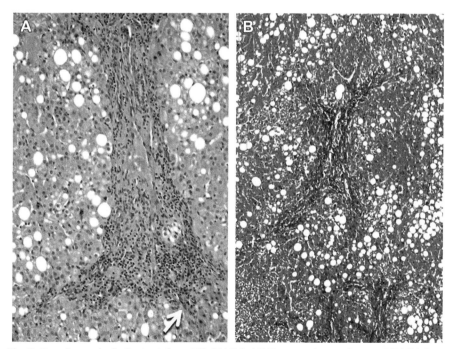

Fig. 6. Type 2 nonalcoholic steatohepatitis (NASH). (*A*) The portal tracts in type 2 NASH show chronic inflammation, sometimes with periportal interface hepatitis (*yellow arrow* at bottom). Note the predilection for large droplet fat in pediatric liver biopsies to accumulate in periportal regions. (*B*) Trichrome stain demonstrates irregular periportal fibrosis (*A*, stain: hematoxylin and eosin; original magnification, ×100; *B*, stain: Masson trichrome; original magnification, ×40).

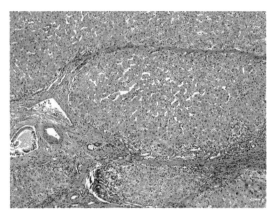

Fig. 7. Late nonalcoholic fatty liver disease (NAFLD) cirrhosis. The regenerative nodule at center is surrounded by fibrosis. However, there is no steatosis present, despite the presence of several NAFLD risk factors in this patient. Such cases often are misdiagnosed as "cryptogenic cirrhosis" and few histologic clues regarding etiology are found (stain: hematoxylin and eosin; original magnification, ×40).

mild, moderate, or severe designations in macrovesicular steatosis, ballooning, and lobular and portal inflammation.[30]

HISTOLOGIC INSIGHTS INTO PATHOGENESIS

The histology of NAFLD is well-described; however, the pathophysiology is not as well-understood. It was initially proposed that NAFLD was the result of 2 "hits."[31] In this model, the first hit is the accumulation of fat in hepatocytes, which is caused by caloric excess and subsequent development of insulin resistance and hyperinsuline-mia.[32,33] In this model, steatosis is the histopathologic manifestation of first hit, which occurs owing to an imbalance between fatty acid uptake and catabolism in liver. Peripheral tissue lipolysis, de novo lipogenesis, and dietary intake of fatty acids produce an overall influx of lipid into hepatocytes and a decrease in fatty acid oxidation, and secretion of free fatty acids as very low-density lipoproteins results in a retention of hepatic lipid. This imbalance produces a net increase in hepatocyte lipid content. His-tology supports this with severity of steatosis seen in nonalcoholic fatty liver.[31] The next hit may be multifactorial. One proposed insult includes increased reactive oxygen species (ROS), which promote hepatocellular damage, perhaps through peroxidation or epoxidation of lipids. Histopathologic findings support this theory with the presence of megamitochondria and microvesicular steatosis.[34] Megamitochondria are a known consequence of ROS accumulation, as a result of mitochondrial membrane fusion. This may decrease oxygen consumption to decrease ROS levels. If ROS decreases, the mitochondria return to normal size and function; however, continuous exposure of cells containing megamitochondria to additional free radicals induces apoptosis.[35] Furthermore, microvesicular steatosis is caused by oxidized phospholipid on surface of small lipid droplets within hepatocytes.[36] Oxidized phospholipid is formed nonen-zymatically by ROS,[37] and products of oxidative damage are often found in zone 3,[38] indicating the potential role of ROS in the pathophysiology of NAFLD. Overexpres-sion of cytochrome P450 2E1 (CYP2E1) has been found in zone 3 in patients with NASH and insulin resistance. CYP2E1 is known to generate ROS.[39]

Glutathione depletion has also been implicated in the development of NASH, owing to its role in recovery from ROS-related stress. Glutathione is a major intracellular antioxidant in the liver and because oxidative stress and lipid peroxidation may contribute to the pathogenesis of NASH, and its depletion may predispose obese individuals to the development of hepatocellular injury in NASH.[40,41] Patients with NASH may have a diet deficient in antioxidant-rich foods. Rodent models of glutathione deficiency have supported this finding,[42] and supplementing with glutathione-enhancing agents have shown some protection against NASH-related liver injury.[43,44]

There is evidence that other hepatocellular metabolic processes are affected. Liver biopsies of patients with NASH exhibit ballooning degeneration and Mallory-Denk bodies, which are ubiquinated (or other protein-bound) intermediate filament proteins.[26] Cellular processes that contribute to Mallory-Denk body formation include chronic stress, stress-induced protein misfolding (promoting endoplasmic reticulum stress), proteasome overload, transamidation of cytokeratin K8, and autophagy. Mallory-Denk bodies, therefore, act as a histologic and potential prognostic marker of NASH.[45]

The progression of disease and development of fibrosis also provides histologic clues to pathogenesis. In 2 separate studies, stellate cell activation was evaluated by immunohistochemistry, and found zone 3 accentuation in human liver biopsies of NASH.[46,47] In humans, fibrosis is also associated with hepatocyte progenitor cell (oval cell) accumulation, and NAFLD is no exception. These cells inhibit mature hepatocyte replication, which results in expansion of the hepatic progenitor cell (oval cell) population. It is thought that the increased number of these immature hepatocytes is, in part, responsible for the increased risk of hepatocellular carcinoma.[48]

The cause of these metabolic derangements and the reason for such varied severity in patients with NAFLD is largely debated. Adipokines have been proposed to have a causal role in the development and progression of disease. Low levels of adiponectin and high levels of leptin in combination have a strong independent association with presumed early stage NASH,[49] and adipokine expression has been associated with regulation of hepatic lipid receptors in obese patients with NAFLD.[50] Twin, familial, and epidemiologic studies have suggested a genetic component to NAFLD[51–53] and genome-wide association studies have identified variants in patatin-like phospholipase domain containing 3 and transmembrane 6 superfamily member 2 genes in NAFLD.[54,55] As with many other inflammatory diseases, the microbiome has also been implicated. There have been a number of recent studies on the intestinal microbiome of obese and NAFLD patients with varying results, but when controlled for exposure to medication known to alter the microbiome, an increase in *Bacteroides/Firmicutes* ratio was found in children who were obese and had NASH compared with lean healthy controls.[56]

Finally, it should be noted that the reason for the different patterns of NAFLD between adults and some children remains unexplained, and it is unclear if these differences are owing to truly different pathogenesis, different phenotypes of a similar pathogenesis, or natural disease progression with age. The recent randomized, placebo-controlled, double-blind trial of delayed release cysteamine as a treatment for NASH, demonstrated that there are significant differences in histology (in post hoc analyses) for children who were younger, less obese, and had "type 2" NASH. This is of importance because it may indicate that the etiopathogenesis is in fact different, and thus natural history and response to treatment may be different.[44] This study serves as a possible example, although further drug and mechanistic studies are needed to confirm this observation.

TREATMENT AND MANAGEMENT

Treatment of NAFLD is directed at a reduction in hepatocyte injury and the prevention of fibrosis. The mainstay of treatment in pediatrics remains lifestyle modification and diet modification. There are several pediatric studies that have shown biochemical and biopsy-proven improvements after these types of interventions.[57] These interventions have included a hypocaloric diet and daily exercise. Marchesini and colleagues[58] found that a 7% to 10% decrease in body weight was necessary for improvement in steatosis and NASH remission.

Because the microbiome has been implicated in the pathogenesis of NAFLD, probiotics as a treatment for this disease have also been studied. Obesity has been shown to alter the gut microbiota,[59] which communicates with the liver via the portal system. Thus, it is thought that, by shifting the microbiome back toward that of a lean person with probiotic therapy, the metabolic effects of the abnormal microbiome on the liver can be reversed. Probiotics are generally considered safe and well-tolerated; however, trials in NAFLD are limited. In 1 small study, obese children were treated with *Lactobacillus rhamnosus* for 8 weeks, resulting in a reduction in ALT.[60] In obese pediatric subjects with NAFLD, those put on probiotic VSL #3 showed evidence of improved steatosis, decreased body mass index, and increased circulating glucagon-like peptide.[61] Studies remain limited, but there is a modicum of evidence that probiotics and synbiotics improve some components of NAFLD and the metabolic syndrome.[62]

Long chain omega-3 fatty acids have also been studied as potential therapy for NAFLD in children. In a Western diet, typically many more omega-6 fatty acids are consumed than omega-3 fatty acids. This change in ratio of omega-6 to omega-3 is thought to increase proinflammatory metabolites.[63] Supplementing with additional omega-3 fatty acids would restore the ratio and decrease production of these metabolites. In a pediatric cohort of 60 patients with biopsy-proven NAFLD, DHA supplementation was associated with improvement in steatosis as well as decreased ALT and triglyceride levels.[64] More recent studies in children[65,66] and adults[67,68] have not been able to replicate the study, so DHA is not used as a therapy.

Elevated oxidative stress is recognized as a contributor to NAFLD severity, so antioxidant augmentation has been tested as a potential therapy. Lavine and colleagues[69] showed a normalization of aminotransferases and alkaline phosphatase in children with NASH on oral vitamin E in a pilot study. In the multicenter, randomized, placebo-controlled, double-blind TONIC trial, it was found that there was significant resolution of NASH on vitamin E (800 IU orally per day for 96 weeks) relative to placebo ($P = .006$), and significant improvement in the NAFLD Activity Score. Metformin, an insulin sensitizer, was also assessed in the TONIC trial (1 g/d), but did not result in improved histology.[70]

Bariatric surgery has been recommended for severely obese adolescents and obese adolescents with major comorbidities. Various bariatric surgeries decrease steatosis and improve inflammation and fibrosis in patients with NASH.[71]

EMERGING THERAPEUTIC TARGETS AND THERAPIES

As new insights are gained with regard to the pathophysiology, new treatment targets become available. Pentoxfylline is a phosphodiesterase inhibitor that antagonizes the proinflammatory cytokine tumor necrosis factor-α. Studies demonstrate improvement in aminotransferases, steatosis, inflammation and fibrosis in adult subjects treated with this drug.[72–75]

Farnesoid X receptor is a bile acid receptor that mediates lipid and glucose homeostasis. In a multicenter, randomized, placebo-controlled trial, the farnesoid X receptor agonist obeticholic acid significantly improved multiple histologic features of NASH, including fibrosis.[76] This drug is now in being tested in a Food and Drug Administration phase III trial.

Most recently, a multicenter, randomized, double-blind trial of delayed release cysteamine for treatment of NAFLD in children has shed light on pathogenesis and new treatment modalities. Cysteamine is a small molecule that reacts with extracellular cystine to form cysteine, which is then taken up into cells and used to support glutathione synthesis.[77,78] ALT reduction by cysteamine in the treatment group was improved significantly compared with placebo, but the primary histology endpoint, reduction in the NAFLD Activity Score by 2 or more points without worsening of fibrosis, did not show significant improvement. A post hoc analysis reveals there was histologic improvement in those who were younger, less heavy, and with type 2 NASH. This demonstrates that surrogate endpoints for clinical trials may not always accurately reflect recognized histologic ones, particularly in children. This study highlights that the etiopathogenesis may be different between pediatric-type and adult-type NASH; therefore, response to treatment may be different. This calls for recognition of the need for appropriate histology-based endpoints for therapeutic trials in pediatrics.[44]

SUMMARY

NAFLD is a spectrum of disease from steatosis to steatohepatitis to fibrosis and cirrhosis and its increasing prevalence is a direct result of historically high rates of obesity. Some children with NAFLD demonstrate distinct histopathologic differences from the pattern found in adults; however, the cause of these differences is unknown. Hepatocyte lipid accumulation is the first step in a cascade of metabolic events that are thought to cause NAFLD, and histologic findings provide insight into these events. There are few well-studied, effective therapies that are successful in treating NAFLD, and lifestyle modification remains the primary therapy in children. Administration of vitamin E in children with NASH has shown to result in significant resolution relative to placebo, and guidelines set forth by the American Gastroenterological Association, American Association for the Study of Liver Disease, and the American College of Gastroenterology recommend vitamin E treatment for children with biopsy-proven NASH.[14] Trials of novel drugs are in multiple phase trials of adults with NASH, and as efficacy and safety are established, these therapies may be tenable for use in children. However, biopsy-driven histology endpoints will be necessary to establish whether future therapies can improve either pediatric or adult-type NASH in children.

REFERENCES

1. Ogden CL, Carroll MD, Curtin LR, et al. Prevalence of high body mass index in US children and adolescents, 2007-2008. JAMA 2010;303(3):242–9.
2. Schwimmer JB, Pardee PE, Lavine JE, et al. Cardiovascular risk factors and the metabolic syndrome in pediatric nonalcoholic fatty liver disease. Circulation 2008;118(3):277–83.
3. Schwimmer JB, Dunn W, Norman GJ, et al. SAFETY study: alanine aminotransferase cutoff values are set too high for reliable detection of pediatric chronic liver disease. Gastroenterology 2010;138(4):1357–64, 1364.e1–e2.
4. Schwimmer JB, Deutsch R, Kahen T, et al. Prevalence of fatty liver in children and adolescents. Pediatrics 2006;118(4):1388–93.

5. Wiegand S, Keller KM, Robl M, et al. Obese boys at increased risk for nonalcoholic liver disease: evaluation of 16,390 overweight or obese children and adolescents. Int J Obes (Lond) 2010;34(10):1468–74.

6. Fraser A, Longnecker MP, Lawlor DA. Prevalence of elevated alanine aminotransferase among US adolescents and associated factors: NHANES 1999-2004. Gastroenterology 2007;133(6):1814–20.

7. Brunt EM, Tiniakos DG. Fatty liver disease. In: Odze RD, Goldblum JR, editors. Pathology of the GI Tract, liver, biliary tract and pancreas. Philadelphia: Elsevier; 2009. p. 1007–14.

8. Brunt EM. Pathology of nonalcoholic fatty liver disease. Nat Rev Gastroenterol Hepatol 2010;7(4):195–203.

9. Gu J, Yao M, Yao D, et al. Nonalcoholic lipid accumulation and hepatocyte malignant transformation. J Clin Transl Hepatol 2016;4(2):123–30.

10. Rockey DC, Caldwell SH, Goodman ZD, et al, American Association for the Study of Liver Diseases. Liver biopsy. Hepatology 2009;49(3):1017–44.

11. Shannon A, Alkhouri N, Carter-Kent C, et al. Ultrasonographic quantitative estimation of hepatic steatosis in children with NAFLD. J Pediatr Gastroenterol Nutr 2011;53(2):190–5.

12. Skelly MM, James PD, Ryder SD. Findings on liver biopsy to investigate abnormal liver function tests in the absence of diagnostic serology. J Hepatol 2001;35(2):195–9.

13. Nalbantoglu IL, Brunt EM. Role of liver biopsy in nonalcoholic fatty liver disease. World J Gastroenterol 2014;20(27):9026–37.

14. Chalasani N, Younossi Z, Lavine JE, et al. The diagnosis and management of non-alcoholic fatty liver disease: practice Guideline by the American Association for the Study of Liver Diseases, American College of Gastroenterology, and the American Gastroenterological Association. Hepatology 2012;55(6):2005–23.

15. Ratziu V, Bellentani S, Cortez-Pinto H, et al. A position statement on NAFLD/NASH based on the EASL 2009 special conference. J Hepatol 2010;53(2):372–84.

16. Feldstein AE, Charatcharoenwitthaya P, Treeprasertsuk S, et al. The natural history of non-alcoholic fatty liver disease in children: a follow-up study for up to 20 years. Gut 2009;58(11):1538–44.

17. Ascha MS, Hanouneh IA, Lopez R, et al. The incidence and risk factors of hepatocellular carcinoma in patients with nonalcoholic steatohepatitis. Hepatology 2010;51(6):1972–8.

18. Starley BQ, Calcagno CJ, Harrison SA. Nonalcoholic fatty liver disease and hepatocellular carcinoma: a weighty connection. Hepatology 2010;51(5):1820–32.

19. Argo CK, Northup PG, Al-Osaimi AM, et al. Systematic review of risk factors for fibrosis progression in non-alcoholic steatohepatitis. J Hepatol 2009;51(2):371–9.

20. Tiniakos DG. Nonalcoholic fatty liver disease/nonalcoholic steatohepatitis: histological diagnostic criteria and scoring systems. Eur J Gastroenterol Hepatol 2010;22(6):643–50.

21. Chalasani N, Wilson L, Kleiner DE, et al. Relationship of steatosis grade and zonal location to histological features of steatohepatitis in adult patients with non-alcoholic fatty liver disease. J Hepatol 2008;48(5):829–34.

22. Schwimmer JB, Behling C, Newbury R, et al. Histopathology of pediatric nonalcoholic fatty liver disease. Hepatology 2005;42(3):641–9.

23. Nobili V, Marcellini M, Devito R, et al. NAFLD in children: a prospective clinical-pathological study and effect of lifestyle advice. Hepatology 2006;44(2):458–65.

24. Roberts EA. Non-alcoholic steatohepatitis in children. Clin Liver Dis 2007;11(1):155–72, x.

25. Patton HM, Lavine JE, Van Natta ML, et al. Clinical correlates of histopathology in pediatric nonalcoholic steatohepatitis. Gastroenterology 2008;135(6): 1961–71.e2.
26. Lackner C, Gogg-Kamerer M, Zatloukal K, et al. Ballooned hepatocytes in steatohepatitis: the value of keratin immunohistochemistry for diagnosis. J Hepatol 2008;48(5):821–8.
27. Hubscher SG. Histological assessment of non-alcoholic fatty liver disease. Histopathology 2006;49(5):450–65.
28. Uppal V, Mansoor S, Furuya KN. Pediatric non-alcoholic fatty liver disease. Curr Gastroenterol Rep 2016;18(5):24.
29. Kleiner DE, Brunt EM, Van Natta M, et al. Design and validation of a histological scoring system for nonalcoholic fatty liver disease. Hepatology 2005;41(6): 1313–21.
30. Brunt EM, Janney CG, Di Bisceglie AM, et al. Nonalcoholic steatohepatitis: a proposal for grading and staging the histological lesions. Am J Gastroenterol 1999; 94(9):2467–74.
31. Day CP, James OF. Steatohepatitis: a tale of two "hits". Gastroenterology 1998; 114(4):842–5.
32. Cali AM, De Oliveira AM, Kim H, et al. Glucose dysregulation and hepatic steatosis in obese adolescents: is there a link? Hepatology 2009;49(6):1896–903.
33. D'Adamo E, Cali AM, Weiss R, et al. Central role of fatty liver in the pathogenesis of insulin resistance in obese adolescents. Diabetes Care 2010;33(8):1817–22.
34. Tandra S, Yeh MM, Brunt EM, et al. Presence and significance of microvesicular steatosis in nonalcoholic fatty liver disease. J Hepatol 2011;55(3):654–9.
35. Wakabayashi T. Megamitochondria formation - physiology and pathology. J Cell Mol Med 2002;6(4):497–538.
36. Ikura Y, Ohsawa M, Suekane T, et al. Localization of oxidized phosphatidylcholine in nonalcoholic fatty liver disease: impact on disease progression. Hepatology 2006;43(3):506–14.
37. Smith WL, Murphy RC. Oxidized lipids formed non-enzymatically by reactive oxygen species. J Biol Chem 2008;283(23):15513–4.
38. Seki S, Kitada T, Yamada T, et al. In situ detection of lipid peroxidation and oxidative DNA damage in non-alcoholic fatty liver diseases. J Hepatol 2002;37(1): 56–62.
39. Farrell GC. Non-alcoholic steatohepatitis: what is it, and why is it important in the Asia-Pacific region? J Gastroenterol Hepatol 2003;18(2):124–38.
40. Malaguarnera L, Madeddu R, Palio E, et al. Heme oxygenase-1 levels and oxidative stress-related parameters in non-alcoholic fatty liver disease patients. J Hepatol 2005;42(4):585–91.
41. Videla LA, Rodrigo R, Orellana M, et al. Oxidative stress-related parameters in the liver of non-alcoholic fatty liver disease patients. Clin Sci (Lond) 2004;106(3): 261–8.
42. Haque JA, McMahan RS, Campbell JS, et al. Attenuated progression of diet-induced steatohepatitis in glutathione-deficient mice. Lab Invest 2010;90(12): 1704–17.
43. Oz HS, Im H-J, Chen TS, et al. Glutathione-enhancing agents protect against steatohepatitis in a dietary model. J Biochem Mol Toxicol 2006;20(1):39–47.
44. Schwimmer JB, Lavine JE, Wilson LA, et al. In Children With Nonalcoholic Fatty Liver Disease, Cysteamine Bitartrate Delayed Release Improves Liver Enzymes but Does Not Reduce Disease Activity Scores. Gastroenterology 2016;151(6): 1141–54.e1149.

45. Zatloukal K, French SW, Stumptner C, et al. From Mallory to Mallory–Denk bodies: what, how and why? Exp Cell Res 2007;313(10):2033–49.
46. Washington K, Wright K, Shyr Y, et al. Hepatic stellate cell activation in nonalcoholic steatohepatitis and fatty liver. Hum Pathol 2000;31(7):822–8.
47. Cortez-Pinto H, Baptista A, Camilo ME, et al. Hepatic stellate cell activation occurs in nonalcoholic steatohepatitis. Hepatogastroenterology 2001;48(37):87–90.
48. Roskams T, Yang SQ, Koteish A, et al. Oxidative stress and oval cell accumulation in mice and humans with alcoholic and nonalcoholic fatty liver disease. Am J Pathol 2003;163(4):1301–11.
49. Zelber-Sagi S, Ratziu V, Zvibel I, et al. The association between adipocytokines and biomarkers for nonalcoholic fatty liver disease-induced liver injury: a study in the general population. Eur J Gastroenterol Hepatol 2012;24(3):262–9.
50. Estep JM, Goodman Z, Sharma H, et al. Adipocytokine expression associated with miRNA regulation and diagnosis of NASH in obese patients with NAFLD. Liver Int 2015;35(4):1367–72.
51. Schwimmer JB, Celedon MA, Lavine JE, et al. Heritability of nonalcoholic fatty liver disease. Gastroenterology 2009;136(5):1585–92.
52. Makkonen J, Pietilainen KH, Rissanen A, et al. Genetic factors contribute to variation in serum alanine aminotransferase activity independent of obesity and alcohol: a study in monozygotic and dizygotic twins. J Hepatol 2009;50(5):1035–42.
53. Guerrero R, Vega GL, Grundy SM, et al. Ethnic differences in hepatic steatosis: an insulin resistance paradox? Hepatology 2009;49(3):791–801.
54. Speliotes EK, Yerges-Armstrong LM, Wu J, et al. Genome-wide association analysis identifies variants associated with nonalcoholic fatty liver disease that have distinct effects on metabolic traits. PLoS Genet 2011;7(3):e1001324.
55. Goffredo M, Caprio S, Feldstein AE, et al. Role of TM6SF2 rs58542926 in the pathogenesis of nonalcoholic pediatric fatty liver disease: a multiethnic study. Hepatology 2016;63(1):117–25.
56. Zhu L, Baker RD, Baker SS. Gut microbiome and nonalcoholic fatty liver diseases. Pediatr Res 2015;77(1–2):245–51.
57. Nobili V, Manco M, Devito R, et al. Lifestyle intervention and antioxidant therapy in children with nonalcoholic fatty liver disease: a randomized, controlled trial. Hepatology 2008;48(1):119–28.
58. Marchesini G, Petta S, Dalle Grave R. Diet, weight loss, and liver health in nonalcoholic fatty liver disease: pathophysiology, evidence, and practice. Hepatology 2016;63(6):2032–43.
59. Parekh PJ, Balart LA, Johnson DA. The influence of the gut microbiome on obesity, metabolic syndrome and gastrointestinal disease. Clin Transl Gastroenterol 2015;6:e91.
60. Vajro P, Mandato C, Licenziati MR, et al. Effects of Lactobacillus rhamnosus strain GG in pediatric obesity-related liver disease. J Pediatr Gastroenterol Nutr 2011;52(6):740–3.
61. Alisi A, Bedogni G, Baviera G, et al. Randomised clinical trial: the beneficial effects of VSL#3 in obese children with non-alcoholic steatohepatitis. Aliment Pharmacol Ther 2014;39(11):1276–85.
62. Saez-Lara MJ, Robles-Sanchez C, Ruiz-Ojeda FJ, et al. Effects of probiotics and synbiotics on obesity, insulin resistance syndrome, type 2 diabetes and nonalcoholic fatty liver disease: a review of human clinical trials. Int J Mol Sci 2016;17(6) [pii: E928].

63. Scorletti E, Byrne CD. Omega-3 fatty acids, hepatic lipid metabolism, and nonalcoholic fatty liver disease. Annu Rev Nutr 2013;33(1):231–48.
64. Nobili V, Alisi A, Della Corte C, et al. Docosahexaenoic acid for the treatment of fatty liver: randomised controlled trial in children. Nutr Metab Cardiovasc Dis 2013;23(11):1066–70.
65. Janczyk W, Lebensztejn D, Wierzbicka-Rucinska A, et al. Omega-3 Fatty acids therapy in children with nonalcoholic Fatty liver disease: a randomized controlled trial. J Pediatr 2015;166(6):1358–63.e1–e3.
66. Janczyk W, Socha P, Lebensztejn D, et al. Omega-3 fatty acids for treatment of non-alcoholic fatty liver disease: design and rationale of randomized controlled trial. BMC Pediatr 2013;13:85.
67. Scorletti E, Bhatia L, McCormick KG, et al. Effects of purified eicosapentaenoic and docosahexaenoic acids in nonalcoholic fatty liver disease: results from the WELCOME* study. Hepatology 2014;60(4):1211–21.
68. Sanyal AJ, Abdelmalek MF, Suzuki A, et al. No significant effects of ethyl-eicosapentanoic acid on histologic features of nonalcoholic steatohepatitis in a phase 2 trial. Gastroenterology 2014;147(2):377–84.e371.
69. Lavine JE. Vitamin E treatment of nonalcoholic steatohepatitis in children: a pilot study. J Pediatr 2000;136(6):734–8.
70. Lavine JE, Schwimmer JB, Van Natta ML, et al. Effect of vitamin E or metformin for treatment of nonalcoholic fatty liver disease in children and adolescents: the TONIC randomized controlled trial. JAMA 2011;305(16):1659–68.
71. Nobili V, Vajro P, Dezsofi A, et al. Indications and limitations of bariatric intervention in severely obese children and adolescents with and without nonalcoholic steatohepatitis: ESPGHAN Hepatology Committee Position Statement. J Pediatr Gastroenterol Nutr 2015;60(4):550–61.
72. Du J, Ma YY, Yu CH, et al. Effects of pentoxifylline on nonalcoholic fatty liver disease: a meta-analysis. World J Gastroenterol 2014;20(2):569–77.
73. Adams LA, Zein CO, Angulo P, et al. A pilot trial of pentoxifylline in nonalcoholic steatohepatitis. Am J Gastroenterol 2004;99(12):2365–8.
74. Zein CO, Lopez R, Fu X, et al. Pentoxifylline decreases oxidized lipid products in nonalcoholic steatohepatitis: new evidence on the potential therapeutic mechanism. Hepatology 2012;56(4):1291–9.
75. Zein CO, Yerian LM, Gogate P, et al. Pentoxifylline improves nonalcoholic steatohepatitis: a randomized placebo-controlled trial. Hepatology 2011;54(5):1610–9.
76. Neuschwander-Tetri BA, Loomba R, Sanyal AJ, et al. Farnesoid X nuclear receptor ligand obeticholic acid for non-cirrhotic, non-alcoholic steatohepatitis (FLINT): a multicentre, randomised, placebo-controlled trial. Lancet 2015;385(9972):956–65.
77. Dohil R, Cabrera BL, Gangoiti JA, et al. Pharmacokinetics of cysteamine bitartrate following intraduodenal delivery. Fundam Clin Pharmacol 2014;28(2):136–43.
78. Maher P, Lewerenz J, Lozano C, et al. A novel approach to enhancing cellular glutathione levels. J Neurochem 2008;107(3):690–700.

Contemporary Evaluation of the Pediatric Liver Biopsy

Deborah A. Schady, MD*, Milton J. Finegold, MD

KEYWORDS

- Liver • Biopsy • Pediatric • Metabolic • Cholestatic

KEY POINTS

- Main histologic patterns of liver injury in children include cholestatic, storage, steatotic, hepatitic, cirrhotic, and neoplastic patterns.
- Ultrastructural examination may be essential for diagnosis in some pediatric liver diseases.
- Hepatic neoplasia may occur in children with metabolic diseases, so investigation for an underlying metabolic disease may be warranted for patient and family.

INTRODUCTION

Liver disease in the pediatric patient encompasses a vast range of disorders that include neonatal cholestasis, disorders of metabolism, drug-induced liver injury, viral diseases, immunologic disorders, nonalcoholic fatty liver disease (NAFLD), and issues affecting the transplanted liver. The liver biopsy is an essential component in the workup of most of these diseases. The most frequent indication for liver biopsy in the native livers of infants is persistent jaundice, whereas in older children hepatomegaly, splenomegaly with gastrointestinal bleeding, incidental discovery of a mass, and elevated serum transaminases are more common indications. Workup in most of these cases typically includes biochemical, genetic, and imaging analysis. Liver biopsies also are performed for prognosis, or monitoring disease progression or response to treatment.[1]

The first percutaneous liver biopsy was performed by Paul Ehrlich in Germany in 1883 but was not widely used until Menghini developed a safer and quicker technique in 1958, leading to widespread use of the liver biopsy in practice.[2,3] This article provides a brief overview of current biopsy procedures and the range of histopathology

Disclosure Statement: The authors have nothing to disclose.
Department of Pathology and Immunology, Texas Children's Hospital, Baylor College of Medicine, Houston, TX, USA
* Corresponding author.
E-mail address: daschady@texaschildrens.org

Gastroenterol Clin N Am 46 (2017) 233–252
http://dx.doi.org/10.1016/j.gtc.2017.01.013
0889-8553/17/© 2017 Elsevier Inc. All rights reserved.

gastro.theclinics.com

in the more common liver diseases affecting the neonatal/pediatric population. NAFLD, autoimmune disorders with their overlap syndromes, and drug-induced liver disease are discussed elsewhere in this issue.

Surgical pathologists are integral players in the evaluation of liver diseases, and their participation begins when the liver biopsy is received in the laboratory. They must have a working knowledge of the patient's history so tissue can be triaged appropriately. Tissue is routinely processed for light microscopy and ultrastructural examination. Tissue can then be set aside for additional studies based on the patient's clinical history and laboratory tests. Portions can be snap frozen in liquid nitrogen for "special" stains, such as Oil Red O for fat and immunofluorescence, reference laboratory assays, direct assessment of enzyme activities (ie, glycogen storage disease type I), specific chemical assays (ie, copper quantification), viral polymerase chain reaction (PCR), and molecular analyses (ie, mitochondriopathies and tumors).[4] Typically two 2.0-cm-long core biopsies are recommended for there to be enough tissue for all required tests.

Neonatal Cholestasis

Neonatal cholestasis can be caused by a heterogeneous group of disorders that present with jaundice and can also include hypocholic/acholic stools, dark urine, and hypoglycemia.[1] The incidence of neonatal liver disease with clinical or biochemical evidence of cholestasis is approximately 1 in 2500 livebirths.[5] Neonatal cholestasis can be divided into cholestatic, which includes extrahepatic biliary atresia, bile duct paucity, cystic fibrosis, and neonatal sclerosing cholangitis, and intrahepatic cholestasis, which includes viruses, bacteria, genetic causes such as alpha-1-antitrypsin (α1AT) deficiency, tyrosinemia, progressive familial intrahepatic cholestasis (PFIC), and Alagille syndrome (ALGS), and total parenteral nutrition (TPN) cholestasis.[5,6] Many of these disorders demonstrate overlap in clinical history and serum liver chemistries, so the clinical evaluation begins with liver function tests, which include aspartate aminotransferase (AST), alanine aminotransferase (ALT), gamma-glutamyl transferase, and levels of direct and conjugated bilirubin, but often require biochemical, genetic, and imaging analyses (**Table 1**).

Biliary atresia (BA) is a congenital fibro-inflammatory obstructive cholangiopathy of the extrahepatic biliary tree and the most common cause of pathologic direct hyperbilirubinemia, with an incidence of 1 in 8000 to 18,000 livebirths.[6,7] It is also the most common cause of progressive liver disease, with approximately 80% of children with BA requiring liver transplantation over the course of their lifetime.[6,8] The underlying pathogenesis of BA remains unclear and may be due to an initial hit by viral infection, such as rotavirus, reovirus-2/3, or cytomegalovirus with a subsequent autoimmune disorder causing the second hit.[9,10] Other hypotheses are based on the role of T, B, and natural killer cells in the destruction of extrahepatic bile ducts mediated by interferon-γ, interleukin (IL)-2, tumor necrosis factor-α, and IL-12.[11] Recently, maternal chimeric CD8$^+$ T cells were discovered in BA infant livers, suggesting graft-versus-host interaction by engrafted maternal effector T cells as the initiating hit.[12,13] The typical biopsy histology consists of a triad of expanded portal ducts with bile plugs, acute pericholangitis and direct cholangitis, and bile ductule proliferation. Portal tract edema is a prominent feature as well, but may be seen in other extrahepatic obstructive conditions. BA may show multinucleated "giant" hepatocytes containing bile, which are not uncommon in all forms of neonatal cholestasis and provide a challenge to the pathologist. Fibrosis develops quickly with rapid progression to cirrhosis, so early recognition and diagnosis are essential. Early intervention with a hepatoportoenterostomy (HPE), initially described by Morio Kasai[3] to redirect the flow of bile directly into the duodenum, provided the basis for survival, and patients who receive an HPE

Table 1
Neonatal cholestatic disorders divided into categories based on etiology

Cholestasis	Metabolic	Infections		Toxins	Immunologic
Biliary atresia	A1AT deficiency	Sepsis	Adenovirus	TPN	Langerhans cell histiocytosis
Choledochal cyst	Gaucher disease	UTIs	Coxsackie	Drugs/Medications	Hemophagocytic lymphohistiocytosis
Neonatal sclerosing cholangitis	Cystic fibrosis	TORCH	Parvovirus B19	Fetal alcohol syndrome	Neonatal lupus erythematosus
Alagille syndrome	Inborn errors of bile acid synthesis	Hepatitis A-E	HHV6-8		Graft-versus-host disease
Caroli disease	Niemann-Pick type C	EBV	VZV		Erythroblastosis fetalis
Gallstones/biliary sludge	Wolman, CESD	HIV	Syphilis		Neonatal leukemia
Idiopathic neonatal giant cell hepatitis	Mitochondriopathies	Echovirus	Leptospirosis		Neonatal alloimmune hepatitis
PFIC	Peroxisomal disorders (Zellweger)				
Gracile syndrome (BCS1L mutation)	Galactosemia				
	Congenital disorders of glycosylation				
	Hypopituitarism				
	Tyrosinemia				
	GSD type IV				
	Urea cycle disorders				

Abbreviations: A1AT, alpha-1-anti-trypsin; CESD, cholesterol ester storage disease; EBV, Epstein-Barr virus; GSD, glycogen storage disease; HHV-6, human herpes virus-6; HIV, human immunodeficiency virus; TORCH, toxoplasmosis, other, rubella, cytomegalovirus, herpes simplex virus; TPN, total parenteral nutrition; UTI, urinary tract infection; VZV, varicella zoster virus.

before 8 weeks of life have better outcomes than those who do not; however, only 25% to 35% of these children will reach 10 years of age with their native livers.[14,15] Recent studies looking at serum bilirubin levels for diagnosis and prognosis suggest that patients with BA have significantly elevated direct/conjugated bilirubin levels shortly after birth in comparison with controls, and these remain elevated at the infant's usual 2-week pediatrician visit. Most patients have normal direct bilirubin to total bilirubin levels ($\leq$0.2 mg/dL).[16] These patients should be evaluated for BA. A study measuring total serum bilirubin levels within 3 months post HPE showed if the total bilirubin was greater than 2.0 mg/dL during this period these patients had an increased risk of complications with progressive liver disease and death or need for liver transplantation within 2 years.[7] Recent studies also show the infrequent occurrence of hepatocellular carcinoma and hepatoblastoma in the explanted livers of patients with BA.[17]

ALGS, or syndromic paucity of bile ducts, was first described in 1975 by Alagille and colleagues,[18,19] who described 15 patients with hypoplastic bile ducts, chronic cholestasis, and a patent extrahepatic biliary tree. These patients also had characteristic facies, vertebral malformations, growth and mental retardation, hypogonadism, and cardiac murmurs. Since then, it has been discovered that it is inherited in an autosomal dominant manner, with most patients demonstrating mutations in the JAGGED1 gene, which encodes a ligand in the Notch signaling pathway.[5,20] Approximately 70% to 98% of cases have a JAG1 mutation, with 30% to 50% of cases demonstrating inherited mutations and up to two-thirds showing de novo mutations.[5,6,20] Mutations in the NOTCH2 gene coding for the receptor of JAG1 have been described at a lower frequency (2% of cases).[6,20] The overall incidence of ALGS is estimated at 1 per 100,000 livebirths. The diagnosis of ALGS consists of demonstrating bile duct paucity (ratio of bile ducts to portal tracts in term infants is 0.9–1.8) defined by a bile duct to portal tract ratio of $\leq$0.5 with evaluation of at least 5 to 10 portal tracts in the presence of 3 or more of 5 major clinical criteria, including characteristic facies, cholestasis, heart disease (most frequent is pulmonary artery branch stenosis without or without Tetralogy of Fallot), vertebral anomalies (most common is butterfly vertebrae), and posterior embryotoxon.[5,6] Early in the disease, paucity of bile ducts may not be present and bile ductular proliferation may be present without bile plug formation. Laboratory testing may show elevations of bile salts up to 100 times normal (manifesting clinically as pruritus), bilirubin levels up to 30 times normal, elevated gamma-glutamyl transferase (GGT), and elevated alkaline phosphatase levels, as well as high cholesterol.[6] The overall outcomes of these patients depends on multiple organ involvement and severity. Patients manifesting liver disease in infancy tend to develop portal hypertension leading to cirrhosis, with the need for possible liver transplantation in 21% to 50% of patients, with relatively good posttransplant survival rates (**Box 1**).[21–23]

PFIC is an evolving group of 5 autosomal recessive disorders involved in intrahepatic bile transport and formation, with an estimated overall incidence of 1 per 50,000 to 1 per 100,000 live births and affects both genders equally.[24] Laboratory testing includes evaluation of the serum GGT, which is low to normal (impaired bile salt secretion) in PFIC 1, PFIC 2, TJP-2, and farnesoid X receptor (FXR) types and elevated (bile acids are secreted in bile) in PFIC 3 cases (**Table 2**). Liver histology is variable among the different PFIC types (**Fig. 1**). PFIC 1 or Byler disease was originally described in the mid-1960s in a group of Amish children, with onset of pruritus, loose stools, and failure to thrive at less than 1 year of age, with jaundice and direct hyperbilirubinemia being common.[25] Canalicular cholestasis with periportal hepatocyte biliary metaplasia and possible biliary plugs without bile ductular proliferation is the typical histology present, and lobular fibrosis is a late finding. PFIC 2 or bile salt export

Box 1
Causes of bile duct paucity
Alagille syndrome
A1AT deficiency
Niemann-Pick Type C
Cystic fibrosis
Zellweger syndrome
Progressive familial intrahepatic cholestasis type 1
Cytomegalovirus
Rubella
Syphilis
Chronic liver allograft rejection
Graft-versus-host-disease
Neonatal sclerosing cholangitis
Down syndrome
Ivemark syndrome
Langerhan cell histiocytosis

pump (BSEP) shows canalicular cholestasis as well, but in a setting of prominent lobular disarray, portal and lobular fibrosis, greater amount of periportal hepatocyte biliary metaplasia, and possible hepatocellular necrosis and giant cell hepatitis. Bile ductular proliferation and portal fibrosis is present in PFIC 3 at diagnosis, with biliary cirrhosis developing later in the disease course. PFIC 4 or TJP2 shows similar histology to PFIC 2, with canalicular cholestasis and prominent bridging fibrosis.[26,27] PFIC 5 or FXR shows canalicular cholestasis with diffuse giant cell transformation, ballooning hepatocytes, and bile ductular proliferation with development of biliary cirrhosis later in the disease course.[28] There appears to be an increased risk of hepatocellular carcinoma (HCC) in patients with PFIC 2 and PFIC 4.[29] Medical management is the first line of treatment in all of the PFICs, with the common medications being ursodeoxycholic acid, rifampicin, and cholestyramine. Surgical treatment options consist of partial external bile diversion in the PFIC types with low to normal GGT.[24]

Alpha-1-antitrypsin (α1AT) deficiency is the most common genetic cause of liver disease, inherited in an autosomal codominant fashion, and can result in neonatal cholestasis.[30] The most common form is due to a homozygous variant of the α1AT gene (SERPINA1), which leads to a Glu342Lys substitution in the gene product ZZ or PiZZ. The incidence of PiZZ is approximately 1 in 2000 live births, but only 10% to 15% of these patients will manifest liver disease by the age of 18 years.[30] Liver histology demonstrates accumulation of α1AT polymers (Z protein insoluble homopolymers) within the endoplasmic reticulum of hepatocytes, with cytoplasmic diastase-resistant periodic acid-Schiff (PAS)-positive inclusion bodies in periportal hepatocytes. Giant cell hepatitis is variably present, and when bile ductular proliferation is noted, it may be misinterpreted as biliary obstruction. Paucity of intralobular bile ducts typically occurs later in the disease course. The clinical presentation is variable, with cholestatic jaundice, hepatomegaly, elevated transaminases, and hepatitis in the newborn and increased liver function tests and hepatosplenomegaly in the late

Table 2
Progressive familial intrahepatic cholestasis

Type	Serum GGT Levels	Genetic Mutation (Protein)	Histology (Early)	Immunohistochemistry	Electron Microscopy Findings	Increased Risk of HCC
PFIC 1	Low to normal	ATP8b1 (FIC1)	Canalicular cholestasis + periportal hepatocyte biliary metaplasia		Granular bile	No
PFIC 2	Low to normal	ABCB11 (BSEP)	Canalicular cholestasis + lobular/portal fibrosis + inflammation + hepatocellular necrosis + giant cell transformation	BSEP is absent from canaliculi	Amorphous bile	Yes
PFIC 3	High	ABCB4 (MDR3)	Canalicular cholestasis + portal fibrosis + ductular proliferation	MDR3 is absent from canaliculi		No
PFIC 4	Low to normal	TJP2 (TJP2)	Canalicular cholestasis + lobular/portal fibrosis + inflammation + hepatocellular necrosis + giant cell transformation	TJP2 is absent from canaliculi with Claudin 1 decreased expression	Tight junctions between hepatocytes and biliary canaliculi elongated and lack the densest part of the zona occludens	Yes
PFIC 5	Low to normal	NR1H4 (FXR)	Canalicular cholestasis + diffuse giant cell transformation + ballooning hepatocytes + ductular proliferation	BSEP is absent from canaliculi and FXR is absent in hepatocyte nuclei		

Abbreviations: BSEP, bile salt export pump; HCC, hepatocellular carcinoma; PFIC, progressive familial intrahepatic cholestasis.

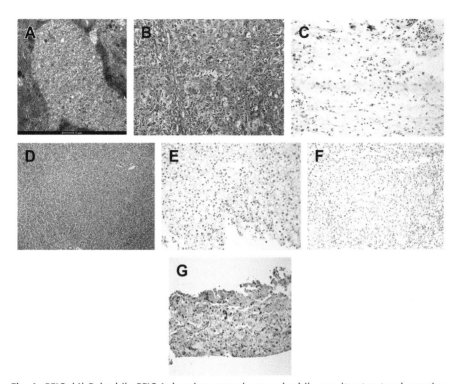

Fig. 1. PFIC. (*A*) Byler bile PFIC-1 showing coarsely granular bile on ultrastructural examination. (*B*) PFIC-2 showing canalicular cholestasis, giant cell transformation, lobular inflammation, and hepatocyte necrosis (×200). (*C*) Complete absence of BSEP protein in the canaliculi in a patient with PFIC-2 (×250). (*D*) TJP2 with canalicular cholestasis, mild lobular/portal fibrosis, mild portal inflammation, and focal acidophil bodies (×100). (*E*) TJP2 immunohistochemical stain demonstrating typical staining of canaliculi (×200), whereas (*F*) shows complete absence of TJP2 in the canaliculi of a patient with PFIC 4 (×200). (*G*) 4 + staining of the nuclei with FXR in a normal control. Patient with NR1H4 mutation shows loss of this nuclear staining (×200).

infancy/childhood period with possible development of esophageal varices.[30] Cirrhosis and acute liver failure are rare and HCC is a rare sequela.

Cholestasis due to TPN in the neonate occurs most often in premature infants of low birthweight with 50% of seriously affected infants having birthweight of less than 1000 g and a duration of TPN longer than 2 weeks.[31] Histologic features include canalicular cholestasis followed by hepatocyte and Kupffer cell cholestasis with variable portal inflammation, and bile ductular proliferation. This can mimic BA in the neonatal period.

HEREDITARY DISORDERS OF BILIRUBIN METABOLISM

The disorders within the group of hereditary nonhemolytic hyperbilirubinemia syndromes are in the differential of pediatric jaundice and include Dubin-Johnson syndrome, Rotor syndrome, Gilbert-Meulengracht syndrome, and Crigler-Najjar syndrome. Most patients are asymptomatic and approximately 50% demonstrate jaundice by puberty, with normal liver transaminases.[32] These can be separated into those presenting as nonconjugated hyperbilirubinemia (Gilbert-Meulengracht and Crigler-Najjar syndromes) and those presenting with predominantly conjugated hyperbilirubinemia with some nonconjugated hyperbilirubinemia (Dubin-Johnson and Rotor syndromes). Urine analysis for coproporphyrin types and levels are different in these 2 categories, with the mixed conjugated/nonconjugated hyperbilirubinemias excreting abundant amounts of coproporphyrin I, whereas the unconjugated hyperbilirubinemias show excretion of the normal coproporphyrin III.[33] Gilbert and Crigler-Najjar syndromes do not show histologic or ultrastructural abnormalities, and both show mutations in the UGT1A1 gene leading to complete absence of the UGT1A1 enzyme, which leads to improper conjugation activity. Dubin-Johnson syndrome has gross, light microscopic, and ultrastructural abnormalities. Grossly the liver core biopsy will appear dark (almost black) with a greenish hue. Light microscopy demonstrates coarse brownish/black pigment in the cytoplasm of the hepatocytes predominantly located in the centrilobular regions and along the biliary poles, while ultrastructurally these coarse granules appear to be lysosomal electron-dense granules composed of lipofuscin and melanin. Additional ultrastructural features include dilation of the rough endoplasmic reticulum, paracrystalline mitochondrial inclusions, and bile canaliculi dilation with patchy loss of microvilli.[34] Kupffer cells also contain thick black pigment granules. Dubin-Johnson syndrome is characterized by mutations in the ABCC2 gene, which leads to defect in the MRP2 protein. Immunohistochemical staining of the liver for MRP2 shows complete absence of staining along the canaliculi. Rotor syndrome has no described genetic defect currently, and shows normal histology on liver biopsy.

METABOLIC DISORDERS

Metabolic disorders affecting the liver consist of diseases involving carbohydrate metabolism (glycogen storage diseases [GSDs] and hereditary fructose intolerance), amino acid metabolism (hereditary tyrosinemia), lipid metabolism (Gaucher disease and Niemann-Pick disease), peroxisome abnormalities (Zellweger syndrome), and the urea cycle (ornithine transcarbamylase deficiency). The primary histologic patterns of liver injury demonstrate overlap between these categories, which include the cholestatic pattern (PFICs, Niemann-Pick disease type C, and Zellweger syndrome), storage patten (Gaucher, Niemann-Pick type A, B, and Wolman), steatotic pattern (hereditary fructose intolerance and cystic fibrosis), hepatitic pattern (α1AT and Wilson disease), and cirrhotic/fibrotic pattern (hereditary tyrosinemia and GSD types I, III, and IV). Many of these also have prominent superimposed secondary histologic patterns and electron microscopy features as well. The workup of the metabolic liver biopsy begins at the grossing bench with appropriate triaging of tissue. Tissue should be distributed for possible electron microscopy in glutaraldehyde, frozen in $-80°C$ liquid nitrogen for possible viral PCR studies or biochemical analysis or molecular analyses, and submitted in formalin for light microscopy studies. Portions also can be placed in OCT and snap frozen for possible histochemical analysis, such as Oil Red O and Sudan black staining.

Disorders of Carbohydrate Metabolism

Disorders of carbohydrate metabolism or disorders of glycogen pathways include the GSDs, which have an overall incidence of 1 in 20,000 to 43,000 live births. Approximately 80% of the GSDs affecting the liver are types I, III, and IX, with type IX being the most common.[35] Most GSDs are inherited in an autosomal recessive pattern, affect the liver and/or muscle, and predominantly present with episodic hypoglycemia and hepatomegaly.[35,36] There are approximately 15 GSDs that have been identified at this time, and all relate to either an abnormal quality of glycogen in cells or an abnormal quantity with different gene defects and enzyme deficiencies.[37] **Table 3** outlines the

Table 3
Glycogen storage diseases

GSD Type	Enzyme Deficiency	Gene Defect	Clinical Features	Light Microscopy	Electron Microscopy
0 (Aglycogenosis)	Glycogen synthase	GYS2 (liver isoform)/GYS1 (muscle isoform)	Hypoglycemia without hepatomegaly	Decreased quantity of hepatocellular cytoplasmic glycogen with moderate microvesicular and macrovesicular steatosis	
I (von Gierke disease)	Glucose-6-phosphatase translocase/transporter	SLC37A4 (types I b, c, d)/G6PC (type Ia)	Hypoglycemia, hyperlipidemia, hyperuricemia, hyperlactatemia with GSD type Ib having neutropenia	Swollen hepatocytes with thick cell membranes, displacement of organelles to the periphery by abundant cytoplasmic glycogen, glycogenated nuclei, and macrovesicular and microvesicular steatosis	Abundant monoparticulate glycogen with enlarged but reduced in number mitochondria
II (Pompe disease)	Alpha-1-4-glucosidase	GAA	Cardiomyopathy and muscular hypotonia; no hypoglycemia	Glycogen accumulation in heart, skeletal and smooth muscle, liver, kidney, endothelial cells, anterior horn cells and motor neurons	Membrane-bound vesicles variably filled with monoparticulate glycogen within lysosomes and glycogen rosettes within the cytoplasm
III (Cori disease, Forbes disease, debranching enzyme disease)	Amylo-1-6-glucosidase	AGL	Hepatomegaly, hypoglycemia, short stature, dyslipidemia	Swollen hepatocytes with thick cell membranes, displacement of organelles to the periphery by abundant cytoplasmic glycogen, glycogenated nuclei, periportal fibrosis, hepatocellular fibrosis and microsteatosis	Abundant and dispersed multiparticulate glycogen and small lipid droplets

(continued on next page)

Table 3
(continued)

GSD Type	Enzyme Deficiency	Gene Defect	Clinical Features	Light Microscopy	Electron Microscopy
IV (Andersen disease, glycogen branching enzyme deficiency)	Amylo-1,4 to 1,6-transglucosidase	GBE1	Variable - FTT, PoHTN, HSM, and cirrhosis	Ground-glass amphophilic to slightly eosinophilic inclusions within hepatocytes which are PASD resistant but digest with pectinase and amylase, and stain with colloidal iron; periportal fibrosis with progression to cirrhosis	Amylopectin-like fibrillar material
V (McArdle disease)	Glycogen phosphorylase	PYGM	Muscle pain, cramps and tenderness with exercise intolerance	No liver findings; muscle shows type 1 fiber atrophy and subsarcolemmal glycogen	Muscle - subsarcolemmal glycogen and ± myofibrillar accumulation
VI (Hers disease)	Liver glycogen phosphorylase E	PYGL	Asymptomatic hepatomegaly and growth retardation	Swollen hepatocytes with abundant glycogen and thick cell membranes; microsteatosis, mild periportal fibrosis and septal fibrosis	Large pools of monoparticulate glycogen with glycogen rosettes and lipid vacuoles; low-density granular material within the glycogen in hepatocytes
VII (Tarui disease)	Phosphofructokinase enzyme	PFKM	Exercise intolerance, muscle cramps, myoglobinuria, mild hyperbilirubinemia and reticulocytosis		

Type	Inheritance/Enzyme	Gene	Clinical features	Liver histology	Ultrastructure
VIII, IX (GSD with phosphorylase activation system defects)	X-linked	PHKA (Type IXa), PHKB (Type IXb), PHKG2 (Type IXc), PHKA1 (Type IXd)	HM, growth retardation, motor skill delay and hypotonia, increased ALT, AST, triglycerides and cholesterol	Swollen hepatocytes with thick cell membranes, displacement of organelles to the periphery by abundant cytoplasmic glycogen, ± septal fibrosis and microsteatosis	Abundant monoparticulate glycogen, glycogen rosettes and frequent lipid vacuoles with glycogen particles
X	Cyclic 3',5' AMP-dependent kinase	PGAM2	Asymptomatic hepatomegaly	Swollen hepatocytes with thick cell membranes, displacement of organelles to the periphery by abundant cytoplasmic glycogen, ± septal fibrosis and microsteatosis	Glycogen rosettes and lipid vacuoles with embedded glycogen particles; ± lysosomal monoparticulate glycogen with associated lipofuscin, cell membranes and other cellular components
XI (Fanconi-Bickel syndrome, GLUT2 deficiency)	Glucose transporter 2		Fasting hypoglycemia, postprandial hyperglycemia and hypergalactosemia, hypophosphatemic rickets with osteoporosis, and marked growth retardation; HM; moon facies and fat deposition in abdomen and shoulders	Increased glycogen and steatosis	Typical glycogen granules
XII (aldolase A deficiency)	Aldolase A		Myopathy with exercise intolerance and nonspherocytic hemolytic anemia; proximal wasting	No liver findings; muscle shows type 1 fiber atrophy and subsarcolemmal glycogen	Muscle - subsarcolemmal glycogen and ± myofibrillar accumulation

Abbreviations: ALT, alanine aminotransferase; AST, aspartate aminotransferase; FTT, failure to thrive; GSD, glycogen storage disorder; HM, hepatomegaly; HSM, hepatosplenomegaly; PASD, PAS with diastase; PoHTN, Portal hypertension.

main clinical, histologic, and ultrastructural features associated with each GSD.[35–37] Two GSDs that typically stand out are Pompe disease (GSD type II) because it is often considered a lysosomal storage disease due to its ultrastructural characteristic of monoparticulate glycogen filling membrane-bound vesicles or lysosomes, and GSD type IV (glycogen branching enzyme disease), which demonstrates amylopectinlike fibrillar material ultrastructurally and PAS diastase-resistant intrahepatocellular inclusions (**Fig. 2**).

Hereditary fructose intolerance (HFI) is another important but rare disorder of carbohydrate metabolism that affects the liver, with an incidence of 1 per 20,000 to 1 per 30,000 in live births. HFI is caused by a mutation in the *ALDOB* gene, which leads to a defect in the aldolase B enzyme and accumulation of fructose-1-phosphate.[38] In the newborn infant, marked macrovesicular steatosis is present with cholestasis and without cirrhosis. Ultrastructurally, there is increased smooth endoplasmic reticulum with concentric and irregular arrays of membranous material. Diagnosis is based on liver enzyme activity and sequencing of the *ALDOB* gene.

Disorders of Amino Acid Metabolism

Disorders of amino acid metabolism are rare and include hereditary tyrosinemia type 1 (HT1), which has an overall incidence of 1 per 100,000 live births but an incidence of 1 per 16,000 to 17,000 live births in Quebec. It is caused by a mutation in the *FAH* gene, leading to fumarylacetoacetate hydrolase deficiency, which leads to elevated levels of tyrosine, urinary succinyl acetone, and persistent elevations of serum a-Fetoprotein, reflecting the strong propensity to hepatocarcinoma.[39] Liver biopsy can be twofold, with an acute picture or a chronic form. Acutely, there is a hepatitic pattern with portal and lobular necroinflammatory foci, varying degrees of steatosis, pseudoacinar formation with occasional giant cell transformation, and iron accumulation within Kupffer

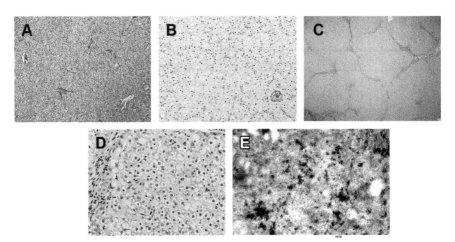

Fig. 2. GSDs. (*A*) Pale swollen hepatocytes with increased cytoplasmic glycogen and accentuated cell membranes in Type 1b GSD (×100). (*B*) PAS with diastase shows complete digestion of cytoplasmic glycogen (×200). (*C*) Delicate portal-to-portal fibrous septa are noted illustrating a nodule pattern without true cirrhosis in a case of GSD IV (×40). (*D*) GSD IV with swollen hepatocytes with glycogenated nuclei that are focally eccentrically positioned and focally amphophilic cytoplasmic material (×200). (*E*) Electron microscopy demonstrating filamentous amylopectinlike material within hepatocytes in GSD IV.

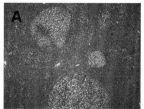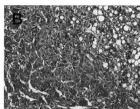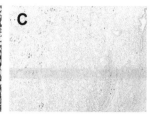

Fig. 3. Tyrosinemia. (*A*) Micronodular cirrhosis in tyrosinemia with focal macrovesicular steatosis (×40). (*B*) Regenerative nodule with reactive hepatocytes, pseudoacinar formation, focal macrovesicular steatosis, canalicular cholestasis, and variable acidophil bodies (×200). (*C*) Complete lack of FAH in the hepatocytes by immunohistochemistry (×100).

cells and periportal hepatocytes (**Fig. 3**B). Micronodular cirrhosis may develop (see **Fig. 3**A). The chronic hepatic phase typically shows a mixed micronodular and macronodular cirrhosis picture with minimal ductular proliferation and mild lymphoplasmacytic infiltrates within the fibrous septa. Steatosis is variably seen. FAH immunohistochemistry is typically negative in tyrosinemia (see **Fig. 3**C). Dysplastic nodules and/or HCC may develop during the chronic stage.[40] Cirrhotic nodules also may undergo "reversion," in which rare regenerative nodules become immunoreactive for FAH protein in a background of FAH-negative nodules.[39,41,42] The risk of HCC in HT1 is considered the highest among all metabolic disorders, with a risk of 13% to 17%.[40,43] Treatment of HT1 with 2-(2-nitro-4-trifluoromethylbenzoyl)-1,3cyclohexanedione (NTBC or nitisinone) has altered the clinical course of this disease and reduced the incidence of acute HT1 to 10% from approximately 75%. It should be noted that liver cirrhosis and hepatocarcinoma may occur without elevated tyrosine or succinylacetone levels in silent HT1.[44]

Disorders of Lipid Metabolism

Disorders of lipid metabolism or lysosomal storage disorders (LSDs) that significantly affect the liver include more than 50 known disorders, with an overall approximate incidence of 1 per 1500 to 1 per 7000 live births and commonly present with hepatomegaly.[45,46] Most are inherited in an autosomal recessive pattern with the exception of Fabry disease, Hunter syndrome (MPS II), and Danon disease, which are X-linked disorders. The histologic pattern of most is the storage pattern, with the exception of Niemann-Pick disease type C, which is primarily cholestatic with a secondary storage pattern. Histologically, the storage pattern consists of swollen and pale hepatocytes as well as Kupffer cells and portal macrophages due to intracellular storage material specific to each disorder. For the purpose of this discussion, Gaucher disease and Niemann-Pick types A, B, and C are discussed in more detail, with the other more common liver-affecting LSDs being outlined in **Table 4**.

Gaucher disease is caused by a mutation in the glucosylceramidase beta (*GBA*) gene with deficient activity of b-glucocerebrosidase resulting in increased accumulation of glucosylceramide in macrophages predominantly in the liver, bone marrow, and spleen. The Ashkenazi Jew population has the highest incidence, with approximately 1 per 450 live births, whereas the overall incidence excluding this population ranges from 1 per 20,000 to 1 per 200,000 live births.[47] Three subtypes have been described and based on neuropathic involvement, with types 2 and 3 having acute and chronic neuropathic features, respectively, and type 1 showing no involvement of the central nervous system.[47,48] Type 1 is the most common subtype and has an overall incidence of 1 per 50,000 to 1 per 75,000 live births in the non-Ashkenazi

Table 4
Lysosomal storage disorders

Disorder	Gene Involved	Protein Affected	Storage Material	Liver Histology	Electron Microscopy
Gaucher disease	GBA (glucosylceramidase beta)	β-glucocerebrosidase	Glucosylceramide	Gaucher cells: macrophages with pale eosinophilic tissue paper–like cytoplasm	Rounded, elongated lysosomes containing twisted or spiraled tubules
Niemann-Pick disease type A, B	SMPD1	Sphingomyelinase	Sphingomyelin	Large foamy lipid-laden PAS-negative histiocytes	Lipid inclusions with concentric laminated myelinlike figures
Niemann-Pick disease type C	NPC1 or NPC2	Lysosoma; cholesterol-binding protein	De-esterified cholesterol/sphingolipid	Cholestatic pattern with a secondary hepatitic pattern	Lipid inclusions with whorled aggregates of myelin
Farber disease	ASAH1	Lysosomal acid ceramidase	Ceramide	Foamy histiocytes and multinucleated cells	Curvilinear structures (Farber bodies)
G$_{M1}$ gangliosidosis	GLB1	β-galactosidase	Glycosphingolipids	Foamy histiocytes and large hepatocytes with fine PAS + vacuoles	Vacuoles - empty or with membrane-bound fibrillogranular material
GSD type II (Pompe disease)	GAA	Alpha-1-4-glucosidase	Glycogen	PAS + vacuoles in hepatocytes	Membrane-bound vesicles variably filled with monoparticulate glycogen within lysosomes and glycogen rosettes within the cytoplasm
Wolman disease/CESD	LIPA	Lysosomal acid lipase	Cholesterol esters	Microvesicular steatosis with/without cirrhosis	Membrane-bound lipid and cholesterol crystals
Mucopolysaccharidoses (MPS)				Colloidal iron +	Vacuoles - empty or with membrane-bound fibrillogranular material
Hurler (MPS type I)	IDUA	a-L-iduronate	Glycosaminoglycans	Vacuolated and swollen Kupffer cells and hepatocytes	
Hunter (MPS type II)	IDS	Iduronate sulfatase	Glycosaminoglycans		
Sanfilippo (MPS type III)	SGSH, NAGLU, HGSNAT, GNS		Glycosaminoglycans		

Abbreviations: CESD, cholesterol ester storage disease; GSD, glycogen storage disorder; PAS, periodic acid-Schiff.

Jew population, with estimates of 1 per 12 live births in this population.[49] Type 1 often presents with hepatosplenomegaly and may present with clinical features of autoimmune hepatitis (elevated immunoglobulin G, positive antinuclear antibodies, elevated anti-smooth muscle antibodies, and elevated ferritin levels). Liver histology demonstrates Gaucher cells (Kupffer cells and macrophages) that contain abundant pale eosinophilic tissue paper–like material with ultrastructural rounded, elongated lysosomes with twisted/spiraled tubules. Pericellular fibrosis is also present and cirrhosis may occur late.

Niemann-Pick disease has 3 subtypes (A, B, and C). Niemann-Pick types A and B are caused by mutations in the *SMPD1* gene, which leads to deficient sphingomyelinase and accumulation of sphingomyelin in cells that correlates into large foamy lipid-laden PAS-negative histiocytes in multiple organs and ultrastructural lipid inclusions with concentric laminated myelinlike figures. Niemann-Pick disease type C (NP-C) is related to mutations in the *NPC1* and *NPC2* genes, leading to deficient cholesterol-binding protein and accumulation of de-esterified cholesterol and sphingolipids in the lysosomes of cells. Liver histology shows a cholestatic pattern with a secondary hepatitic pattern. Ultrastructural examination reveals phospholipid inclusions with whorled aggregates of myelin. The overall incidence of NP-C is approximately 1 per 120,000 live births with 95% of causes being caused by mutations ion the *NPC1* gene with the remaining in the *NPC2* gene. Clinical presentation includes persistent hepatosplenomegaly with a neonatal hepatitis picture and an elevated GGT.

Disorders of Peroxisomes

Disorders of peroxisomes result from defects in the structure or function of peroxisomes and include a genetically heterogeneous group of congenital disorders involving mutations in the *PEX* genes that encode the peroxins proteins.[50] This group of disorders includes Zellweger syndrome, neonatal adrenoleukodystrophy, and infantile Refsum disease, with Zellweger syndrome being the most severe form with death typically occurring within the first 2 years of life. Zellweger syndrome presents in the neonatal period with hypotonia, characteristic facies, seizures, poor feeding, and hepatic dysfunction.[51] Liver histology noted in Zellweger syndrome includes mild cholestasis, increased iron within hepatocytes, and mild hepatocellular injury. A lesion of cholangioles also may be present with cholangiole and bile duct bile plugs, as well as biliary epithelial cell swelling, attenuation, or absence of cytoplasm in these foci. Septal and intralobular fibrosis may be present, and ultrastructural examination reveals an absence of peroxisomes.[52]

Disorders of the Urea Cycle

Disorders of the urea cycle typically present with hyperammonemia and consist of disorders with genetic defects in enzymes comprising the hepatic ammonia detoxification pathway.[53] This group includes ornithine transcarbamylase (OTC) deficiency, carbamoylphosphate synthetase 1 (CPS-1) deficiency, N-acetylglutamate synthase deficiency, argininosuccinate synthetase deficiency, argininosuccinate lyase (ASL) deficiency, and arginase deficiency. The overall incidence of these disorders is approximately 1 per 35,000 live births, with OTC being the most common with an incidence of approximately 1 per 56,500.[54] Liver histology is variable, ranging from normal to cirrhosis. OTC deficiency shows small aggregates of enlarged and pale/clear hepatocytes composed of increased glycogen with minimal fibrosis, which are also seen in ASL deficiency. Livers in CPS-1 deficiency typically show only mild fatty change without significant ultrastructural abnormalities.

INBORN ERRORS OF COPPER AND IRON METABOLISM

Wilson disease is a disorder of copper metabolism and storage that results in abundant copper accumulation in many organs but predominantly involves the liver, brain, and corneas. It is due to a loss of function mutation in the *ATP7B* gene, which encodes a hepatocyte canalicular membrane ATP-dependent metal transporter and leads to decreased biliary copper excretion and incorporation into ceruloplasmin leading to accumulation of copper within the liver. The overall incidence is 1 per 30,000 with a carrier rate of 1 in 86. Clinical presentation is markedly variable, but hepatic manifestations tend to develop within the first decade and neurologic manifestations tend to develop in the third decade.[55] Liver histology is also variable, ranging from mild features to overt macronodular cirrhosis at time of presentation. Typical early histologic features consist of mild to moderate macrovesicular steatosis, vacuolization of periportal hepatocyte nuclei, periportal mononuclear inflammatory infiltrates, cholestasis, and variable degrees of hepatocyte necrosis. Copper staining of the liver may be performed using rhodanine (copper appears red-orange) or orcein (copper appears black/brown) stains. Copper is not typically present in the liver, so presence of copper should alert the pathologist to the possibility of Wilson disease; however, copper may be seen in cholestatic disorders, so overinterpretation in cholestatic livers should be avoided and a negative copper stain does not rule out Wilson disease. Copper in Wilson disease is seen early in the periportal hepatocytes, and with time distributes throughout the lobular parenchyma. Ultrastructural features include large, pleomorphic mitochondria with dilated intracristal spaces and large electron-dense granular inclusions.[56] Quantitative assessment of hepatic copper content is still the gold standard for diagnosis, and a copper content of greater than 250 µg/g dry weight of liver is diagnostic.

Hereditary hemochromatoses (HH) are disorders of iron overload and can be separated into HFE-associated HH and non–HFE-associated HH, with HFE-associated HH accounting for 85% to 90% of patients with HH. Most patients with HFE-associated HH carry a homozygous mutation in C282Y, with the remaining smaller subset demonstrating a compound heterozygosity for C282Y/H63D mutations.[57] HH is typically not a disorder of the pediatric population, but is a disorder resulting in progressive iron overload. Liver histology shows iron deposition predominantly within periportal, zone 1 hepatocytes in a pericanalicular distribution with progressive gradation into zones 2 and 3. Later in the disease, iron can be identified in Kupffer cells, portal macrophages, biliary epithelial cells, and vascular endothelium and culminating into cirrhosis.[58] One of the non–HFE-associated HH disorders occurs in utero and is a main primary cause of neonatal hemochromatosis, and is termed gestational alloimmune liver disease (GALD). GALD typically presents with severe liver disease and extrahepatic siderosis involving pancreas, thyroid, and cardiac myocytes, but conspicuously absent reticuloendothelial (spleen, bone marrow) siderosis. Histologic findings noted in the liver are variable, ranging from marked hepatocyte necrosis with siderosis, giant cell or pseudoacinar transformation, and canalicular bile plugs to cirrhosis. The morphology of the iron on light microscopy is coarse granules and spares the reticuloendothelial cell system. This disease has a very high mortality and morbidity, and diagnosis is additionally important due to risk for subsequent pregnancies.[59]

LIVER TUMORS

Hepatic neoplasia is a rare complication of metabolic diseases in children. Chronic injury due to toxic metabolites may accumulate in the liver from these metabolic disorders and cirrhosis and/or hepatic neoplasia may occur.[40,60] The most common neoplasm to occur in this setting is HCC, which is typically rare in the pediatric patient

Table 5
Metabolic disorders associated with hepatocellular carcinoma

Disorder	Gene	Inheritance	Neoplasia	Background Cirrhosis	RR
Hereditary tyrosinemia	*FAH*	AR	HCC	++	ND
AAT deficiency	*SERPINA1*	AR	HCC, CC, CHCC	+/−	5
Hereditary hemochromatosis	*HFE*	AR	HCC	++	20
Wilson disease	*ATP7B*	AR	HCC, CC	+	ND
Acute intermittent porphyria	*HMBS*	AD	HCC	+	>30
PFIC-2	*ABCB11 (BSEP)*	AR	HCC, CC, CHCC	+/−	ND
Mitochondrial ETC disorders	Multiple	AR	HCC	+	ND
GSD-I	*G6PC, G6PT*	AR	HA, HCC	−	ND
GSD-III	*AGL*	AR	HCC, HA	+	ND
GSD IV	*GBE1*	AR	HCC	+	ND
NASH	Multiple	Complex	HCC	+	ND

Abbreviations: AAT, α-1 antitrypsin; ABCB11, ATP-binding cassette, subfamily B, member 11; AD, autosomal dominant; AGL, amylo-1, 6-glucosidase, 4-alpha-glucanotransferase (glycogen debrancher enzyme); AR, autosomal recessive; ATP7B, ATPase, Cu++ transporting, beta polypeptide; BSEP, bile salt export pump; CC, cholangiocarcinoma; CHCC, mixed cholangio-hepatocellular carcinoma; ETC, electron transport chain; FAH, fumarylacetoacetate hydrolase; G6PC, glucose-6-phosphatase, catalytic subunit; G6PT, glucose-6-phosphatase transporter; GBE1, glucan (1,4-alpha-), branching enzyme 1 (glycogen branching enzyme); GSD, glycogen storage disorder; HA, hepatic adenoma; HCC, hepatocellular carcinoma; HFE, hemochromatosis; HMBS, hydroxymethylbilane synthase; NASH, nonalcoholic steatohepatitis; ND, not determined; PFIC, progressive familial intrahepatic cholestasis; RR, relative risk; SERPINA1, serine protease inhibitor, alpha 1.

but common in cirrhosis. However, HCC does not necessarily occur in the setting of cirrhosis in this population, with an example being GSD type 1 in which malignant transformation of hepatic adenomas may occur. The most common malignant hepatic tumor to occur in children is hepatoblastoma, which typically is not associated with metabolic disorders but may occur with other heritable defects such as Beckwith-Wiedemann syndrome, Down syndrome, familial polyposis coli, and other chromosomal abnormalities. Boys are affected twice as much as girls.

Biopsies offer diagnostic challenges for a multitude of reasons. Histologic diversity, often present in hepatoblastomas, may lead to misinterpretations. Other challenges are related to nonrepresentative sampling or small sample sizes in small children/infants. Benign regeneration, focal nodular hyperplasia, and adenomas may appear very similar histologically on needle core biopsies, and pathologists must depend very heavily on their radiology colleagues with imaging modalities that include MRI, magnetic resonance angiography, and PET scans (**Table 5**).

SUMMARY

Liver disease in the neonate, infant, child, and adolescent may manifest differently depending on the type of disorder. These disorders show marked overlap clinically and on light microscopy. For example, neonatal cholestasis has a more broad differential diagnosis than in older children. Histologically, it is also variable and may show features of a giant cell hepatitis or prominent cholestasis, whereas in the older child giant cells are rare. Metabolic disorders also affect the liver differently based on the age of onset of hepatic injury. Histology and ultrastructural examination are used in tandem for the diagnosis of most of these disorders. However, these are rare, and more common etiologies, such as infection, specifically viruses, toxins, drugs such as acetaminophen or antibiotics or dietary supplements, TPN, and prematurity should be ruled out first. A final diagnosis or interpretation of the pediatric liver biopsy depends on appropriate and adequate clinical history, laboratory test results, biochemical assays, and molecular analyses, as indicated by the light microscopic and ultrastructural examination.

REFERENCES

1. Dezsofi A, Baumann U, Dhawan A, et al. Liver biopsy in children: position paper of the ESPGHAN hepatology committee. J Pediatr Gastroenterol Nutr 2015;60(3):408–20.
2. Menghini G. One-second biopsy of the liver—problems of its clinical application. N Engl J Med 1970;283(11):582–5.
3. Kasai M, Kimura S, Asakura Y, et al. Surgical treatment of biliary atresia. J Pediatr Surg 1968;3:665–75.
4. Roy A, Finegold MJ. Biopsy diagnosis of inherited liver disease. Surg Pathol Clin 2010;3:743–68.
5. Li L, Krantz ID, Deng Y, et al. Alagille syndrome is caused by mutations in human Jagged1, which encodes a ligand for Notch1. Nat Genet 1997;16(3):243–51.
6. Oda T, Elkahloun AG, Pike BL, et al. Mutations in the human Jagged1 gene are responsible for Alagille syndrome. Nat Genet 1997;16(3):235–42.
7. Shneider BL, Magee JC, Karpen SJ, et al. Total serum bilirubin within 3 months of hepatoportoenterostomy predicts short-term outcomes in biliary atresia. J Pediatr 2016;170:211–7.
8. Zagory JA, Nguyen MV, Wang KS. Recent advances in the pathogenesis and management of biliary atresia. Curr Opin Pediatr 2015;27(3):389–94.
9. Mohanty SK, Donnelly B, Bondoc A, et al. Rotavirus replication in the cholangiocyte mediates the temporal dependence of murine biliary atresia. PLoS One 2013;8(7):3690969.
10. Nakashima T, Hayashi T, Tomoeda S, et al. Reovirus type-2-triggered autoimmune cholangitis in extrahepatic bile ducts of weanling DBA/1J mice. Pediatr Res 2014; 75(1–1):29–37.
11. Shivakumar P, Campbell KM, Sabla GE, et al. Obstruction of extrahepatic bile ducts by lymphocytes is regulated by IFN-gamma in experimental biliary atresia. J Clin Invest 2004;114(3):322–9.
12. Muraji T. Maternal microchimerism in biliary atresia: are maternal cells effector cells, targets, or just bystanders? Chimerism 2014;5(1):1–5.
13. Muraji T, Hosaka N, Irie N, et al. Maternal microchimerism in underlying pathogenesis of biliary atresia: quantification and phenotypes of maternal cells in the liver. Pediatrics 2008;121(3):517–21.
14. Iwaisako K, Jiang C, Zhang M, et al. Origin of myofibroblasts in the fibrotic liver in mice. Proc Natl Acad Sci U S A 2014;111(32):E3297–305.
15. Verkade HJ, Bezerra JA, Davenport M, et al. Biliary atresia and other cholestatic childhood diseases: advances and future challenges. J Hepatol 2016;65(3):631–42.
16. Harpavat S, Ramraj R, Finegold MJ, et al. Newborn direct or conjugated bilirubin measurements as a potential screen for biliary atresia. J Pediatr Gastroenterol Nutr 2016;62(6):799–803.
17. Amir AZ, Sharma A, Cutz E, et al. Hepatoblastoma in explanted livers of patients with biliary atresia. J Pediatr Gastroenterol Nutr 2016;63(2):188–94.
18. Subramaniam P, Knisely A, Portmann B, et al. Diagnosis of Alagille syndrome—25 years of experience at King's College Hospital. J Pediatr Gastroenterol Nutr 2011; 52(1):84–9.

19. Alagille D, Odievre M, Gautier M, et al. Hepatic ductular hypoplasia associated with characteristic facies, vertebral malformations, retarded physical, mental, and sexual development, and cardiac murmur. J Pediatr 1975;86:63–71.

20. McDaniell R, Warthen DM, Sanchez-Lara PA, et al. Notch2 mutations cause Alagille syndrome, heterogeneous disorder of the Notch signaling pathway. Am J Hum Genet 2006;79(1):169–73.

21. Hoffenberg EJ, Narkewicz MR, Sondheimer JM, et al. Outcome of syndromic paucity of interlobular bile ducts (Alagille syndrome) with onset of cholestasis in infancy. J Pediatr 1995;127(2):220–4.

22. Emerick KM, Rand EB, Goldmuntz E, et al. Features of Alagille syndrome in 92 patients: frequency and relation to prognosis. Hepatology 1999;29(3):822–9.

23. Cardona J, Houssin D, Gauthier F, et al. Liver transplantation in children with Alagille syndrome–a study of twelve cases. Transplantation 1995;60(4):339–42.

24. Davit-Spraul A, Gonzales E, Baussan C, et al. Progressive familial intrahepatic cholestasis. Orphanet J Rare Dis 2009;4:1.

25. Clayton RJ, Iber FL, Ruebner BH, et al. Byler disease. Fatal familial intrahepatic cholestasis in an Amish kindred. J Pediatr 1965;67:1025–8.

26. Sambrotta M, Strautnieks S, Papouli E, et al. Mutations in TJP2 cause progressive cholestatic liver disease. Nat Genet 2014;46(4):326–8.

27. Sambrotta M, Thompson RJ. Mutations in TJP2, encoding zona occludens 2, and liver disease. Tissue Barriers 2015;3(3):e1026537.

28. Gomez-Ospina N, Potter CJ, Xiao R, et al. Mutations in the nuclear bile acid receptor FXR cause progressive familial intrahepatic cholestasis. Nat Commun 2016;7:10713.

29. Zhou S, Hertel PM, Finegold MJ, et al. Hepatocellular carcinoma associated with tight junction protein 2 deficiency. Hepatology 2015;62(6):1914–6.

30. Nelson D, Teckman J, Di Bisceglie A, et al. Diagnosis and management of patients with a1-antitrypsin (A1AT) deficiency. Clin Gastroenterol Hepatol 2012; 10(6):575–80.

31. Suchy FJ. Neonatal cholestasis. Pediatr Rev 2004;25(11):388–96.

32. Lee JH, Chen HL, Chen HL, et al. Neonatal Dubin-Johnson syndrome: long-term follow-up and MRP2 mutations study. Pediatr Res 2006;59(4 Pt 1):584–9.

33. Strassburg CP. Hyperbilirubinemia syndromes (Gilbert-Meulengracht, Crigler-Najjar, Dubin-Johnson, and Rotor syndrome). Best Pract Res Clin Gastroenterol 2010;24(5):555–71.

34. Sobaniec-Lotowska ME, Lebensztein DM. Ultrastructure of Kupffer cells and hepatocytes in Dublin-Johnson syndrome: a case report. World J Gastroenterol 2006;12(6):987–9.

35. Ozen H. Glycogen storage diseases: new perspectives. World J Gastroenterol 2007;13(18):2541–53.

36. Hicks J, Wartchow E, Mierau G. Glycogen storage diseases: a brief review and update on clinical features, genetic abnormalities, pathologic features, and treatment. Ultrastruct Pathol 2011;35(5):183–96.

37. Filimann MW, Oldfors A. Glycogen pathways in disease: new developments in a classical field of medical genetics. J Inherit Metab Dis 2015;38:483–7.

38. Bouteldja N, Timson DJ. The biochemical basis of hereditary fructose intolerance. J Inherit Metab Dis 2010;33:105–12.

39. Demers SI, Russo P, Lettre F, et al. Frequent mutation reversion inversely correlates with clinical severity in a genetic liver disease, hereditary tyrosinemia. Hum Pathol 2003;34:1313–20.

40. Schady DA, Roy A, Finegold MJ. Liver tumors in children with metabolic disorders. Transl Pediatr 2015;4(4):290–3.
41. Kvittingen EA, Rootwelt H, Brandtzaeg P, et al. Hereditary tyrosinemia type I: self-induced correction of the fumarylacetoacetase. J Clin Invest 1993;91:1816–21.
42. Kvittingen EA, Rotwelt H, Berger R, et al. Self-induced correction of the genetic defect in tyrosinemia type I. J Clin Invest 1994;94:1657–61.
43. Russo PA, Mitchell GA, Tanguay RM. Tyrosinemia: a review. Pediatr Dev Pathol 2001;4:212–21.
44. Blackburn PR, Hickey RD, Nace RA, et al. Silent tyrosinemia type I without elevated tyrosine or succinylacetone associated with liver cirrhosis and hepatocellular carcinoma. Hum Mutat 2016;37(10):1097–105.
45. vom Dahl S, Mengel E. Lysosomal storage disease as differential diagnosis of hepatosplenomegaly. Best Pract Res Clin Gastroenterol 2010;24:619–28.
46. Staretz-Chacham O, Lang TC, LaMarca ME, et al. Lysosomal storage disorders in the newborn. Pediatrics 2009;123(4):1191–207.
47. Zhang H-F, Yang X-J, Zhu S-S, et al. Pathological changes and clinical manifestations of 1020 children with liver disease confirmed by biopsy. Hepatobiliary Pancreat Dis Int 2004;3:395–8.
48. Saadi T, Rosenbaum H, Veitsman E, et al. Gaucher's disease type I: a disease masked by the presence of abnormal laboratory tests common to primary liver disease. Eur J Gastroenterol Hepatol 2010;22(8):1019–21.
49. Beutler E. Gaucher disease: multiple lessons from a single gene disorder. Acta Paediatr Suppl 2006;95(451):103–9.
50. Al-Dirbashi OY, Shaheen R, Al-Sayed M, et al. Zellweger syndrome caused by PEX13 deficiency: report of two novel mutations. Am J Med Genet Part A 2009; 149A:1219–23.
51. Braverman NE, Raymond GV, Rizzo WB, et al. Peroxisome biogenesis disorders in the Zellweger spectrum: an overview of current diagnosis, clinical manifestations, and treatment guidelines. Mol Genet Metab 2016;117(3):313–21.
52. Bove KE, Daugherty CC, Tyson W, et al. Bile acid synthetic defects and liver disease. Pediatr Dev Pathol 2004;7(4):315–34.
53. Yaplito-Lee J, Chow CW, Boneh A. Histopathological findings in livers of patients with urea cycle disorders. Mol Genet Metab 2013;108(3):161–5.
54. Mew NA, Lanpher BC, Gropman A, et al. Urea cycle disorders overview. In: Pagon RA, Adam MP, Ardinger HH, et al, editors. Gene reviews. Seattle (WA): University of Washington; 2003. p. 1993–2016. April 9, 2015.
55. Cope-Yokoyama S, Finegold MJ, Sturniolo GC, et al. Wilson disease: histopathological correlations with treatment on follow-up liver biopsies. World J Gastroenterol 2010;16(12):1487–94.
56. Jevon GP, Dimmick JE. Histopathologic approach to metabolic liver disease: part 1. Pediatr Dev Pathol 1998;1(3):179–99.
57. Cheng R, Barton JC, Morrison ED, et al. Differences in hepatic phenotype between hemochromatosis patients with HFE C282Y homozygosity and other HFE genotypes. J Clin Gastroenterol 2009;43(6):569–73.
58. Brunt EM, Olynyk JK, Britton BS, et al. Histological evaluation of iron in liver biopsies: relationship to HFE mutations. Am J Gastroenterol 2000;95(7):1788–93.
59. Whitington PF. Gestational alloimmune liver disease and neonatal hemochromatosis. Semin Liver Dis 2012;32(4):325–32.
60. Jevon GP, Dimmick JE. Histopathologic approach to metabolic liver disease: part 2. Pediatr Dev Pathol 1998;1(4):261–9.

Hepatocellular Adenomas
Morphology and Genomics

Paulette Bioulac-Sage, MD[a],*, Christine Sempoux, MD, PhD[b], Charles Balabaud, MD[a]

KEYWORDS

- Hepatocellular adenomas • Genomics • Genoptye/phenotype
- Hepatocellular adenoma classification • Malignant transformation

KEY POINTS

- Hepatocellular adenoma (HCA) is a global entity encompassing several subtypes identified by specific mutations.
- Immunomarkers, liver-type fatty acid binding protein (LFABP) and C-reactive protein (CRP), allow the identification of the 2 major subtypes, hepatocyte nuclear factor (HNF) 1α-inactivated HCA (H-HCA) and inflammatory HCA (IHCA).
- Glutamine synthetase (GS) is a surrogate marker to identify β-catenin–activated HCA (β-HCA): homogeneous and diffuse for exon 3 mutation (outside S45) and heterogeneous and diffuse for exon 3 S45, both linked to potential malignancy.
- IHCA can be β-catenin mutated.
- β-Catenin mutation alone is not sufficient to induce malignancy. A second hit is necessary, such as telomorase reverse transcriptase promoter mutation.
- HCA classification using immunomarkers may require expertise, particularly on liver biopsy, and, if necessary, molecular confirmation.

HCAs are rare benign monoclonal liver tumors, described for the first time by Edmondson in 1953.[1] HCAs have since been linked to the use of oral contraceptives by Baum and colleagues in 1973.[2] The understanding of HCA was completely renewed when the 2 first underlying gene mutations were discovered in 2002, soon followed by others. These mutations are the basis of the genotype/phenotype classification of HCA discussed in this article.

Disclosures: The authors have no conflict of interest and nothing to disclose.
[a] Inserm U 1053, Université Bordeaux, 146 rue Léo Saignat, 33076 Bordeaux, France; [b] Service of Clinical Pathology, Lausanne University Hospital, Institute of Pathology, Rue du Bugnon 25, CH-1011 Lausanne, Switzerland
* Corresponding author.
E-mail address: paulette.bioulac-sage@u-bordeaux2.fr

Gastroenterol Clin N Am 46 (2017) 253–272
http://dx.doi.org/10.1016/j.gtc.2017.01.003
0889-8553/17/© 2017 Elsevier Inc. All rights reserved.

HEPATOCELLULAR ADENOMAS: GENOMICS—THE GENOTYPE CLASSIFICATION

The first mutations responsible for the development of HCA were described in 2002, in Taiwan and in France. The first one is an activating mutation of *CTNNB1* gene coding for β-catenin[3] and the second corresponds to a biallelic inactivating mutation of *HNF1A*.[4] Consequently, HCAs are classified today into 3 main categories[5]: (1) *HNF1A*-mutated HCA [H-HCA] (35%–40%); (2) IHCA (40%–50%), with multiple mutated genes identified, mainly *IL6*[6]; and (3) β-catenin–mutated HCA (β-HCA) (15%–20%). An additional important leap forward was made recently, in 2014 and 2016, when β-HCA was subdivided into several subgroups according to the degree of activation of β-catenin.[7,8] β-Catenin mutation is also found in 10% of IHCA (β-IHCA). So far, fewer than 10% of HCAs remain unclassified HCAs (UHCAs).

HCAs, mainly β-HCA (discussed later), have a malignant potential and can evolve into hepatocellular carcinoma (HCC). The transformation depends on the occurrence of additional mutations. Telomerase reverse transcriptase (TERT) promoter mutations have been identified as responsible for this complication in half of the β-HCAs (mainly those showing mutations in exon 3).[9] In HCC derived from HCA, the observed number of genetic alterations is much lower than in classic HCC.[7]

The different mutated genes in HCA identified to date, in 2016, are presented in **Box 1**.[5–8,10–19]

Despite the great achievements, the underlying mutated genes are still unidentified in 15% of IHCA, and 10% of HCAs are still unsolved (UHCAs). In 2016, microarray analysis revealed an additional subgroup of HCAs previously unclassified, associated with dysregulation of the prostaglandin pathway, therefore named prostaglandin HCAs.[20] The genetic alterations, however, have not yet been identified. In multiple HCAs, different subtypes are occasionally observed and remain puzzling.[21] An intriguing and important question is why, within the large number of women taking oral contraceptives, only a few develop HCA. This is also observed in patients with genetic diseases associated with HCA development, such as maturity-onset diabetes of the young type 3 (MODY3) or glycogen storage disease (GSD).[12,18] This suggests that different genetic and environmental factors predispose to the development of HCAs, which are, therefore, often multiple.[5] In less than 20 years, molecular biology has made tremendous progress to understand HCA. At present, in practice, hematoxylin-eosin stain (H&E) combined with immunohistochemistry (IHC) allows classification and has largely replaced the need for molecular biology. When there is doubt about interpretation, this molecular analysis can be performed on frozen but also fixed tissue.

HEPATOCELLULAR ADENOMAS: MORPHOLOGY—THE GENOTYPE/PHENOTYPE CLASSIFICATION

The genotype/phenotype classification has been a great step forward in recognizing the different HCA subtypes. Several reviews on the subject have been published in the literature.[22–32]

Technical Considerations

A correct interpretation of the histologic and immuno-histochemical data can only be performed if the sampling and the techniques are adequate. Advice (through slides or virtual slides) are more and more common. Interpretation is facilitated when the techniques are of good quality and requires the comparison with the nontumoral liver. The size of the biopsy is still a major problem. The main considerations are presented in **Box 2** and **Table 1**.

Box 1
Hepatocellular adenoma subtypes: genomics

First hit

H-HCA — *HNF1A* gene belongs to the hepatocyte nuclear factor family, a key transcription factor involved in the development of the liver; also controls hepatocyte differentiation as well as glucose and lipid metabolism[4,11,12]
    In H-HCA mutations are biallelic, somatic in 90%, germline in 10% of cases
    In H-HCA occurring in MODY3 patients, in addition to a germline monoallelic monogenic type 2 diabetes mutation, there is another somatic mutation inactivating the second allele in the tumor
    Somatic monoallelic mutations are rarely identified in any kind of HCA

IHCA — several genes mutated, all promoting the constitutive activation of STAT 3 pathway[6,7,13–15]:
- IL6-signal transducer (*IL6ST* coding gp130): 65%
- Fyn-related kinase (*FRK*): 10%
- *STAT3*: 5%
- *GNAS* complex locus: 5%
- Janus kinase 1 (*JAK1*): 2%

In fewer than 15% of IHCAs, the mutations are still unknown.

β-HCA — *CTNNB1* gene. Three classes of mutations according to the β-catenin activation[8]:
- Highly active mutations: exon 3 deletions and amino acid substitutions in the β-TRCP binding site (D32-S37)
- Moderately active: exon3 T41
- Weakly active: exon 3 S45; exon 7/8 (K335, N 387)

Second hit (in the process of malignant transformation for β-HCA AND β-IHCA)[8]

- TERT promoter mutations. These mutations create a potential binding site for ETS (E-26)/ternary complex factor transcription factors and are predicted to increase promoter activity and TERT transcription. Observed in 60% of HCA with malignant transformation (in association with CTNNB1 mutations).

- Other second activating hit: *CTNNB1* mutant allele duplication (60%); second *CTNNB1* highly activating mutation (33%); *APC* inactivating mutation (6%)

Morphology Hematoxylin-eosin

HNF1α-inactivated hepatocellular adenoma (35%–40%)

Typical aspect with steatosis H-HCA is mainly a homogenous group of tumors (**Fig. 1**A). The classic aspect is a steatotic tan nodule, with a various amount of macrovesicular and microvesicular steatosis. Intermingling clear cells are found, usually sparing the arterial zones that appear composed of thin strands of smaller eosinophilic cells. This leads to a packeting aspect, characteristic of H-HCA. Contours of the tumor are often lobulated, sometimes isolating small tumoral areas in the immediate surrounding parenchyma. There are often numerous glycogenic nuclei.

A few unusual misleading features can be associated. Few rosettes or pseudo-glandular aspects can be found in the nonsteatotic areas and most probably related to cholestasis. Foci of sinusoidal dilatation, congestion, peliosis, or fibrinoid deposits can also be present.

Steatosis is a good argument for the diagnosis of H-HCA, allowing its recognition already by imaging, but alone it is insufficient to diagnose H-HCA; steatosis can also be observed in other HCA subtypes.

Box 2
Technical considerations

Surgical specimen: gross pathology

- Tumor: sampling of different areas: homogeneous, heterogeneous (avoiding large areas of hemorrhage/necrosis)
- Sampling of interface T/NT
- NT
  - Sampling with at least 1 block at distance of the tumor(s) if normal, homogeneous NT
  - Sampling of all abnormal foci/nodules (color, consistence, etc.)
- Pictures of tumoral slices and/or scheme of the different sampled areas
- Fixation of sliced specimen in 10% formalin (at least 24 hours), followed by the same different steps of sampling and pictures, as described previously

Biopsy

- T and NT fragments are mandatory (clearly labeled)

Stainings

- At least H&E, reticulin on T; + Masson trichrome and Perls on NT
- IHC on T and/or junction T/NT: usual panel of antibodies, step by step (see **Table 1** and **Fig. 6**)

Abbreviations: NT, nontumoral liver; T, tumoral liver.

Atypical case without steatosis In rare cases, H-HCA cannot be recognized with certainty on H&E (**Fig. 1**B). This is due to the absence or the scarcity of steatosis (macro, micro) within the lesion. It is rare to observe this phenomenon on the entire HCA as well as to see it on several lesions in the same patient. At high magnification, some well-limited areas show tiny droplets of steatosis. In this situation, the diagnosis relies only on IHC, that is, the absence of LFABP (discussed later). In the total absence of fat, molecular analysis may be warranted.

Inflammatory hepatocellular adenoma (40%–50%)

Typical features IHCAs are characterized by a variable degree of sinusoidal dilatation/peliosis, associated with the presence of inflammatory infiltrates and numerous and often thickened arteries surrounded by small amount of connective tissue and more or less obvious ductular reaction (**Fig. 2**A, B). These 2 last features can be particularly prominent, especially when the IHCAs are remodeled secondary to severe necrosis/hemorrhage, and they can be misleading, giving the impression of a focal nodular

---

Table 1
Antibodies used for subclassification of hepatocellular adenoma

Antibody	Clone	Dilution	Retrieval	Company
Anti-LFABP	Rabbit polyclonal	1/400	pH 9	LSBIO (Seattle, USA)
Anti-CRP	Mouse monoclonal Y284	1/1500	pH 6	ABCAM (Cambridge, UK)
Anti-SAA	Mouse monoclonal MC1	1/200	pH 9	DAKO (Courtaboeuf, France)
Anti-GS	Mouse monoclonal 6GS	1/400	pH 6	BD Biosciences (Le Pont de Claix, France)
Anti–β-catenin	Mouse monoclonal 14	1/100	pH 6	BD Biosciences (Le Pont de Claix, France)

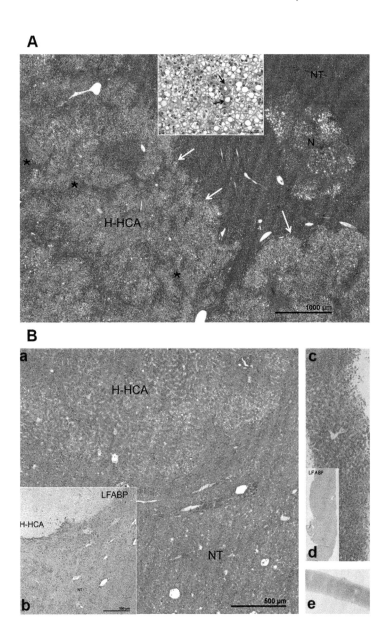

Fig. 1. (A) H-HCA — H&E: areas of more or less steatotic and clear cells, separated by thin strands of nonsteatotic cells (*asterisk*) leading to a typical packeting aspect; the tumor has lobulated contours (*white arrows*) and a small tumoral nodule (N) is isolated in the surrounding nontumoral parenchyma (NT). (*Inset*) Mixture of macrosteatosis and microsteatosis and 2 rosettes (*black arrows*). (B) H-HCA — (*left*) (a) H&E: this resected tumor exhibiting very mild steatosis is difficult to differentiate from the nontumoral liver (NT); IHC showing lack of LFABP is mandatory to make the diagnosis of H-HCA (b); (*right*) biopsy of another case showing a benign hepatocellular tumor (c, H&E), lacking LFABP (d), which is normally expressed in a fragment of NT liver (e).

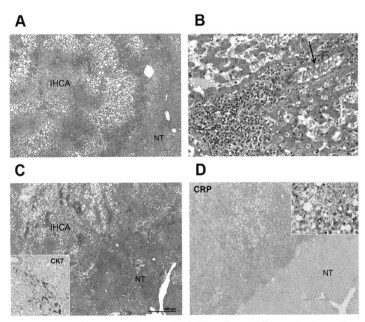

Fig. 2. IHCA (*A, B*) typical aspect with sinusoidal dilatation, thick arteries (*arrow*) and inflammatory foci, contrasting with normal nontumoral (NT) liver; (*C, D*) this other case exhibited in addition obvious steatosis, CK7 underlined the ductular reaction (*inset* [C]); CRP is highly expressed in all tumoral cells, steatotic or not (*inset* [D]), with sharp demarcation from the surrounding NT; LFABP is normally expressed in the tumor (not shown).

hyperplasia (FNH). Inflammatory infiltrates are polymorphous but composed mainly of lymphocytes.

In some cases, these cardinal features can be absent, with few or no sinusoidal dilatations and weak inflammation. In this case, diagnosis is made only by IHC (discussed later). Furthermore, IHCAs can exhibit steatosis (**Fig. 2**C), mainly irregularly dispersed; when the steatosis is more pronounced, this can be misleading for the radiologists who diagnosed H-HCA.

Atypical features The percentage of the different histologic items varies from case to case but commonly not interfering with the diagnosis feasibility. In rare instances, however, in the absence of inflammation and of sinusoidal dilatation, diagnosis of IHCA is difficult, particularly if there is no ductular reaction but a detectable steatosis. IHC is necessary to confirm the diagnosis of IHCA (**Fig. 2**D).

β-catenin–activated hepatocellular adenoma (15%–20%)
β-HCA can exhibit mild cytologic/architectural abnormalities, which can be sometimes difficult to differentiate from well differentiated HCC, especially if associated with cholestasis.

These features are inconstant, however, and no specific histologic aspects can reliably predict a diagnosis of β-HCA. In this case, it is necessary to perform IHC (**Fig. 3**).

β-Catenin–activated inflammatory hepatocellular adenoma
Approximately 10% of IHCA harbor mutations in *CTNNB1* gene and 50% of β-HCA displayed inflammatory features (β-IHCA). Their morphologic features associate those of IHCA and β-HCA, typical or not (**Fig. 4**).

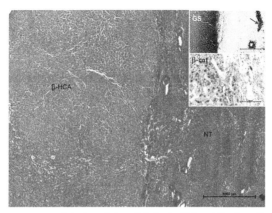

Fig. 3. β-HCA: the nonencapsulated nodule exhibited mild architectural/cytologic abnormalities (not visible at this magnification), a strong/diffuse expression of GS, contrasting with normal expression around centrolobular veins (*arrow*) in nontumoral liver (NT) and aberrant nuclear staining of β-catenin (β-cat) (*insets*).

Both β-HCA and β-IHCA have a risk of malignant transformation (discussed later).

Unclassified hepatocellular adenoma

UHCAs (7%–10%), by definition, do not exhibit any particular morphologic feature and lack the immunophenotypic characteristics of the other subtypes (described later) (**Fig. 5**).

Morphology Immunohistochemistry

The different subtypes are presented in **Table 2a, b** and **Fig. 6**.

Markers

Liver-type fatty acid binding protein, the key marker to identify HNF1α-inactivated hepatocellular adenoma In all H-HCAs, the absence of LFABP expression by IHC is an excellent diagnostic marker, irrespective of the degree of steatosis, the presence of unusual features, or the size of the nodule, contrasting with the normal diffuse expression observed within the surrounding nontumoral parenchyma that serves as internal positive control (see **Fig. 1B**). LFABP immunostaining belongs to the panel of IHC markers used to classify HCA.

C-reactive protein and/or serum amyloid A, the key markers to identify inflammatory hepatocellular adenoma The inflammatory proteins have an intense diffuse expression specific to this subtype of HCA, restricted to tumor cells, with a sharp demarcation from the nontumoral parenchyma (see **Figs. 2D and 4**). It is not useful to use the 2 markers. In the authors' institution, CRP is preferably used. When the staining is weak or when it is difficult to interpret because expressed both within the tumor and outside the tumor, both markers are used and compared.

Glutamine synthetase, an excellent surrogate marker to identify β-catenin mutation If GS staining is diffuse and homogeneous within the HCA, it can reasonably be concluded that there is a *CTNNB1* exon 3 mutation (see **Fig. 3**).[7,8] This interpretation is reinforced when there is aberrant β-catenin nuclear staining (discussed later). In 2014 and 2016, more mutations were described in *CTNNB1* in HCA, showing that HCA mutated in exon 3 S45 or in exon 7/8 have different patterns of GS staining compared with the classic one. The correlation between molecular data and GS staining

A

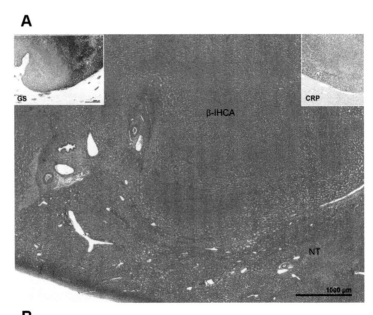

B

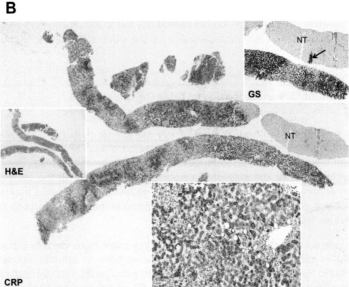

Fig. 4. (*A*) β-IHCA: this tumor does not exhibit specific features on H&E; strong positivity of CRP (*right inset*) and GS (*left inset*) with sharp demarcation from nontumoral liver (NT) allows diagnosing a β-IHCA. (*B*) β-IHCA, biopsy: the precise diagnosis cannot be made on H&E (*left inset*) but is easy on CRP showing a strong and diffuse expression, restricted to tumoral hepatocytes (*middle inset*) with sharp demarcation from nontumoral liver (NT); in addition, GS is also strongly expressed (*right inset*) in the same area as CRP; in the small fragment of NT, there is only a positivity of a few hepatocytes around a central vein (*arrow*).

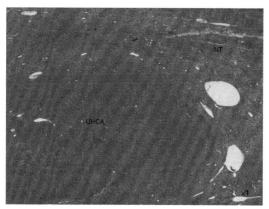

Fig. 5. UHCA: this nonencapsulated tumor does not exhibit any specific feature or cytologic anomalies; LFABP was normally expressed; there were no CRP or abnormal GS stainings (not shown). NT, non tumoral liver.

concerning S45 and exon 7/8 has not been published yet in detail (only in abstract form by the American Association for the Study of Liver Disease in 2016). Briefly, in the presence of exon 3 S45 mutation, a pattern of diffuse heterogeneous expression of GS is observed (**Fig. 7**), whereas when exon 7/8 is mutated, a patchy GS expression around veins and/or forming small positive foci is seen. In classic IHCA, GS staining is either absent or present focally around some veins in limited amount. Occasionally GS around hepatic veins is more pronounced, raising the question of a *CTNNB1* mutation that needs to be verified using molecular tools.

β-Catenin, a specific marker for β–hepatocellular adenoma but with low sensitivity It is not necessary to perform β-catenin staining if GS staining is completely normal. Aberrant nuclear staining (see **Fig. 3**) confirms the diagnosis of *CTNNB1* mutations (exon 3, including S45) but it can be scarce or focal. Positivity has so far not been observed when mutations are in exon 7/8. Negativity does not rule out the diagnosis of β-catenin mutation.

Additional markers
- In HCA, CD34 staining can be normal, expanded, or diffuse. The interpretation of abnormal staining is difficult. Diffuse CD34 can be seen in malignant transformation but also around congestive, peliotic area and, surprisingly, in many β-HCAs/β-IHCAs with S45 mutation (see **Fig. 7**).
- CK7-positive cells are seen within HCA either in ductules (ductular reaction of IHCA) or in hepatocytes, reflecting cholestasis. Small ovoid CK7-positive cells interpreted as progenitor cells are frequently observed in β-HCA and β-IHCA but have not been yet carefully investigated.

When and how to perform immunohistochemistry
There is no consensus on how to proceed and in which sequence. The guidelines used in the authors' institution are discussed (see **Fig. 6**). The most important message is that a diagnosis of UHCA subtype cannot be made prior to having done all the markers and finding them inconclusive.

Limits of the interpretation
There are numerous limitations to the interpretation of IHC.[33–39] They are linked to the techniques themselves and then they are avoidable. Interpretation of IHC on a

Table 2a	
Hepatocellular adenoma subtypes: immunohistochemistry interpretation (surgical specimen, no liver disease)	
H-HCA	**IHCA**
Hepatocyte markers	
LFABP	**CRP/SAA**
Results	
T absent NT present	T present NT absent
Interpretation	
Sensitivity/specificity excellent IHC cannot be interpreted in necrotic, hemorrhagic, burned areas (including their vicinity) It is recommended to have on the same block T and NT	
LFABP neg is not an absolute criteria of mutation in HCC thin bands LFABP+ may be observed in T (mainly at the periphery; this is due to a yet incomplete coalescence of nearby H-HCA).	Data may be not interpretable in liver disease.
Limits	
T faint staining should not be interpreted as negative. NT weak staining: the differential intensity between T and NT may be difficult to interpret. T staining may be difficult to analyze in massive steatosis and in small H-HCA.	T positivity limited to inflammatory areas should not be considered as IHCA. Occasionally heterogeneous, or very faint (use of the 2 markers) NT positivity: necrosis, hemorrhage, portal vein embolisation, inflammatory syndrome preclude the interpetation NT mild centrolobular positivity may be observed: no consequence on the interpretation.
When to perform the stainings?	
Whenever the diagnosis (H&E) is a possibility, specific markers allow ascertaining the diagnosis. All markers are mandatory before saying UHCA.	
Additional markers	
GS	
If strongly positive, molecular analysis is mandatory.	Frequently positive around hepatic veins, especially at the periphery of the nodule and occasionally well beyond (can sometimes be difficult to differentiate from β-IHCA)
CD34	
Normal or extended	
CK7	
Few to moderate number of positive cells (cholestatic pattern) and/or small progenitor cells	

biopsy[40] is possible and often of good performance (see **Figs. 1**B and **4**B) but can be difficult and occasionally impossible, particularly for GS staining. It requires imperatively the presence of nontumoral tissue for comparison.

Borderline hepatocellular adenoma and hepatocellular carcinoma

HCA can give rise to HCC.[41–49] It is primarily β-HCA or β-IHCA, however, with mutations in exon 3, including S45 who harbor the highest risk.[8,23] For this reason, these

Table 2b
Hepatocellular adenoma subtypes: immunohistochemistry interpretation (surgical specimen, no liver disease)

β-HCA, β-IHCA

Hepatocyte markers: GS

Results: different patterns

GS1 — homogenous and diffuse, intensity: strong or moderate
GS2 — heterogeneous and ± diffuse, intensity: +/− strong, number of positive cells: from few to many (starry sky)
GS3 — GS around some or many hepatic veins, +/− packs of labeled hepatocytes

Interpretation

• Easy for GS1. Activation of the β-catenin pathway, however, is not always related to β-catenin mutation. Other pathways can be responsible (ie, axin).
• Easy for GS2, when the number of stained hepatocytes look like a starry sky but could be more difficult if faint staining; the presence of a GS border, often irregular (thickness and density), is an important additional criterion.
• Easy for GS3 when the perivascular/motted pattern is obvious, but this pattern could be difficult to interpret; the presence of a GS border (usually less dense than in GS2) is also an important additional criterion in β-IHCA; the diagnosis is more difficult than in β-HCA for GS2 and GS3 pattern because GS can be over-expressed in some IHCA (**Table 2a**); all these data are part on an ongoing investigation.

Limits

Each time GS interpretation is equivocal, molecular analysis is mandatory, particularly concerning GS2 pattern.
The GS border should not be misinterpreted as the GS over-expression in NT liver.

When to perform the stainings?

In all cases

Additional markers

β-catenin

Aberrant β-catenin nuclear staining is always focal; the number depends of the GS pattern.
  GS1: usually positive, from few to many labeled nuclei
  GS2: from no to rare labeled nuclei
  GS3: no labeled nuclei
Some are faint/rare nuclear staining can be difficult to interpret.
β-Catenin staining is not necessary when GS is strictly normal.

CD34

Diffuse expression in T with GS2 and GS3 pattern, to the noticeable exception in the border
Interestingly, CD34 is not diffuse in GS1 pattern.

CK7

As described (see **Table 2a**)

---

subgroups need to be correctly identified. HCA occurring in specific context, such as GSD,[18,50] and male hormone administration[51] are more prone to transform into HCC. Recently H-HCA, previously considered benign, has been associated with HCC.[52–54]

The criteria on H&E to favor a borderline HCA are (1) cell atypia: variation in size of the cells and of the nuclei, (2) increased cell thick plates, (3) presence of pseudoglands, (4) abnormal reticulin network, and (5) pigmented nodule.[4,55] Typical foci of HCC (unique or multiple) can also be identified in some cases (**Fig. 8**). Additional markers, such as GPC3 and HSP70, can theoretically be useful but in practice they are not expressed in well-differentiated lesions. When the HCC covers the entire area of the nodule, it is not possible anymore to trace the putative benign origin of

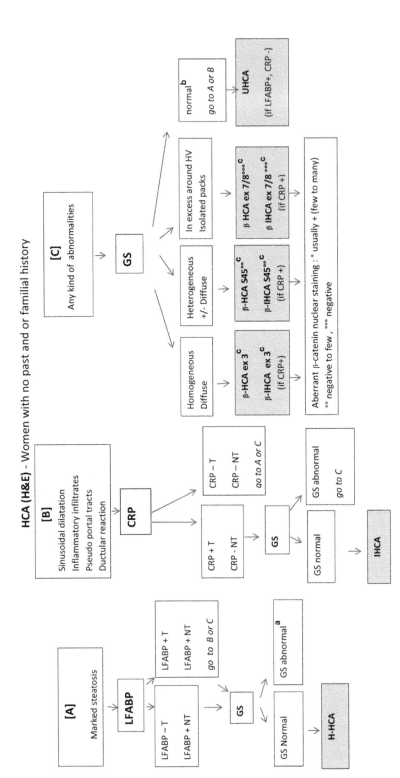

Fig. 6. HCA. Identification of subtypes using immunomarkers. Algorithm. [a] H-HCA: in the absence of well documented β-catenin mutation, whatever the expression of abnormal GS, molecular analysis is recommended. [b] No staining or staining limited to some hepatic veins at the periphery. [c] When GS is difficult to interpret: β-HCA (S45 or 7/8); IHCA or β-IHCA (S45 or 7/8); UHCA or β-HCA (S45 or 7/8); it is recommended to perform molecular analysis (frozen or fixed tissue).

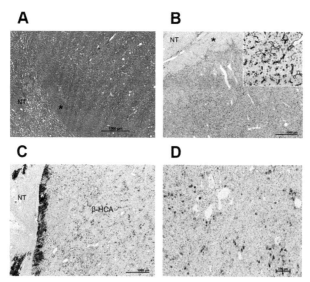

Fig. 7. β-HCA exon 3 S45: (*A*) the nodule presented at its interface with nontumoral liver (NT), a border (*asterisk*), still visible on H&E; (*B*) CD34 is diffusely expressed except at the border (higher magnification in inset); (*C*) GS is heterogeneous and diffuse in the tumor, stronger in the border; (*D*) at higher magnification: starry sky pattern with hepatocytic GS expression of various intensity: strong, moderate, mild, or negative.

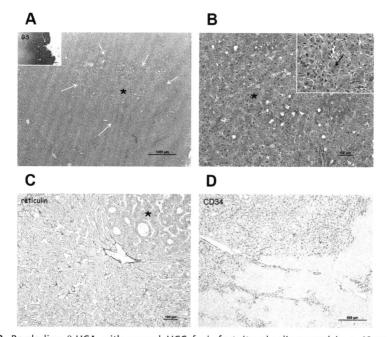

Fig. 8. Borderline β-HCA with several HCC foci, fortuitously discovered in a 40-year-old woman; (*A*) well-differentiated hepatocellular tumor with several atypical foci (*asterisk, white arrows*); strong/diffuse GS expression in the whole tumor (*inset*); (*B*) HCC foci with glandular features, canalicular cholestasis (*arrow in inset*); (*C*) reticulin network is focally decreased (*asterisk*), whereas it is normal otherwise; (*D*) CD34 is expanded but not diffuse.

the tumor. HCC can be LFABP negative without any underlying *HNF1 A* mutation or be CRP positive or β-catenin mutated without any link to a prior benign tumor. When there is still a rim of what looks like benign HCA at the periphery, it is often difficult to be sure that the rim is not malignant. It could correspond just to a better differentiated area of the same malignant tumor. The best way to solve the problem is to test by molecular biology several areas. It is admitted that HCCs derived from HCA have fewer numerous mutations than classic HCCs[7] and have better prognosis.

Multiple Nodules

Multiple nodules are often of the same phenotype. Their H&E appearance may vary, however, that is, H-HCA can show different steatosis content; H-HCA and IHCA can be found within the same liver[21] as well as IHCA and β-IHCA; β-HCA can have different mutations, some in exon 3, others in exons 7/8, and so forth. It is also not rare to observe a combination with other types of nodules, such as FNH[56] or hemangiomas.

The number of nodules is difficult to determine; it depends on the quality of the imaging techniques and whether the number of micro-HCAs not seen on imaging but identified on tissue sections on microscope analysis is taken into account.[57] When the number of nodules exceeds 10 by imaging, the term, *adenomatosis*, is used.[58–60] Adenomatosis is not a specific entity. It is encountered most frequently in H-HCA and IHCA. Adenomatosis related to H-HCA is not observed in male patients, except in the background of genetic diseases (MODY3 and GSD). Adenomatosis

---

Box 3
Should we use the hepatocellular adenoma classification?

No

Classification not used in most clinical practice for the diagnosis before resection (no need of biopsy)
- HCAs greater than 5 cm: resection to avoid the risk of bleeding and malignant transformation in the great majority of cases
- HCAs in men: resected independently of the size because of the risk of malignant transformation
- All HCAs showing evidence of growth on successive imaging, even after stopping OC: resection

Yes

Classification an important tool for pathologists to confirm the diagnosis of HCA, to make the differential diagnosis between FNH and HCA and even sometimes between HCA and HCC, to identify HCA in rare circumstances (cirrhosis and vascular diseases).

Classification is a potent research tool for clinical and fundamental progress in HCA understanding.

IHC: natural partnership with the molecular analysis, the driving force to understand the disease, and to support the recommendations within guidelines. Examples:
- Correlation between imaging and pathology to improve the accuracy of imaging (identification of subtypes either on resected specimen or on biopsy)
- To understand the complexity of the disease in terms of multiplicity of nodules (same phenotype with different aspect ie, H-HCA and IHCA, associations with other nodules: FNH, hemangiomas, and so forth)

HCAs are rare, so there is a need to collect data worldwide to have enough number to be able to study the significance and role of age, gender, oral contraception, genetic diseases, underlying liver diseases, metabolic diseases, vascular diseases, and so forth.

does not usually require a specific management except in rare cases (great number and large tumors).

The Background Liver and Clinical Context

The study of the background liver is essential for the interpretation of IHC data of all HCA subtypes.

In a classic situation of HCA development, the background liver is usually normal. Steatosis, from mild to severe, is often observed, particularly in cases of IHCA[61–66] and UHCA. In MODY3, HCAs are H-HCAs, whereas in patients taking male hormones, HCAs are β-HCAs, and in GSD all HCA subtypes can be observed except H-HCA.[18] All subtypes can exist for HCA developed on vascular liver diseases.[53] In cirrhotic livers, IHCAs have been recently described.[67,68] More and more cases of HCA are discovered in liver diseases: nonalcoholic steatohepatiatis,[64–66] cirrhosis (alcoholic),[67–69] and liver vascular diseases[53] in addition to genetic diseases GSD[18] and MODY3.[12]

Box 4
Pathologic report

Surgical specimen, biopsy
   Concordance between H&E features and IHC results (LFABP, CRP, GS diffuse/homogeneous), easy interpretation of the IHC: straightforward answer of H-HCA, IHCA, β-HCA, or β-IHCA
   Discordance between H&E features and IHC results
    -H-HCA and IHCA
    Before reporting H-HCA or IHCA with unusual histologic features, make sure the IHC technique is reliable in terms of protocol of the staining and in terms of analysis of the results (comparison with NT liver is mandatory for LFABP and CRP).
    -β-HCA/β-IHCA. GS interpretation
    Apart from a homogeneous/diffuse staining for GS or for a typical heterogeneous/diffuse GS positivity reliably related to specific *CTNNB1* mutations, GS may be difficult to interpret. Due to the consequence of this interpretation (higher risk of malignant transformation when mutations are located in exon 3, but not when they involve exon 7/8), it is reasonable to mention that molecular analysis is required to confirm the diagnosis of β-HCA or β-IHCA.
   Reporting borderline HCA and raising the diagnosis of a focal area of HCC within the HCA
    Surgical specimen: in the absence of evidence of HCC on H&E, it is preferable to be cautious (describe the lesions without mentioning the term HCC without other explanation), because this diagnosis may be detrimental to the patient in terms of insurance, quality of life, and so forth, although the borderline HCA/HCC is mainly of good prognosis once it has been removed entirely. If the tumor has not been removed entirely, it is important to mention the potential risk to leave atypical tissue in place.
    Biopsy: without using the term HCC (discussed later) it is reasonable — at the present stage of knowledge — particularly if GS is diffuse (homogeneous or heterogeneous) to call attention on the potential malignancy of the tumor and to advice for resection.
   Conclusion
    Surgical specimen: reporting is simple when the diagnosis is self-evident, such as in typical H-HCA and IHCA, which represent approximately 70% of HCA cases. The diagnosis is also simple for β-HCA and β-IHCA with diffuse and homogeneous GS, usually related to exon 3 mutations (outside S45), associated often with some positive β-catenin nuclei, and often also when GS expression is clearly diffuse and heterogeneous, usually related to exon 3 S45 mutations. More difficult whenever there is doubt in GS expression or inconclusive results by IHC. In this situation, it is important to ask for a second opinion and/or to require molecular data.
    Biopsy: the difficulty can be greater between subtypes of β-HCA because GS interpretation can be even more complicated and this can also be the case to differentiate between UHCA and FNH, with consequently a more frequent need to confirm the data on secondary resection and/or by molecular analysis.

Malignant transformation seems to be more frequent when the background liver is abnormal or when the clinical context is unusual.

The Report

Writing a precise report (**Box 3**) is an essential step in HCA work-up. Its interpretation is easy if a pathologist works closely with surgeons, hepatologists, radiologists, and molecular biologists in a specialized multidisciplinary team. If it is not the case, which is the most frequent situation, and/or if the pathologist is not a specialist in liver diseases, it is recommended to be as simple as possible and to give sharp data within a short report or in case of difficulties in interpretation to ask for advice.

HEPATOCELLULAR ADENOMA: WHY SHOULD WE CLASSIFY AND DO WE HAVE TO?

The question, is important and reasonable. Looking at the European Association for the Study of the Liver clinical practice guidelines on the management of benign liver tumors, guidelines written by expert liver radiologists, pathologists, surgeons, and molecular biologists, the recommendation for presumed HCA does not mention the phenotype classification as mandatory but underlines the positive identification of H-HCA or IHCA with MRI, with more than 90% specificity.[70] This is in contrast to what is found in articles written under the guidance of specialists of the HCA classification. HCA subtyping has not yet had an impact in general clinical practice, but when a biopsy is performed, the aim is to rule out an FNH (if imaging is doubtful) and to check for β-catenin subtype. To see a clinical impact, more longitudinal observational studies, registry building, and multidisciplinary cooperation are needed (**Box 4**). Pathologists need to know the size of the tumor, its content (steatosis and hemorrhage/necrosis), and if there are arguments for malignancy or underlying genetic or liver diseases. It is also important to mention if the tumor has been entirely removed or not. The multidisciplinary approach is essential (radiologist, surgeon, and hepatologist) in this field, as in many others.

SUMMARY

The main advantage of the genotype/phenotype classification is to identify and recognize the HCA entity, which is different from FNH and different from the majority of HCCs developed on normal liver. Furthermore, it has broadened the scope of the disease from women taking oral contraceptives to men, children, and aging persons, from normal liver to diseased livers, and from somatic to constitutional abnormalities.

ACKNOWLEDGMENTS

We would like to thank clinician Jean Frédéric Blanc; surgeons Christophe Laurent, Jean Saric, and Laurence Chiche; radiologists Nora Frulio and Hervé Trillaud; liver pathologists Brigitte le Bail and Claire Castain (all from CHU Bordeaux); and molecular biologists David Cappellen (CHU Bordeaux), Gabrielle Couchy, Sandra Rebouissou, and Jessica Zucman-Rossi (U 1624 Paris) for their contribution in the diagnosis and classification of hepatocellular adenomas.

REFERENCES

1. Edmondson HA. Tumors of the liver and intrahepatic bile ducts. Washington, DC: Armed Forces Institute of Pathology; 1958.

2. Baum JK, Bookstein JJ, Holtz F, et al. Possible association between benign hepatomas and oral contraceptives. Lancet 1973;2(7835):926–9.
3. Chen YW, Jeng YM, Yeh SH, et al. P53 gene and Wnt signaling in benign neoplasms: beta-catenin mutations in hepatic adenoma but not in focal nodular hyperplasia. Hepatology 2002;36:927–35.
4. Bluteau O, Jeannot E, Bioulac-Sage P, et al. Bi-allelic inactivation of TCF1 in hepatic adenomas. Nat Genet 2002;32:312–5.
5. Nault JC, Bioulac-Sage P, Zucman-Rossi J. Hepatocellular benign tumors-from molecular classification to personalized clinical care. Gastroenterology 2013; 144:888–902.
6. Pilati C, Zucman-Rossi J. Mutations leading to constitutive active gp130/JAK1/STAT3 pathway. Cytokine Growth Factor Rev 2015;26:499–506.
7. Pilati C, Letouzé E, Nault JC, et al. Genomic profiling of hepatocellular adenomas reveals recurrent FRK-activating mutations and the mechanisms of malignant transformation. Cancer Cell. 2014;25:428–41.
8. Rebouissou S, Franconi A, Calderaro J, et al. Genotype-phenotype correlation of CTNNB1 mutations reveals different ß-catenin activity associated with liver tumor progression. Hepatology 2016;64(6):2047–61.
9. Nault JC, Mallet M, Pilati C, et al. High frequency of telomerase reverse-transcriptase promoter somatic mutations in hepatocellular carcinoma and preneoplastic lesions. Nat Commun 2013;4:2218.
10. Jeannot E, Poussin K, Chiche L, et al. Association of CYP1B1 germ line mutations with hepatocyte nuclear factor 1 alpha-mutated hepatocellular adenoma. Cancer Res 2007;67:2611–6.
11. Jeannot E, Mellottee L, Bioulac-Sage P, et al, Groupe d'étude Génétique des Tumeurs Hépatiques (INSERM Network). Spectrum of HNF1A somatic mutations in hepatocellular adenoma differs from that in patients with MODY3 and suggests genotoxic damage. Diabetes 2010;59:1836–44.
12. Bacq Y, Jacquemin E, Balabaud C, et al. Familial liver adenomatosis associated with hepatocyte nuclear factor 1alpha inactivation. Gastroenterology 2003;125:1470–5.
13. Rebouissou S, Amessou M, Couchy G, et al. Frequent in-frame somatic deletions activate gp130 in inflammatory hepatocellular tumours. Nature 2009;457:200–4.
14. Pilati C, Amessou M, Bihl MP, et al. Somatic mutations activating STAT3 in human inflammatory hepatocellular adenomas. J Exp Med 2011;208:1359–66.
15. Nault JC, Fabre M, Couchy G, et al. GNAS-activating mutations define a rare subgroup of inflammatory liver tumors characterized by STAT3 activation. J Hepatol 2012;56:184–91.
16. Poussin K, Pilati C, Couchy G, et al. Biochemical and functional analyses of gp130 mutants unveil JAK1 as a novel therapeutic target in human inflammatory hepatocellular adenoma. Oncoimmunology 2013;2:e27090.
17. Gupta A, Sheridan RM, Towbin A, et al. Multifocal hepatic neoplasia in 3 children with APC gene mutation. Am J Surg Pathol 2013;37:1058–66.
18. Calderaro J, Labrune P, Morcrette G, et al. Molecular characterization of hepatocellular adenomas developed in patients with glycogen storage disease type I. J Hepatol 2013;58:350–7.
19. Ladeiro Y, Couchy G, Balabaud C, et al. MicroRNA profiling in hepatocellular tumors is associated with clinical features and oncogene/tumor suppressor gene mutations. Hepatology 2008;47:1955–63.
20. Nault JC, Couchy G, Bioulac-Sage P, et al. Nosology and molecular classification of hepatocellular adenomas [abstract]. J Hepatol 2016;64:S160.

21. Castain C, Sempoux C, Brunt EM, et al. Coexistence of inflammatory hepatocellular adenomas with HNF1α-inactivated adenomas: is there an association? Histopathology 2014;64:890–5.

22. Bioulac-Sage P, Balabaud C, Wanless IR. Focal nodular hyperplasia and hepatocellular adenoma. In: Bosman FT, Carneiro F, Hruban RH, et al, editors. WHO classification of tumours of the digestive system. 4th edition. Lyon: IARC; 2010. p. 198–204.

23. Zucman-Rossi J, Jeannot E, Nhieu JT, et al. Genotype-phenotype correlation in hepatocellular adenoma: New classification and relationship with HCC. Hepatology 2006;43:515–24.

24. Bioulac-Sage P, Rebouissou S, Thomas C, et al. Hepatocellular adenoma subtype classification using molecular markers and immunohistochemistry. Hepatology 2007;46:740–8.

25. Shanbhogue A, Shah SN, Zaheer A, et al. Hepatocellular adenomas: current update on genetics, taxonomy, and management. J Comput Assist Tomogr 2011;35: 159–66.

26. Dhingra S, Fiel MI. Update on the new classification of hepatic adenomas: clinical, molecular, and pathologic characteristics. Arch Pathol Lab Med 2014;138: 1090–7.

27. Bellamy CO, Maxwell RS, Prost S, et al. The value of immunophenotyping hepatocellular adenomas: consecutive resections at one UK centre. Histopathology 2013;62:431–45.

28. Bioulac-Sage P, Cubel G, Balabaud C, et al. Revisiting the pathology of resected benign hepatocellular nodules using new immunohistochemical markers. Semin Liver Dis 2011;31:91–103.

29. Raft MB, Jørgensen EN, Vainer B. Gene mutations in hepatocellular adenomas. Histopathology 2015;66:910–21.

30. Goltz D, Fischer HP. Current proceedings in the molecular dissection of hepatocellular adenomas: review and hands-on guide for diagnosis. Int J Mol Sci 2015; 16:20994–1007.

31. Margolskee E, Bao F, de Gonzalez AK, et al. Hepatocellular adenoma classification: a comparative evaluation of immunohistochemistry and targeted mutational analysis. Diagn Pathol 2016;11:27.

32. Fonseca S, Hoton D, Dardenne S, et al. Histological and immunohistochemical revision of hepatocellular adenomas: a learning experience. Int J Hepatol 2013; 2013:398308.

33. Kakar S, Torbenson M, Jain D, et al. Immunohistochemical pitfalls in the diagnosis of hepatocellular adenomas and focal nodular hyperplasia: accurate understanding of diverse staining patterns is essential for diagnosis and risk assessment. Mod Pathol 2015;28:159–60.

34. Joseph NM, Ferrell LD, Jain D, et al. Diagnostic utility and limitations of glutamine synthetase and serumamyloid-associated protein immunohistochemistry in the distinction of focal nodular hyperplasia and inflammatory hepatocellular adenoma. Mod Pathol 2014;27:62–72.

35. Evason KJ, Grenert JP, Ferrell LD, et al. Atypical hepatocellular adenoma-like neoplasms with β-catenin activation show cytogenetic alterations similar to well-differentiated hepatocellular carcinomas. Hum Pathol 2013;44:750–8.

36. Liu L, Shah SS, Naini BV, et al. Immunostains Used to Subtype Hepatic Adenomas Do Not Distinguish Hepatic Adenomas From Hepatocellular Carcinomas. Am J Surg Pathol 2016;40:1062–9.

37. Hale G, Liu X, Hu J, et al. Correlation of exon 3 β-catenin mutations with glutamine synthetase staining patterns in hepatocellular adenoma and hepatocellular carcinoma. Mod Pathol 2016;29(11):1370–80.

38. Shafizadeh N, Genrich G, Ferrell L, et al. Hepatocellular adenomas in a large community population, 2000 to 2010: reclassification per current World Health Organization classification and results of long-term follow-up. Hum Pathol 2014;45: 976–83.

39. Kondo F, Fukusato T, Kudo M. Pathological diagnosis of benign hepatocellular nodular lesions based on the new World Health Organization classification. Oncology 2014;87(Suppl 1):37–49.

40. Bioulac-Sage P, Cubel G, Taouji S, et al. Immunohistochemical markers on needle biopsies are helpful for the diagnosis of focal nodular hyperplasia and hepatocellular adenoma subtypes. Am J Surg Pathol 2012;36:1691–9.

41. Foster JH, Berman MM. The malignant transformation of liver cell adenomas. Arch Surg 1994;129:712–7.

42. Stoot JH, Coelen RJ, De Jong MC, et al. Malignant transformation of hepatocellular adenomas into hepatocellular carcinomas: a systematic review including more than 1600 adenoma cases. HPB (Oxford) 2010;12:509–22.

43. Farges O, Dokmak S. Malignant transformation of liver adenoma: an analysis of the literature. Dig Surg 2010;27:32–8.

44. Farges O, Ferreira N, Dokmak S, et al. Changing trends in malignant transformation of hepatocellular adenoma. Gut 2011;60:85–9.

45. Kudo M. Malignant transformation of hepatocellular adenoma: how frequently does it happen? Liver Cancer 2015;4:1–5.

46. Kakar S, Grenert JP, Paradis V, et al. Hepatocellular carcinoma arising in adenoma: similar immunohistochemical and cytogenetic features in adenoma and hepatocellular carcinoma portions of the tumor. Mod Pathol 2014;27:1499–509.

47. Hechtman JF, Raoufi M, Fiel MI, et al. Hepatocellular carcinoma arising in a pigmented telangiectatic adenoma with nuclear β-catenin and glutamine synthetase positivity: case report and of the literature. Am J Surg Pathol 2011;35:927–32.

48. Burri E, Steuerwald M, Cathomas G, et al. Hepatocellular carcinoma in a liver-cell adenoma within a non-cirrhotic liver. Eur J Gastroenterol Hepatol 2006;18: 437–41.

49. Sorkin T, Strautnieks S, Foskett P, et al. Multiple β-catenin mutations in hepatocellular lesions arising in Abernethy malformation. Hum Pathol 2016;53:153–8.

50. Cassiman D, Libbrecht L, Verslype C, et al. An adult male patient with multiple adenomas and a hepatocellular carcinoma: mild glycogen storage disease type Ia. J Hepatol 2010;53:213–7.

51. Stueck AE, Qu Z, Huang MA, et al. Hepatocellular carcinoma arising in an HNF-1α-mutated adenoma in a 23-year-old woman with maturity-onset diabetes of the young: a case report. Semin Liver Dis 2015;35:444–9.

52. Gupta S, Naini BV, Munoz R, et al. Hepatocellular Neoplasms Arising in Association With Androgen Use. Am J Surg Pathol 2016;40:454–61.

53. Sempoux C, Paradis V, Komuta M, et al. Hepatocellular nodules expressing markers of hepatocellular adenomas in Budd-Chiari syndrome and other rare hepatic vascular disorders. J Hepatol 2015;63(5):1173–80.

54. Arrivé L, Zucman-Rossi J, Balladur P, et al. Hepatocellular adenoma with malignant transformation in a patient with neonatal portal vein thrombosis. Hepatology 2016;64:675–7.

55. Souza LN, de Martino RB, Thompson R, et al. Pigmented well-differentiated hepatocellular neoplasm with beta-catenin mutation. Hepatobiliary Pancreat Dis Int 2015;14(6):660–4.
56. Mounajjed T, Yasir S, Aleff PA, et al. Pigmented hepatocellular adenomas have a high risk of atypia and malignancy. Mod Pathol 2015;28:1265–74.
57. Laurent C, Trillaud H, Lepreux S, et al. Association of adenoma and focal nodular hyperplasia: experience of a single French academic center. Comp Hepatol 2003;2:6.
58. Frulio N, Chiche L, Bioulac-Sage P, et al. Hepatocellular adenomatosis: what should the term stand for! Clin Res Hepatol Gastroenterol 2014;38:132–6.
59. Lepreux S, Laurent C, Blanc JF, et al. The identification of small nodules in liver adenomatosis. J Hepatol 2003;39:77–85.
60. Han J, van den Heuvel MC, Kusano H, et al. How normal is the liver in which the inflammatory type hepatocellular adenoma develops? Int J Hepatol 2012;2012:805621.
61. Bioulac-Sage P, Laumonier H, Cubel G, et al. Hepatic resection for inflammatory hepatocellular adenomas: pathological identification of micronodules expressing inflammatory proteins. Liver Int 2010;30:149–54.
62. Bioulac-Sage P, Rebouissou S, Sa Cunha A, et al. Clinical, morphologic, and molecular features defining so-called telangiectatic focal nodular hyperplasias of the liver. Gastroenterology 2005;128:1211–8.
63. Paradis V, Champault A, Ronot M, et al. Telangiectatic adenoma: an entity associated with increased body mass index and inflammation. Hepatology 2007;46:140–6.
64. Bioulac-Sage P, Taouji S, Possenti L, et al. Hepatocellular adenoma subtypes: the impact of overweight and obesity. Liver Int 2012;32:1217–21.
65. Lefkowitch JH, Antony LV. The evolving role of nonalcoholic fatty liver disease in hepatic neoplasia: inflammatory hepatocellular adenoma in a man with metabolic syndrome. Semin Liver Dis 2015;35:349–54.
66. Watkins J, Balabaud C, Bioulac-Sage P, et al. Hepatocellular adenoma in advanced-stage fatty liver disease. Eur J Gastroenterol Hepatol 2009;21:932–6.
67. Nascimbeni F, Ballestri S, Di Tommaso L, et al. Inflammatory hepatocellular adenomatosis, metabolic syndrome, polycystic ovary syndrome and non-alcoholic steatohepatitis: chance tetrad or association by necessity? Dig Liver Dis 2014;46:288–9.
68. Sasaki M, Yoneda N, Sawai Y, et al. Clinicopathological characteristics of serum amyloid A-positive hepatocellular neoplasms/nodules arising in alcoholic cirrhosis. Histopathology 2015;66:836–45.
69. Calderaro J, Nault JC, Balabaud C, et al. Inflammatory hepatocellular adenomas developed in the setting of chronic liver disease and cirrhosis. Mod Pathol 2016;29(1):43–50.
70. EASL Clinical Practice Guidelines on the management of benign liver tumours. J Hepatol 2016;65:386–98.

Drug-induced Liver Injury

The Hepatic Pathologist's Approach

David E. Kleiner, MD, PhD

KEYWORDS

- Hepatotoxicity • Acute liver failure • Acute hepatitis • Hepatic necrosis • Cholestasis

KEY POINTS

- Hepatic pathology in drug-induced liver injury is complex, but may be approached systematically.
- Biopsy assessment begins with objective evaluation of the character and severity of histologic changes.
- The histologic findings are summarized as a pattern of injury that generates the histologic differential diagnosis.
- The pathologist provides an expert interpretation of the findings in light of the patient's medical and drug history.

INTRODUCTION

Evaluation of a liver biopsy in a suspected case of drug-induced liver injury (DILI) can be a daunting experience. Unlike the well-defined and commonly encountered patterns of chronic hepatitis and fatty liver disease, a biopsy in a case of DILI can show a wide variety of histologic findings, including inflammation, necrosis, cholestasis, fibrosis, nodular regeneration, vascular injury, and duct destruction. These histologic lesions can be arranged in combinations that can be difficult to classify into recognizable patterns of liver injury. Nevertheless, the determination that a drug is or is not involved in liver injury has real clinical consequences and a liver biopsy can provide a wealth of information on both the pattern of injury and its severity, guiding both determination of the cause of the injury as well as subsequent clinical decision making.

Because of the inherent complexity of the pathology, the pathologist must approach the biopsy with a systematic evaluation plan. This article outlines one possible method, beginning with objective assessment of the extent and pattern of hepatic

Disclosure: This article was supported by the Intramural Research Program of the NIH, National Cancer Institute.
Laboratory of Pathology, National Cancer Institute, 10 Center Drive, Building 10, Room 2S235, MSC 1500, Bethesda, MD 20892, USA
E-mail address: kleinerd@mail.nih.gov

injury, followed by correlation with the clinical history and laboratory findings and then an assessment of both the likelihood and the specific cause of DILI. Although most of the discussion relates to evaluation of injury related to prescription and nonprescription medications, these same principles apply to the evaluation of injury related to environmental and occupational toxins and injury caused by herbal and dietary supplements. Therefore, although it is not explicitly stated in every instance, the term DILI should also be understood to include these other causes as appropriate.

USE OF THE LIVER BIOPSY IN DRUG-INDUCED LIVER INJURY

A liver biopsy is not required to evaluate a patient with suspected DILI. In the US Drug-Induced Liver Injury Network (DILIN), only 50% of patients enrolled in the prospective protocol underwent liver biopsy during the course of their evaluation.[1] Unlike autoimmune hepatitis, in which the published algorithms incorporate liver biopsy as part of the diagnosis,[2,3] the most widely used clinical algorithm for DILI determination (the RUCAM [Roussel Uclaf Causality Assessment Method])[4] does not have a place for including the findings of liver biopsies. Nevertheless, when a liver biopsy is performed, there are several questions the pathologist may be asked to address: are the patient's liver abnormalities caused by DILI or some other cause of liver disease? If DILI is likely, can the liver biopsy help define which drug is causing the patient's injury? How severe is the injury and does the inflammatory pattern suggest steroid responsiveness by analogy to autoimmune hepatitis? Can it inform clinicians with respect to mechanism of injury or prognosis?

Once the clinical decision to perform a biopsy has been made, it is important that a plan for biopsy evaluation be made before the procedure. A portion of the biopsy may need to be sent for culture or for viral polymerase chain reaction testing. If mitochondrial injury is suspected, a 1-mm to 2-mm segment may be fixed in glutaraldehyde and sent for ultrastructural examination. Saving a piece frozen for cryostat sections is unlikely to be necessary because most specialized tests can be performed on the formalin-fixed tissue. If staining for fat is desired (as in the case of microvesicular steatosis), a formalin-fixed piece can be cut on a cryostat before processing and stained with oil red O or Sudan black. Contacting the pathologist before the biopsy can be helpful to decide how best to triage the specimen.

The more clinical questions that need to be addressed, the more critical it is to have an adequate biopsy to work with, both for the separate specialized testing outlined earlier and for routine histologic assessment. There have not been studies of biopsy adequacy in DILI, but some answers can be inferred from studies of biopsy adequacy in chronic viral hepatitis and fatty liver disease. Most of these studies have focused on the effects of biopsy size on the staging and grading of chronic hepatitis C. Sampling error is increased with shorter biopsies as well as with those taken with a narrow-gauge needle with a significant underestimation of both grade and stage in biopsies less than 1.5 cm in length or with 10 portal areas.[5–7] Studies of biopsy size in fatty liver disease have shown similar findings.[8] It should be remembered that these studies were performed to identify size limitations with respect to specific biopsy features or for making a specific diagnosis (steatohepatitis). In biopsies performed to evaluate a broad clinical differential diagnosis, these biopsy size estimates should be considered as lower estimates. In order to adequately evaluate injury to ducts[9] and veins, 10 to 20 complete portal areas and a similar number of central veins may be necessary. Given the dependence of observing complete structures on the width of the biopsy and the total number of structures on the biopsy length[10,11] it is reasonable to follow the guidance of the American Association for the Study of Liver Diseases position paper on liver biopsy and obtain at least 3 cm of core using a 16-gauge nee-dle.[12] Biopsies obtained using a transvenous approach using narrower gauge needles may require additional length of biopsy.

CONSIDERATIONS IN THE HISTOLOGIC ASSESSMENT OF DRUG-INDUCED LIVER INJURY

Fig. 1 outlines a general approach to the evaluation of liver biopsies in DILI. The initial review should be as objective as possible, without regard to clinical information. True blinded review, in which the biopsy is evaluated in the absence of any clinical

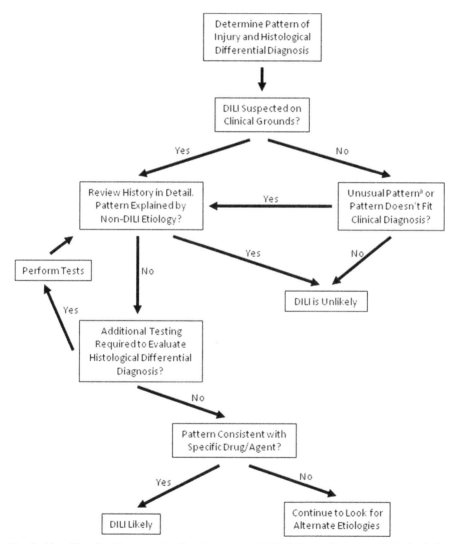

Fig. 1. Algorithm for biopsy evaluation in suspected DILI. [a] Unusual patterns include chole-static hepatitis, combination pattern (eg, cholestasis with steatohepatitis), and patterns with eosinophils, granulomas, and necrosis. (*From* Kleiner DE. Liver histology in the diagnosis and prognosis of drug-induced liver injury. Clinical Liver Disease 2014;4(1):13; with permission.)

information, has the greatest chance to identify subtle unexpected findings but is difficult to achieve in a typical practice setting. Pathologists should be ready to use all of the available histochemical and immunohistochemical tools so as to provide as much information as possible. In cases in which the cause of liver injury is unclear or potentially multifactorial, the evaluation begins with examination of multiple levels stained with hematoxylin and eosin and includes routine special stains (**Table 1**). Masson trichrome and reticulin stains are used to assess hepatic architecture and fibrosis. Staining for iron helps to distinguish the various pigments in the liver as well as to assess iron overload. Although Wilson disease sometimes enters the differential diagnosis of DILI, the copper stain is better used to identify evidence of chronic cholestasis. Periodic acid–Schiff (PAS) staining performed following diastase digestion is mainly useful for identifying clusters of macrophages that may remain as the only evidence of injury following an episode of acute hepatitis, although occult storage diseases such as alpha1-antitrypsin deficiency may also be revealed. Stains for bile (if not clearly seen on the other stains) and infectious organisms can be used as needed. Fat stains are only useful on tissue that has not undergone tissue processing, although, as noted earlier, the tissue can be formaldehyde fixed before cryostat sectioning and still be stained for fat.

Immunoperoxidase stains can also be helpful in the evaluation of suspected DILI. Acute viral infection with herpes simplex virus (HSV) or adenovirus can mimic toxic acute hepatitis and the viral inclusions can be difficult to identify without specific stains. Similarly, patients with acute reactivation of hepatitis B secondary to immunosuppressive medications often have positive reactions to immunostains for hepatitis B. The immunostains for keratin 7 and 19 as well as for the endothelial cell marker CD34 may be the most useful. The keratin stains can help identify residual ductal epithelial cells in portal areas with marked inflammation and duct injury. The absence of staining can confirm the loss of bile ducts. In cases with chronic cholestatic injury, keratin 7 may be expressed in periportal hepatocytes.[13] CD34 is normally not expressed in the sinusoidal endothelial cells, but in situations in which arterial blood flow is increased relative to portal vein flow, the sinusoidal endothelial cells express CD34 aberrantly.[14] Epstein-Barr virus (EBV) is detected through the use of an in situ hybridization reaction, allowing EBV-related hepatitis to be detected or excluded from consideration.

CHARACTERISTIC PATTERNS OF INJURY

The result of this initial evaluation should be an accurate and detailed description of the histologic lesions as well as characterization of the injury into 1 or more of the stereotypical patterns of hepatic injury. Although drugs and herbals have been associated with all types of liver injury, any individual agent has a limited range of injury patterns.[15] For example, the combination drug amoxicillin-clavulanate most often causes a cholestatic hepatitis with mild to moderate inflammation, prominent cholestasis, and duct injury.[16,17] It sometimes causes a chronic cholestatic injury with bile duct loss[18] and has only rarely been implicated in cases of true acute hepatitis. It does not cause fatty liver disease of any sort and has not been associated with vascular injury patterns or cirrhosis. Thus, classification of the injury pattern can be correlated with the known range of injury patterns for particular suspect agents, allowing pathologists to limit the differential diagnosis and comment on the likelihood that a particular agent caused the patient's liver injury.

Despite the wide range of potential patterns, most suspected drug injuries that come to biopsy seem to be in one of the necroinflammatory or cholestatic patterns

Table 1
Special histochemical stains and immunoperoxidase stains useful in the evaluation of liver injury

Core Stains[a]

Masson trichrome	Distinguishes necrotic collapse from fibrosis and identifies early perisinusoidal fibrosis; helps to identify occluded or narrowed veins (portal and central)
Reticulin	Allows assessment of the hepatocyte plate architecture, including detection of nodular regenerative hyperplasia, collapse of reticulin network in necrosis, peliotic dilatations
Iron	Identifies iron deposits and helps to distinguish pigments (iron, lipofuscin, bile)
Copper (rhodanine)	Identifies copper accumulation in chronic cholestasis and copper storage diseases
Periodic acid–Schiff with diastase	Highlights macrophages containing cell debris as well as glycoprotein/glycolipid storage diseases. Also stains some forms of bile and lipofuscin

Discretionary Histochemical Stains[b]

Oil red O, Sudan black	Fat stains; must be performed on fixed or frozen tissue before processing
Bile	Directly identifies bile
Periodic acid–Schiff	Dark purple stain highlights hepatocytes against areas of necrosis or fibrosis as well as outlining hepatocellular fat vacuoles; secondary stain for fungi
Elastin	Identifies vessels and elastin deposits in fibrosis
Acid fast (Ziehl-Nielsen or Fite)	Identifies mycobacteria
Methenamine silver	Identifies fungal organisms
Warthin-Starry, Steiner, and Dieterle	Identifies atypical bacterial infection

Immunoperoxidase Stains[c]

Keratin 7	Bile ducts and ductules, cholestatic hepatocytes
Keratin 19	Bile ducts and ductules, canals of Hering
CD34	Normally stains endothelium of arteries and veins and aberrantly expressed in sinusoidal endothelium exposed to increased arterial blood flow
Ubiquitin	Mallory-Denk bodies
Hepatitis B surface and core antigens	Detection of hepatitis B in viral carriers
CMV, HSV, adenovirus	Identification of specific viral infection

In Situ Hybridization

EBER	Identification of EBV-infected lymphocytes

Abbreviations: CMV, cytomegalovirus; EBER, in situ hybridization for Epstein-Barr virus RNA; EBV, Epstein-Barr virus; HSV, herpes simplex virus.
[a] Used in all cases in which the cause is unclear or the clinical scenario is complex.
[b] Optional stains for particular applications.
[c] Used to identify specific proteins.

of injury (**Table 2**). In Popper and colleagues'[19] landmark article on liver injury induced by drugs and toxins, acute viral hepatitis–like injury and cholestatic hepatitis accounted for 39% and 32% of the cases, respectively. A more recent analysis of biopsies from 249 cases of suspected drug-induced and herbal-induced liver injury by the DILIN found that more than half of the biopsies could be classified into one of 6 necroinflammatory and cholestatic injury patterns. These patterns included cholestatic hepatitis (29%), acute hepatitis (21%), chronic hepatitis (14%), chronic cholestasis (10%), and acute cholestasis (9%).[15] Zonal necrosis, the typical pattern of acetaminophen injury, accounted for only 3% of cases, probably because cases of acetaminophen DILI were excluded from enrollment in the DILIN.

For most cases, an initial categorization of the inflammatory pattern into acute hepatitis–like or chronic hepatitis–like can be made at low magnification. **Fig. 2** shows schematic diagrams of the combinations of inflammation and necrosis that can be seen. Acute hepatitis–like inflammation predominantly affects the lobular parenchyma and can be associated with either zonal or nonzonal necrosis (**Fig. 3**). Foci of lobular inflammation, composed of small aggregates of lymphocytes and macrophages, can be so numerous that they disrupt the normal lobular sinusoidal architecture, a phenomenon known as lobular disarray. The inflammation is often accompanied by evidence of cytologic injury of hepatocytes, including cytoplasmic swelling, clumping, and clearing, as well as apoptosis or necrosis. There may be evidence of hepatocyte regeneration, including variation in the size of hepatocytes, hepatocyte rosette formation, and reactive nuclear changes. Portal inflammation and interface hepatitis are often present as well, but they are not dominant in the inflammatory pattern. Portal-dominant inflammation with only mild to moderate lobular inflammation is more characteristic of chronic hepatitis–like injury, such as is seen in cases of chronic viral or autoimmune hepatitis (**Fig. 4**). Other features may also help in this categorization. Necrosis, particularly large areas of confluent necrosis or hepatocyte dropout, is more consistent with acute hepatitis, whereas advanced fibrosis (more than fibrotic expansion of portal areas) is more consistent with chronic hepatitis. Note that, in the context of DILI, a patient presenting with acute hepatitis may show a chronic hepatitis pattern of inflammation. For example, both minocycline[20,21] and the statins[22,23] may show portal-predominant inflammation similar to chronic viral hepatitis, but present with an acute onset of aminotransferase level increases and jaundice. Other features, including microgranulomas and mild to moderate steatosis, may be present without affecting the categorization as either acute or chronic hepatitis. The presence of hepatocellular or canalicular bile accumulation should prompt consideration of one of the cholestatic patterns of injury, discussed later. The differential diagnosis for both acute and chronic hepatitis patterns mainly includes the hepatitis viruses and autoimmune hepatitis, but consideration should also be given to less common causes of hepatitis, including EBV-related hepatitis,[24] hepatitis associated with collagen vascular diseases,[25] and hepatitis associated with immunodeficiencies.[26]

When large epithelioid granulomas dominate the inflammation, the pattern should be classified as granulomatous hepatitis. This pattern was uncommon in the DILIN series, accounting for only 1% of the cases, although epithelioid granulomas were noted in almost 5% of cases.[15] Granulomas may be an indication of a hypersensitivity type of drug reaction and their presence has been associated with a better prognosis.[15] Certain drugs have granulomas or granulomatous hepatitis as a typical pattern of injury. These drugs include the sulfonamides, dapsone, allopurinol, and phenytoin, all of which have been associated with systemic syndrome of rash, eosinophilia, and other systemic symptoms of hypersensitivity.[27] The differential diagnosis includes infection (including unusual bacterial and rickettsial infections as well and those from

Table 2
Common necroinflammatory and cholestatic injury patterns

Pattern	Characteristic Features	Non-DILI Differential	ALT/ULN[a]	AP/ULN[a]	Frequency (%)[b]
Acute (lobular) hepatitis	Lobular-dominant inflammation with/without confluent or bridging necrosis; no cholestasis	Acute viral hepatitis, acute autoimmune hepatitis	13–27	1–3	21
Chronic (portal) hepatitis	Portal-dominant inflammation, interface hepatitis (also includes mononucleosis pattern), with or without portal-based fibrosis; no cholestasis	Chronic viral or autoimmune diseases, early PBC/PSC, mononucleosis-associated hepatitis, reactive hepatitis from systemic disease, common variable immunodeficiency	3–10	1–2	14
Zonal coagulative necrosis	Zone 3 or 1 coagulative necrosis, usually without significant inflammation	Hypoxic-ischemic injury (zone 3)	6–47	1–2	3
Cholestatic hepatitis	Acute or chronic hepatitis pattern plus zone 3 cholestasis	Acute viral hepatitis, large duct obstruction, GVHD	2–13	1–3	29
Acute cholestasis (intrahepatic, canalicular)	Hepatocellular and/or canalicular cholestasis in zone 3; may show duct injury, but little inflammation	Sepsis, acute large duct obstruction, benign recurrent intrahepatic cholestasis	2–10	1–4	9
Chronic cholestasis	Periportal cholate stasis, periportal fibrosis, copper accumulation, duct sclerosis or injury, duct loss	PSC, PBC, chronic cholestatic injury/AIH overlap, chronic large duct obstruction, idiopathic adulthood ductopenia, ductopenic GVHD, IgG4 related systemic sclerosis	3–12	2–8	10

Abbreviations: AIH, autoimmune hepatitis; ALT, alanine aminotransferase; AP, alkaline phosphatase; GVHD, graft-versus-host disease; PBC, primary biliary cirrhosis; PSC, primary sclerosing cholangitis; ULN, upper limits of normal.
[a] ALT/ULN and AP/ULN: ranges of ratios of alanine aminotransferase and alkaline phosphatase to their respective upper limits of normal at the time of biopsy.[15]
[b] Frequencies of pattern among in a recent series of cases from the DILIN.[15]

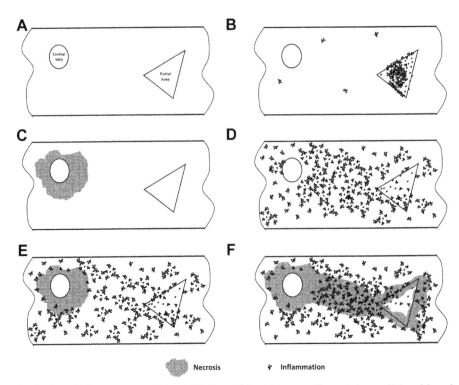

Fig. 2. Necroinflammatory patterns. (*A*) Normal liver biopsy with portal area (*triangle*) and central vein (*oval*). (*B*) Chronic hepatitis pattern with portal-predominant inflammation. (*C*) Zone 3 necrosis without significant portal or parenchymal inflammation. (*D*) Acute hepatitis with diffuse inflammation but no confluent necrosis. (*E*) Acute hepatitis with zone 3 necrosis. (*F*) Acute hepatitis with bridging necrosis involving portal areas and central veins.

fungi and mycobacteria), sarcoidosis, and primary biliary cholangitis. Although drug-induced granulomatous injury can mimic the discrete, round, well-formed granulomas of sarcoidosis (eg, with interferon alfa[28]), they are usually less well-defined, irregular aggregates of epithelioid histiocytes admixed with lymphocytes and eosinophils.

Confluent necrosis centered on the central vein (zone 3) that mimics hypoxic-ischemic liver injury is the characteristic injury pattern of acetaminophen. **Fig. 5** contrasts this zonal type of necrosis with the more irregular necrosis that follows severe acute hepatitis. Although the diagnosis is usually clinically apparent, pathologists may see a biopsy when the diagnosis is not suspected or when there are other potential causes of liver injury. Early in the injury there is coagulative necrosis of hepatocytes in zone 3 extending to involve zones 2 and 1 as the injury becomes more severe. The sinusoidal cells remain mainly intact because the toxic injury is specific to the hepatocytes. Macrophages and neutrophils may be present, particularly within and around the edges of the necrotic zone.[29,30] Although uncommon, similar patterns of zonal necrosis without an inflammatory infiltrate suggestive of acute hepatitis may be seen with other drugs and toxins. Necrosis may also be observed in veno-occlusive disease (VOD)/sinusoidal obstruction syndrome (SOS),[31] so careful review of central veins for occlusive lesions is necessary because the treatments are very different. The main nontoxic cause of bland zonal necrosis is hypoxic/ischemic injury. Irregular patches of nonzonal necrosis should prompt a search for viral inclusions at the edges of the necrotic foci and immunostains for herpes simplex and adenovirus may be helpful.

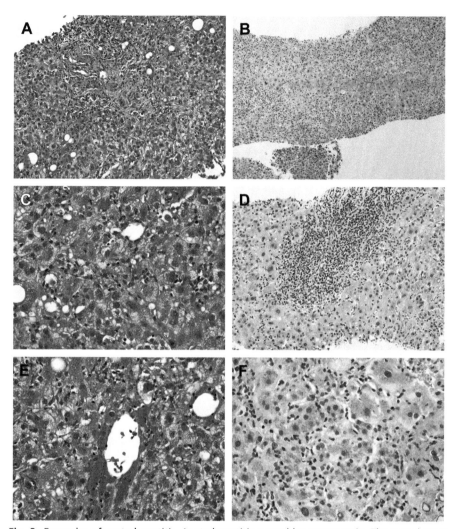

Fig. 3. Examples of acute hepatitis. Acute hepatitis caused by atorvastatin. The portal areas show sparse inflammation although the portal-parenchymal interface is disrupted (hematoxylin-eosin, original magnification ×200) (*A*). Numerous foci of lobular inflammation as well as scattered acidophil bodies are present (hematoxylin-eosin, original magnification ×400) (*C*). Hemorrhage was present around the central veins (hematoxylin-eosin, original magnification ×400) (*E*). Acute hepatitis caused by ipilimumab. At low magnification the biopsy looks cellular, mainly from infiltrates of inflammatory cells. The portal areas do not stand out in panel (*B*) (hematoxylin-eosin, original magnification ×100) but a few showed dense lymphocytic inflammation with circumferential interface hepatitis (*D*) (hematoxylin-eosin, original magnification ×200). At high magnification there is extensive disruption of the hepatocyte plates and the sinusoidal architecture by inflammation (*F*) (hematoxylin-eosin, original magnification ×400).

The cholestatic patterns of injury include acute (or bland) cholestasis, cholestatic hepatitis, and chronic cholestasis. Cholestatic hepatitis was a common pattern of injury in both Popper and colleagues'[19] original study and the DILIN study, accounting for 32% and 29% of cases respectively.[15,19] In the DILIN study, this diagnostic category included all cases with a combination of inflammation and cholestasis that was

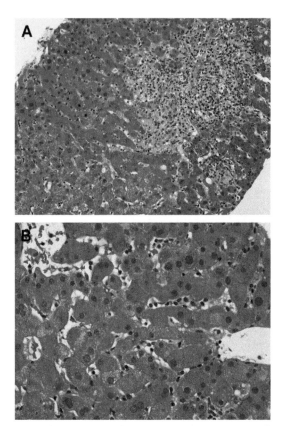

Fig. 4. Chronic hepatitis–like injury caused by 6-mercaptopurine. The inflammation is mainly in the portal areas, with only occasional foci of lobular inflammation (*A*) (hematoxylin-eosin, original magnification ×200). Sinusoidal lymphocytosis is present, but the sinusoidal architecture is intact (*B*) (hematoxylin-eosin, original magnification ×400).

visible on routine stains. The inflammatory component in cholestatic hepatitis varies from very mild portal and lobular inflammation to patterns that mimic acute and chronic hepatitis (**Fig. 6**A–D). Bile plugs are seen in canaliculi and often can be recognized in hepatocyte cytoplasm or in sinusoidal macrophages. The presence of canalicular bile is diagnostic, but bile pigment in hepatocytes and macrophages must be distinguished from iron and lipofuscin. Bile accumulates first in zone 3, and may be accompanied by hepatocyte swelling and infiltration of foamy macrophages in the sinusoids. Although duct injury is a common finding (seen in 52% of cases), it may also be seen in acute hepatitis (40%) and chronic hepatitis (24%) patterns in which no bile stasis was identified.[15] Cholestatic hepatitis is the main pattern of injury for multiple drugs, including most antibiotics and psychotropic drugs. As the degree of inflammation becomes very mild, cholestatic hepatitis patterns merge with acute cholestatic injury (**Fig. 6**E, F). In acute cholestatic injury (also called bland or intrahepatic cholestasis), there is zone 3 cholestasis as described earlier, but with little or no inflammatory reaction either in the portal areas or parenchyma. Acute cholestatic injury is the characteristic injury pattern of the anabolic steroids and oral contraceptives.[32] Such injury from oral contraceptives has become less common as the doses of estrogens and progestins have been reduced in more recent formulations, but anabolic steroid

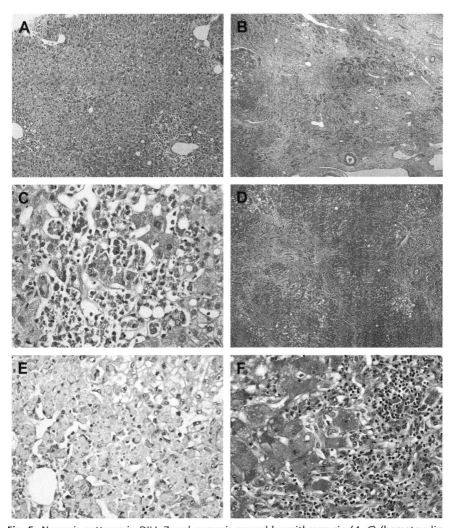

Fig. 5. Necrosis patterns in DILI. Zonal necrosis caused by mithramycin (*A*, *C*) (hematoxylin-eosin, original magnification ×100 and ×400) and acetaminophen (*E*) (hematoxylin-eosin, original magnification ×400). In both of these examples there is some combination of coagulative necrosis and apoptosis in zone 3 without much inflammation beyond an infiltrate of macrophages. In the case of acetaminophen, the coagulative necrosis mainly affects the hepatocytes because the sinusoidal lining cells remain intact (*E*). Submassive necrosis caused by isoniazid injury. The necrosis in this case is irregular, with large areas of complete multi-acinar necrosis (*B*) (hematoxylin-eosin, original magnification ×40) next to areas that show some necrosis along with regenerative nodules (*D*) (hematoxylin-eosin, original magnification ×40). Inflammation remains in residual portal areas and along the edges of the regenerative nodules (*F*) (hematoxylin-eosin, original magnification ×400).

jaundice remains a clinical problem, particularly among young men using bodybuilding supplements.[33–35] These supplements can be easily obtained without a prescription and often contain steroid derivatives.[36] The differential diagnosis for cholestatic hepatitis and acute cholestasis depends heavily on the other histologic features in the biopsy, particularly the inflammatory pattern. With severe acute hepatitis–like

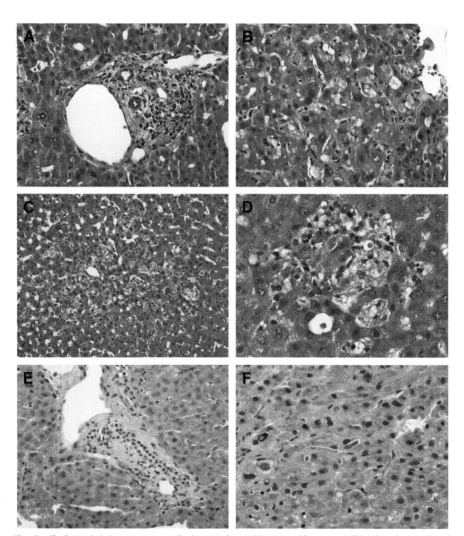

Fig. 6. Cholestatic injury patterns. Cholestatic hepatitis caused by amoxicillin-clavulanate (*A*, *B*) and azathioprine (*C*, *D*). In the amoxicillin-clavulanate case, the portal areas show mild inflammation and duct injury (*A*) (hematoxylin-eosin, original magnification ×400). Canalicular and hepatocellular cholestasis is present in zone 3, associated with mild lobular inflammation (*B*) (hematoxylin-eosin, original magnification ×400). In the azathioprine case, there is zone 3 cholestasis with clusters of pigmented macrophages in the sinuses (*C*) (hematoxylin-eosin, original magnification ×200). Scattered foci of inflammation with hepatocyte apoptosis are also present (*D*) (hematoxylin-eosin, original magnification ×600), whereas the portal areas had little inflammation (not shown). Acute cholestasis caused by anabolic steroids. In this case the portal areas are normal without duct injury or loss (*E*) (hematoxylin-eosin, original magnification ×400). There is prominent canalicular cholestasis with bile plugs in zone 3, but little associated inflammation or hepatocyte injury (*F*) (hematoxylin-eosin, original magnification ×600).

inflammation and hepatocellular injury, the differential mainly includes acute viral hepatitis. Fulminant variants of autoimmune hepatitis are also a consideration, particularly if there is prominent portal inflammation and plasma cells. With acute cholestasis and mild cholestatic hepatitis, acute large duct obstruction and sepsis/postoperative cholestasis should be considered. Cholangiolar cholestasis (bile plugs within dilated ductules) strongly suggests sepsis or sepsislike inflammatory syndromes.[37] Cholestatic hepatitis with moderate degrees of inflammation has a more limited differential diagnosis, but other types of inflammation-associated cholestasis may show this pattern.[38] Cholestatic hepatitis may also be the result if more than 1 cause is present; for example, chronic viral hepatitis with acute large duct obstruction.

Chronic cholestatic injury (**Fig. 7**) is less common than cholestatic hepatitis, accounting for only about 10% of cases,[15] but it is clinically important because it is the most common pattern of injury in patients with evidence of chronic liver injury caused by drugs.[39] Chronic cholestatic injury is recognized by the characteristic hepatocellular change of periportal cholatestasis (pseudoxanthomatous change) often accompanied by copper accumulation or keratin 7 expression in periportal hepatocytes. Duct injury is common, found in 78% of cases, whereas one-third have some degree of bile duct paucity.[15] There may be prominent ductular reaction, but this is not a specific finding. The histologic changes of duct injury are variable, from reactive epithelial changes to infiltration of ducts by inflammatory cells to periductal sclerosis. Although there are some specific drugs that cause chronic cholestasis, most notably hepatic arterial infusion with floxuridine,[40] chronic cholestasis is minor pattern of injury for many drugs that cause cholestatic hepatitis. Vanishing bile duct syndrome (VBDS) may present acutely or may be found on follow-up biopsies in patients with prolonged jaundice. Recent additions to the list of drugs causing VBDS include multiple members from the fluoroquinolone antibiotics[41,42] and the oncological agent temozolomide.[43] Temozolomide seems to cause VBDS as its primary pattern, although it is possible that there is bias toward biopsy of only severe prolonged injury in patients with cancer. The differential diagnosis of chronic cholestatic DILI mainly includes chronic large duct obstruction, primary biliary cholangitis, and the various nondrug causes of sclerosing cholangitis.

Drug-induced fatty liver disease is well reported but, because the nondrug causes of fatty liver disease are very common, caution should be taken before ascribing steatosis to DILI. There are 3 basic patterns of fatty liver disease caused by drugs and other agents: macrovesicular steatosis (with or without inflammation and fibrosis), steatohepatitis, and microvesicular steatosis. In drug-induced macrovesicular steatosis and steatohepatitis, the changes may be similar to the changes of nonalcoholic fatty liver disease (NAFLD) and nonalcoholic steatohepatitis (NASH). Specific drugs may cause histologic changes that are subtly different than common NAFLD and NASH. Methotrexate can be associated with portal fibrosis[44] and lack the ballooning injury of typical NASH, although the typical pattern of steatohepatitis can also be observed.[45] Of note, alcohol use, obesity, and diabetes all increase the risk of methotrexate injury, suggesting synergistic injury.[46,47] In amiodarone-related injury, the Mallory-Denk bodies tend to be periportal rather than perivenular.[48] In contrast, tamoxifen-associated steatohepatitis is indistinguishable from NASH.[49] Steatosis and steatohepatitis may also result from secondary drug effects, such as weight gain or drug-associated lipodystrophy.

The pattern of microvesicular steatosis should be distinguished from other forms of fatty liver disease because of its clinical and prognostic significance. Microvesicular steatosis is not merely small vacuole fat but a foamy change of the hepatocyte cytoplasm resulting from innumerable small fat vacuoles (**Fig. 8**). Cells with larger fat vacuoles may be present but the foamy change should dominate the histologic picture to classify the case as microvesicular steatosis. This pattern is almost always associated with mitochondrial injury, typically with uncoupling of oxidative phosphorylation (aspirin)[50] or damage to mitochondrial DNA (fialuridine).[51,52] A distinctive clinical syndrome of lactic acidosis and hepatic failure results from the mitochondrial injury. The mere presence of patches of microvesicular steatosis (without the full pattern)

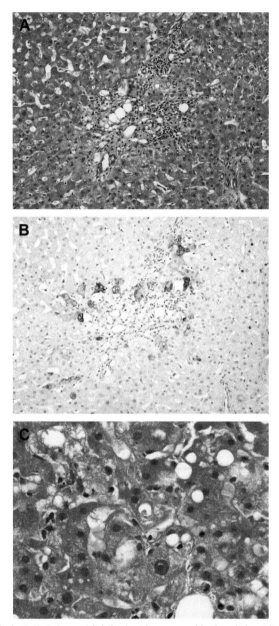

Fig. 7. Chronic cholestatic injury with bile duct loss caused by lenalidomide. The portal areas have mild inflammation and lack either a bile duct or ductular reaction (*A*) (hematoxylin-eosin, original magnification ×200). The absence of duct structures is confirmed by keratin 7 staining, which also shows the aberrant expression of keratin 7 in periportal hepatocytes that occurs in chronic cholestasis (*B*) (antikeratin 7 immunostain, original magnification ×200). As with the other cholestatic patterns, there is often cholestasis in zone 3 (*C*) (hematoxylin-eosin, original magnification ×600).

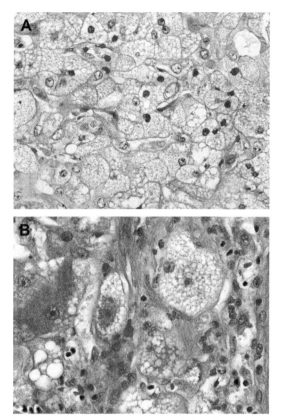

Fig. 8. Microvesicular steatosis in DILI. In fialuridine injury there is diffuse microvesicular steatosis because the drug interferes with mitochondrial DNA replication in all of the hepatocytes. The cells have a uniform, foamy appearance (A) (hematoxylin-eosin, original magnification ×600). Microvesicular steatosis can also be seen as a focal injury in other forms of DILI. (B) This small cluster of foamy cells is seen in a case of isoniazid injury (hematoxylineosin, original magnification ×600).

was associated with worse outcome in the DILIN study.[15] The list of agents in clinical use associated with microvesicular steatosis is short, but includes the anti–human immunodeficiency virus medications zidovudine, didanosine, stavudine, and indinivir,[53–55] as well as the antibiotic linezolid.[56] The differential diagnosis of diffuse microvesicular steatosis is short, including only fatty liver of pregnancy. It should be assumed that diffuse microvesicular steatosis is caused by a drug or toxin unless proved otherwise.

A variety of vascular injury patterns have been attributed to drugs and some, like VOD/SOS, are almost always caused by a drug or toxin (**Fig. 9**). Among the drugs commonly associated with vascular injury are the oncotherapeutic agents and immunosuppressive agents (particularly the purine analogues). The anabolic and contraceptive steroids have also been associated with vascular injury,[32] although the frequency of such injury is probably less than the frequency of cholestatic injury caused by these steroids. It is most helpful to think of the various vascular injuries by the part of the hepatic vasculature affected. Budd-Chiari syndrome results from thrombosis of the major veins. VOD/SOS affects the small veins and distal sinusoids. Peliosis hepatis and sinusoidal dilatation are sinusoidal injuries; sinusoidal dilatation may also be the result of hepatoportal sclerosis.

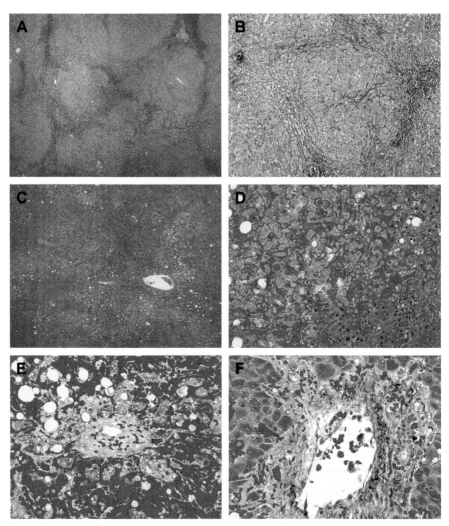

Fig. 9. Examples of vascular injury. Nodular regenerative hyperplasia caused by oxaliplatin injury. There is congestion of dilated sinuses between the regenerative nodules (*A*) (hematoxylin-eosin, original magnification ×40). The reticulin stain shows the irregular liver cells plates more clearly, with widened, 2-cell-thick plates of enlarged hepatocytes within the nodules and compressed plates of atrophic hepatocytes between the nodules (*B*) (reticulin, original magnification ×100). VOD/SOS following hematopoietic stem cell transplant. There is extensive hemorrhage and necrosis (*C*) (hematoxylin-eosin, original magnification ×40), with only a few groups of residual hepatocytes (*D*) (hematoxylin-eosin, original magnification ×200), mainly in zone 1. Trichrome stains show that the central veins are narrowed by loose, pale-staining connective tissue (*E*) (masson trichrome, original magnification ×400). Some of the portal veins also showed partial occlusion with loose connective tissue (*F*) (masson trichrome, original magnification ×400).

Nodular regenerative hyperplasia is observed in the parenchyma but probably results from injury to portal veins. Hepatoportal sclerosis is defined by alterations and loss of small and medium-sized portal veins. True arteritis is rare in the liver, but has been reported as part of a syndrome of drug-induced systemic vasculitis.[57,58] The other changes observed in the liver with vascular injury vary from subtle, in the case of hep-atoportal sclerosis and nodular regenerative hyperplasia, to dramatic, with extensive hemorrhage and necrosis in the case of VOD/SOS and Budd-Chiari. The differential diagnosis varies with the particular vascular pattern. Budd-Chiari may be caused by hy-percoagulable states and central venous stasis, and is associated with a variety of sys-temic disorders. VOD/SOS is mainly observed in the context of stem cell transplantation or exposure to toxins like pyrrolizidine alkaloids[59] and is rarely seen in other than drug/toxin contexts. Nodular regenerative hyperplasia and hepatoportal sclerosis have been associated with collagen vascular diseases,[60] lymphoproliferative diseases,[61] and some immunodeficiency states like common variable immunodeficiency[26] independent of the drugs used to treat these conditions.

Sometimes the changes in the liver biopsy are unremarkable. There may be mild de-grees of portal or lobular inflammation, rare apoptotic bodies, or mild steatosis. This finding may reflect the timing of the biopsy; if the liver biopsy is done because the injury is slow to resolve, there may be only a little residual injury left. Some patterns of injury, like hepatoportal sclerosis or nodular regenerative hyperplasia, are very sub-tle, with nearly normal architecture and no inflammation or fibrosis to suggest injury. VBDS may also be subtle, with no inflammation or ductular reaction and only minimal cholestasis. Resolving acute hepatitis may leave little evidence of its passage. Clus-ters of pigmented, PAS-positive macrophages may be the only remaining evidence of prior injury. Other patterns of injury may be characterized mainly by an alteration of hepatocyte cytoplasm such as inclusions, lipofuscin accumulation, or glycogeno-sis. Glycogenosis may be associated with high-dose corticosteroid therapy, and high aminotransferase levels may prompt a biopsy. The differential diagnosis includes poorly controlled type I diabetes[62] and glycogen storage diseases.

DIFFICULT DIFFERENTIALS

Once the biopsy has been thoroughly reviewed for the pattern and severity of injury, as described, the pathologist must consider the histologic changes in light of the pa-tient's history (see **Fig. 1**). There may already be a differential diagnosis that the clinical team would like assessed and the pathology may suggest other possibilities. It may be, after consideration of the history, that the pathologic changes are not only consis-tent with injury from a drug but that the particular agent can be identified with the pa-thology providing an even greater level of certainty for the diagnosis. In contrast, the histologic changes may be inconsistent with the agents under consideration or may even suggest an alternative cause for the injury. More testing may be required to exclude possible alternative explanations. It is important to remember that the diag-nosis of DILI is always a diagnosis of exclusion, so a conclusion of DILI should be reached only after careful consideration of other possibilities.

If the diagnosis of DILI seems obvious on clinical grounds alone, it is probably less likely that the team will require a liver biopsy merely to confirm their suspicions. It is more likely that a point has been reached in the clinical evaluation where the findings need clarifica-tion and so a decision to perform a liver biopsy is made. **Box 1** lists some of the possible reasons to perform a liver biopsy in a case of suspected DILI. The situations of known underlying liver disease and autoimmune hepatitis deserve further consideration.

Given the prevalence of chronic viral hepatitis and fatty liver disease (both alcoholic and nonalcoholic), it is common for patients with a possible drug injury to have a known (or suspected) underlying liver disease. After an objective review of the histo-logic findings the pathologist must decide whether there are histologic features pre-sent that are not consistent with the underlying liver disease. For example, neither

> **Box 1**
> **Possible reasons to perform a liver biopsy in drug-induced liver injury**
>
> Multiple candidates as the causal agent
>
> Experimental agent or agents for which there is little prior record for injury
>
> Gain insight into potential mechanism of injury
>
> Assessment of the severity of injury to enable clinical decision
>
> Known underlying liver disease
>
> Alternative possible causes (eg, sepsis, graft-versus-host disease)
>
> Exclusion of autoimmune hepatitis

NASH nor chronic viral hepatitis should have canalicular or hepatocellular bile stasis unless there is advanced cirrhosis. Although cholestasis is clearly out of place in most early-stage chronic liver diseases, there may be other findings, such as obvious duct injury or loss, granulomas, vascular injury, or microvesicular steatosis that might suggest a superimposed injury. It may even be possible to distinguish a superimposed acute hepatitis from the underlying disease. These aberrant features can be considered in light of the drug history. Prior biopsies can be helpful in defining a preexisting level of disease severity that can be compared with the current biopsy. One possible outcome is that no histologic features can be identified that are not explained by the known underlying liver disease. Although it is still possible that DILI may be present, the pathologist must conclude that the histologic changes do not support a diagnosis of DILI.

Autoimmune hepatitis (AIH) presents a particularly difficult challenge to both clinicians and pathologists. Because there are no definitive tests for AIH, this diagnosis is also a diagnosis of exclusion. Even in the absence of suspected DILI, a liver biopsy is often performed to confirm the clinical suspicion of AIH. Drug-induced AIH (DIAIH) has been reported in association with several drugs and also has been the subject of larger clinical studies.[20,63] Drugs that have been associated with an AIH-like syndrome include nitrofurantoin, minocycline, hydralazine, methyldopa, and the statins. In a study of 261 Mayo Clinic patients with AIH, 24 were thought have evidence of DIAIH.[63] Nitrofurantoin and minocycline were the main drugs implicated in this study. There were few histologic differences between DIAIH cases and AIH cases. Both showed evidence of chronic hepatitis of similar grade and stage, but there were no cases of cirrhosis in the DIAIH group. Both groups responded similarly to corticosteroid therapy, although the patients with DIAIH could be weaned from steroids more successfully than the patients with AIH. A study from the DILIN analyzed cases of DILI from patients taking drugs typically associated with DIAIH, including nitrofurantoin, minocycline, hydralazine, and methyldopa.[20] Clinical features of AIH were found in most of the cases of nitrofurantoin and minocycline injury and about half of the cases of hydralazine and methyldopa injury. A variety of patterns of injury were observed on histologic examination, including acute hepatitis (43%) and cholestatic hepatitis (29%). Cholestasis is an unusual finding in idiopathic AIH and a separate blinded evaluation of cases of AIH and DIAIH found that cholestasis was helpful in diagnosing DIAIH.[64] Liver biopsies performed to diagnose graft-versus-host disease (GVHD) offer similar difficulties. GVHD, like AIH, is a diagnosis of exclusion and often the diagnosis that must be excluded is DILI. The main histologic change in GVHD is bile duct injury, often without ductular reaction and little inflammation, but hepatitic variants also exist.[65]

Although this differential diagnosis has not been subjected to rigorous study, recent work has been presented that may eventually prove useful.[66]

FINAL ANALYSIS AND CONSULTATIVE OPINION

The assessment should not stop with the assessment of pattern and severity, as **Fig. 1** shows. After the initial evaluation, the pathologist should proceed to interpret the histologic findings in light of the patient's medical history, laboratory tests, and available imaging. Dr. Irey,[67] a toxicologic pathologist at the Armed Forces Institute of Pathology, outlined a series of considerations that are important when evaluating any histologic injury related to a drug, herbal supplement, or toxic agent (**Table 3**). These considerations may be divided into factors purely related to the patient's history and the agents in question, such as temporal eligibility and toxicologic analysis, and factors in which the pathologic changes may play a role. Temporal eligibility refers to the fact that drugs have windows of exposure during which they are most likely to cause injury. For most agents this window is between a few days and several months before the onset of injury. However, some drugs may cause injury even after many months to years of exposure. In particular, the agents associated with autoimmune hepatitis–like reactions, such as nitrofurantoin, minocycline, and the statins, are in this category.[20,22] The injury also may not be recognized until weeks after the drug has been stopped; this is especially true of antibiotics, which are often given in limited courses. Amoxicillin-clavulanate, typically given as a 10-day course, is associated with a cholestatic hepatitis that may not been seen for 1 to 3 weeks after the drug is stopped.[16] A single dose of cefazolin, given as antibacterial prophylaxis before surgery, is associated with cholestatic injury that manifests up to 3 weeks later.[68] Toxicologic analysis may be helpful in the follow-up evaluation of DILI, but, with the exception of tests for acetaminophen adducts, may not be available in real time.

Table 3
Factors to consider in the histologic evaluation of drug-induced liver injury

Factor	Questions
Temporal eligibility	What agents were taken and over what time period? Do those exposures match the known risk profile of the agents?
Exclusion of competing causes	Given the histologic pattern of injury, have all the appropriate clinical tests been performed to exclude other possibilities?
Known potential for injury	What is the evidence that the agents cause liver injury? Are the potential agents common or rare causes of injury?
Precedent for pathologic injury pattern	Given the histologic changes, how do they compare with the reported injury patterns of the agent? If the agent's injury pattern is unknown because the agent is novel or recently introduced, can the injury pattern be explained by the agent's mechanism of action or by relation to other agents in the same class?
Dechallenge/rechallenge	What is the natural history of the injury associated with the agents in question? Are the histologic changes consistent with ongoing/resolving injury?
Toxicologic analysis	Are there laboratory studies that can be done to check for drug levels or accumulation of toxic by-products?

The remaining factors require pathologists to consider clinical information in light of what is seen under the microscope. Key among these factors is the exclusion of competing causes of injury. No matter how suggestive the history, pathologists should assume that there is some alternative, nondrug explanation for the injury. The histologic findings may eliminate some possibilities among the clinical differential diagnoses and raise other possibilities that need to be excluded by additional testing. This possibility applies particularly to the common patterns of injury, chronic hepatitis, and fatty liver disease, as well as cases in which the injury is mild and the cause nonspecific. With these patterns there may always remain some uncertainty as to the cause. Pathologists should be alert to overlapping patterns of injury, particularly if the patient has a known underlying liver disease, such as viral hepatitis or NASH. Once competing causes of injury have been thoroughly evaluated, consideration can turn to the patient's list of medications, including any over-the-counter drugs and herbal or nutritional supplements. A detailed history of such agents may be lacking, in which case the pathologist may need to contact the patient's physician for additional information. Each agent should be considered in turn for the likelihood of causing the particular histologic injury observed. Agents that cause similar histologic patterns of injury can be stratified based on their overall propensity to cause injury,[69,70] but even rare causes of DILI cause injury sometimes.

There are a variety of resources available to help pathologists deal with the complexity of evaluating potential cases of DILI. The hepatotoxicity Web site maintained by the US National Library of Medicine, LiverTox (http://livertox.nlm.nih.gov/), can be helpful as both a summary of clinical presentations by individuals and as a key to the primary literature. Tables of injury caused by particular drugs can be found in DILI-specific chapters of the major textbooks of liver pathology as well as the pathology chapters of hepatotoxicity references. The results of the analysis outlined earlier should be reflected in the pathologist's report. The report should not only include information on the histologic changes and pattern of injury but should comment on the histologic differential diagnosis and the likelihood that the injury is related to particular agents.

FINAL THOUGHTS

A liver biopsy is not like a simple laboratory test or even an imaging evaluation. A biopsy is informative because it provides a comprehensive and direct view of the physical relationships of all of the cell types and pathologic processes in the biopsied organ. Hepatic pathologists are true expert medical consultants, whose job includes the careful assessment of the patient's clinical history in light of these complex histologic changes and to provide an interpretation based on their understanding of hepatic pathophysiology. Additional clinical testing may be required to exclude non-DILI causes that are suggested by the biopsy. Hepatic pathologists may be asked to disentangle contributions to injury from multiple causes; a difficult task requiring experience in the biopsy changes over a wide range of liver diseases. The final report should therefore contain an assessment of pathologic changes in light of the patient's drug exposures as well as whatever clinical evaluation has been performed to exclude competing causes of injury. DILI may be the price paid for pharmacologic progress,[19] but to the individual patient it is an unwanted and potentially lethal complication of therapy. When a liver biopsy is performed in these circumstances, the pathologist should make full use of the opportunity this provides to show the power of careful histologic analysis to illuminate difficult clinical problems.

ACKNOWLEDGMENT

Dr Kleiner prepared this article, including all figures and tables. This work was supported by the Intramural Research Program of the NIH, National Cancer Institute.

REFERENCES

1. Chalasani N, Fontana RJ, Bonkovsky HL, et al. Causes, clinical features, and outcomes from a prospective study of drug-induced liver injury in the United States. Gastroenterology 2008;135(6):1924–34, 1934.e1–4.
2. Alvarez F, Berg PA, Bianchi FB, et al. International Autoimmune Hepatitis Group Report: review of criteria for diagnosis of autoimmune hepatitis. J Hepatol 1999;31(5):929–38.
3. Hennes EM, Zeniya M, Czaja AJ, et al. Simplified criteria for the diagnosis of autoimmune hepatitis. Hepatology 2008;48(1):169–76.
4. Danan G, Benichou C. Causality assessment of adverse reactions to drugs–I. A novel method based on the conclusions of international consensus meetings: application to drug-induced liver injuries. J Clin Epidemiol 1993;46(11):1323–30.
5. Fontana RJ, Kleiner DE, Bilonick R, et al. Modeling hepatic fibrosis in African American and Caucasian American patients with chronic hepatitis C virus infection. Hepatology 2006;44(4):925–35.
6. Colloredo G, Guido M, Sonzogni A, et al. Impact of liver biopsy size on histological evaluation of chronic viral hepatitis: the smaller the sample, the milder the disease. J Hepatol 2003;39(2):239–44.
7. Schiano TD, Azeem S, Bodian CA, et al. Importance of specimen size in accurate needle liver biopsy evaluation of patients with chronic hepatitis C. Clin Gastroenterol Hepatol 2005;3(9):930–5.
8. Ratziu V, Charlotte F, Heurtier A, et al. Sampling variability of liver biopsy in nonalcoholic fatty liver disease. Gastroenterology 2005;128(7):1898–906.
9. Moreira RK, Chopp W, Washington MK. The concept of hepatic artery-bile duct parallelism in the diagnosis of ductopenia in liver biopsy samples. Am J Surg Pathol 2011;35(3):392–403.
10. Crawford AR, Lin XZ, Crawford JM. The normal adult human liver biopsy: a quantitative reference standard. Hepatology 1998;28(2):323–31.
11. Rocken C, Meier H, Klauck S, et al. Large-needle biopsy versus thin-needle biopsy in diagnostic pathology of liver diseases. Liver 2001;21(6):391–7.
12. Rockey DC, Caldwell SH, Goodman ZD, et al, American Association for the Study of Liver Diseases. Liver biopsy. Hepatology 2009;49(3):1017–44.
13. Pai RK, Hart JA. Aberrant expression of cytokeratin 7 in perivenular hepatocytes correlates with a cholestatic chemistry profile in patients with heart failure. Mod Pathol 2010;23(12):1650–6.
14. Delladetsima I, Sakellariou S, Kokkori A, et al. Atrophic hepatocytes express keratin 7 in ischemia-associated liver lesions. Histol Histopathol 2016;31(10):1089–94.
15. Kleiner DE, Chalasani NP, Lee WM, et al. Hepatic histological findings in suspected drug-induced liver injury: systematic evaluation and clinical associations. Hepatology 2014;59(2):661–70.
16. deLemos AS, Ghabril M, Rockey DC, et al. Amoxicillin-clavulanate-induced liver injury. Dig Dis Sci 2016;61(8):2406–16.
17. Larrey D, Vial T, Micaleff A, et al. Hepatitis associated with amoxycillin-clavulanic acid combination report of 15 cases. Gut 1992;33(3):368–71.

18. Smith LA, Ignacio JR, Winesett MP, et al. Vanishing bile duct syndrome: amoxicillin-clavulanic acid associated intra-hepatic cholestasis responsive to ursodeoxycholic acid. J Pediatr Gastroenterol Nutr 2005;41(4):469–73.

19. Popper H, Rubin E, Cardiol D, et al. Drug-induced liver disease: a penalty for progress. Arch Intern Med 1965;115:128–36.

20. de Boer YS, Kosinski AS, Urban TJ, et al. Features of autoimmune hepatitis in patients with drug-induced liver injury. Clin Gastroenterol Hepatol 2017;15(1): 103–12.e2.

21. Gough A, Chapman S, Wagstaff K, et al. Minocycline induced autoimmune hepatitis and systemic lupus erythematosus-like syndrome. BMJ 1996;312(7024): 169–72.

22. Russo MW, Hoofnagle JH, Gu J, et al. Spectrum of statin hepatotoxicity: experience of the drug-induced liver injury network. Hepatology 2014;60(2):679–86.

23. Alla V, Abraham J, Siddiqui J, et al. Autoimmune hepatitis triggered by statins. J Clin Gastroenterol 2006;40(8):757–61.

24. Suh N, Liapis H, Misdraji J, et al. Epstein-Barr virus hepatitis: diagnostic value of in situ hybridization, polymerase chain reaction, and immunohistochemistry on liver biopsy from immunocompetent patients. Am J Surg Pathol 2007;31(9): 1403–9.

25. Abraham S, Begum S, Isenberg D. Hepatic manifestations of autoimmune rheumatic diseases. Ann Rheum Dis 2004;63(2):123–9.

26. Fuss IJ, Friend J, Yang Z, et al. Nodular regenerative hyperplasia in common variable immunodeficiency. J Clin Immunol 2013;33(4):748–58.

27. Kardaun SH, Sekula P, Valeyrie-Allanore L, et al. Drug reaction with eosinophilia and systemic symptoms (DRESS): an original multisystem adverse drug reaction. Results from the prospective RegiSCAR study. Br J Dermatol 2013;169(5): 1071–80.

28. Hoffmann RM, Jung MC, Motz R, et al. Sarcoidosis associated with interferon-alpha therapy for chronic hepatitis C. J Hepatol 1998;28(6):1058–63.

29. Antoniades CG, Quaglia A, Taams LS, et al. Source and characterization of hepatic macrophages in acetaminophen-induced acute liver failure in humans. Hepatology 2012;56(2):735–46.

30. Cover C, Liu J, Farhood A, et al. Pathophysiological role of the acute inflammatory response during acetaminophen hepatotoxicity. Toxicol Appl Pharmacol 2006; 216(1):98–107.

31. Shulman HM, Fisher LB, Schoch HG, et al. Veno-occlusive disease of the liver after marrow transplantation: histological correlates of clinical signs and symptoms. Hepatology 1994;19(5):1171–81.

32. Ishak KG. Hepatic lesions caused by anabolic and contraceptive steroids. Semin Liver Dis 1981;1(2):116–28.

33. Ampuero J, Garcia ES, Lorenzo MM, et al. Stanozolol-induced bland cholestasis. Gastroenterol Hepatol 2014;37(2):71–2.

34. El Sherrif Y, Potts JR, Howard MR, et al. Hepatotoxicity from anabolic androgenic steroids marketed as dietary supplements: contribution from ATP8B1/ABCB11 mutations? Liver Int 2013;33(8):1266–70.

35. Elsharkawy AM, McPherson S, Masson S, et al. Cholestasis secondary to anabolic steroid use in young men. BMJ 2012;344:e468.

36. Nieschlag E, Vorona E. Doping with anabolic androgenic steroids (AAS): adverse effects on non-reproductive organs and functions. Rev Endocr Metab Disord 2015;16(3):199–211.

37. Lefkowitch JH. Bile ductular cholestasis: an ominous histopathologic sign related to sepsis and "cholangitis lenta." Hum Pathol 1982;13(1):19–24.

38. Crawford JM, Boyer JL. Clinicopathology conferences: inflammation-induced cholestasis. Hepatology 1998;28(1):253–60.

39. Fontana RJ, Hayashi PH, Barnhart H, et al. Persistent liver biochemistry abnormalities are more common in older patients and those with cholestatic drug induced liver injury. Am J Gastroenterol 2015;110(10):1450–9.

40. Ludwig J, Kim CH, Wiesner RH, et al. Floxuridine-induced sclerosing cholangitis: an ischemic cholangiopathy? Hepatology 1989;9(2):215–8.

41. Levine C, Trivedi A, Thung SN, et al. Severe ductopenia and cholestasis from levofloxacin drug-induced liver injury: a case report and review. Semin Liver Dis 2014;34(2):246–51.

42. Orman ES, Conjeevaram HS, Vuppalanchi R, et al. Clinical and histopathologic features of fluoroquinolone-induced liver injury. Clin Gastroenterol Hepatol 2011;9(6):517–23.e3.

43. Grant LM, Kleiner DE, Conjeevaram HS, et al. Clinical and histological features of idiosyncratic acute liver injury caused by temozolomide. Dig Dis Sci 2013;58(5):1415–21.

44. Dahl MG, Gregory MM, Scheuer PJ. Liver damage due to methotrexate in patients with psoriasis. Br Med J 1971;1(5750):625–30.

45. Rau R, Karger T, Herborn G, et al. Liver biopsy findings in patients with rheumatoid arthritis undergoing longterm treatment with methotrexate. J Rheumatol 1989;16(4):489–93.

46. Nyfors A, Poulsen H. Liver biopsies from psoriatics related to methotrexate therapy. 2. Findings before and after methotrexate therapy in 88 patients. A blind study. Acta Pathol Microbiol Scand A 1976;84(3):262–70.

47. Yeo CM, Chong VH, Earnest A, et al. Prevalence and risk factors of methotrexate hepatoxicity in Asian patients with psoriasis. World J Hepatol 2013;5(5):275–80.

48. Lewis JH, Mullick F, Ishak KG, et al. Histopathologic analysis of suspected amiodarone hepatotoxicity. Hum Pathol 1990;21(1):59–67.

49. Oien KA, Moffat D, Curry GW, et al. Cirrhosis with steatohepatitis after adjuvant tamoxifen. Lancet 1999;353(9146):36–7.

50. Fromenty B, Pessayre D. Inhibition of mitochondrial beta-oxidation as a mechanism of hepatotoxicity. Pharmacol Ther 1995;67(1):101–54.

51. Kleiner DE, Gaffey MJ, Sallie R, et al. Histopathologic changes associated with fialuridine hepatotoxicity. Mod Pathol 1997;10(3):192–9.

52. Lewis W, Levine ES, Griniuviene B, et al. Fialuridine and its metabolites inhibit DNA polymerase gamma at sites of multiple adjacent analog incorporation, decrease mtDNA abundance, and cause mitochondrial structural defects in cultured hepatoblasts. Proc Natl Acad Sci U S A 1996;93(8):3592–7.

53. Arenas-Pinto A, Grant AD, Edwards S, et al. Lactic acidosis in HIV infected patients: a systematic review of published cases. Sex Transm Infect 2003;79(4):340–3.

54. Mokrzycki MH, Harris C, May H, et al. Lactic acidosis associated with stavudine administration: a report of five cases. Clin Infect Dis 2000;30(1):198–200.

55. Lichterfeld M, Fischer HP, Spengler U, et al. Fatty liver and increased serum lactate in a woman with HIV. Dtsch Med Wochenschr 2003;128(3):81–4.

56. De Bus L, Depuydt P, Libbrecht L, et al. Severe drug-induced liver injury associated with prolonged use of linezolid. J Med Toxicol 2010;6(3):322–6.

57. Gaffey CM, Chun B, Harvey JC, et al. Phenytoin-induced systemic granulomatous vasculitis. Arch Pathol Lab Med 1986;110(2):131–5.

58. Mullick FG, Ishak KG. Hepatic injury associated with diphenylhydantoin therapy. A clinicopathologic study of 20 cases. Am J Clin Pathol 1980;74(4):442–52.

59. Gao H, Li N, Wang JY, et al. Definitive diagnosis of hepatic sinusoidal obstruction syndrome induced by pyrrolizidine alkaloids. J Dig Dis 2012;13(1):33–9.

60. Reynolds WJ, Wanless IR. Nodular regenerative hyperplasia of the liver in a patient with rheumatoid vasculitis: a morphometric study suggesting a role for hepatic arteritis in the pathogenesis. J Rheumatol 1984;11(6):838–42.

61. Al-Mukhaizeem KA, Rosenberg A, Sherker AH. Nodular regenerative hyperplasia of the liver: an under-recognized cause of portal hypertension in hematological disorders. Am J Hematol 2004;75(4):225–30.

62. Torbenson M, Chen YY, Brunt E, et al. Glycogenic hepatopathy: an underrecognized hepatic complication of diabetes mellitus. Am J Surg Pathol 2006;30(4): 508–13.

63. Bjornsson E, Talwalkar J, Treeprasertsuk S, et al. Drug-induced autoimmune hepatitis: clinical characteristics and prognosis. Hepatology 2010;51(6):2040–8.

64. Suzuki A, Brunt EM, Kleiner DE, et al. The use of liver biopsy evaluation in discrimination of idiopathic autoimmune hepatitis versus drug-induced liver injury. Hepatology 2011;54(3):931–9.

65. Stift J, Baba HA, Huber E, et al. Consensus on the histopathological evaluation of liver biopsies from patients following allogeneic hematopoietic cell transplantation. Virchows Arch 2014;464(2):175–90.

66. Stueck AE, Schiano T, Fiel MI. A novel histologic diagnostic algorithm for hepatic graft versus host disease. Mod Pathol 2016;29(S2):426A.

67. Irey NS. Teaching monograph. Tissue reactions to drugs. Am J Pathol 1976;82(3): 613–47.

68. Alqahtani SA, Kleiner DE, Ghabril M, et al. Identification and characterization of cefazolin-induced liver injury. Clin Gastroenterol Hepatol 2015;13(7):1328–36.e2.

69. Bjornsson ES, Hoofnagle JH. Categorization of drugs implicated in causing liver injury: critical assessment based on published case reports. Hepatology 2016; 63(2):590–603.

70. Kleiner DE. Liver histology in the diagnosis and prognosis of drug-induced liver injury. Clin Liver Dis 2014;4(1):12–6.

Antibody-Mediated Rejection After Liver Transplant

 CrossMark

Michael Lee, MD

KEYWORDS

- Liver • Antibody-mediated rejection • Transplant

KEY POINTS

- Antibody-mediated rejection of the allograft liver is a diagnosis that requires both clinical and histologic correlation.
- The criteria for diagnosing acute antibody-mediated rejection include serum donor–specific antibodies, C4d staining, specific histologic findings, and exclusion of other entities.
- There are several treatment options for acute and chronic antibody-mediated rejection.

INTRODUCTION

The first liver transplant was successfully performed in the late 1960s[1]; however, medical knowledge about operative techniques, postoperative complications, organ preservation, immunosuppressive therapies, and graft rejection were in its infancy and the 1-year survival rate was less than 30% for the first decade with this new experimental procedure.[2,3] With improvements in surgical technique, addressing the complications that commonly arose in the first year posttransplant, and the introduction of cyclosporine in the 1980s,[4] the survival rate markedly improved with 5-year and 10-year survival rates at 70% and 50% respectively.[5–7] According to the World Health Organization, there are more than 20,000 liver transplants performed worldwide across 104 countries, which is representative of 90% of the population.[8] There was a rapid surge in liver transplants over the course of the next 2 decades, which gradually slowed because the frequency of the operation outpaced the availability of donor organs. This shortage was addressed by using cadaveric livers, splitting livers for multiple recipients, living related liver transplantation, and extending the donor criteria to organs that were once considered unsuitable.[9,10]

Conflicts of Interest: The author has no conflicts of interest and nothing to disclose.
Department of Pathology and Cell Biology, Columbia University, 630 West 168th Street, VC14-238, New York, NY 10032, USA
E-mail address: mjl2197@cumc.columbia.edu

Gastroenterol Clin N Am 46 (2017) 297–309
http://dx.doi.org/10.1016/j.gtc.2017.01.005
0889-8553/17/© 2017 Elsevier Inc. All rights reserved.

gastro.theclinics.com

PATHOBIOLOGY

The introduction of a foreign organ into a patient creates an environmental milieu for a robust immunologic response. This vigorous immune response is predominantly T cell–mediated and all nucleated cells in the liver, including hepatocytes, endothelium, and bile ducts, are targets.[11-14] The transplanted liver contains numerous major histocompatibility antigens that are present on every nucleated cell. There are also many minor histocompatibility antigens involved in the immunologic reaction, but to a lesser extent.[15,16] All cell types in the liver (hepatocytes, endothelial cells, biliary epithelium) express strong and high levels of class I human leukocyte antigens (HLA). HLA class II antigens are variably expressed, ranging from negative to focally positive on central, sinusoidal, and portal capillary endothelial cells. Portal vein endothelial cells are usually negative for HLA class II antigens.[17-21] However, liver microvascular endothelial cells can be stimulated to strongly express HLA class II antigens under the appropriate environmental impetus, which includes coexistent disorders (ie, medication effect from gamma-interferon, recurrent hepatitis C, autoimmune hepatitis, T cell–mediated rejection [TCMR]).[17,22,23] This ability leads to strong expression of HLA class II (on the magnitude of DR>DP>DQ) in all liver tissue cells (hepatocytes, biliary epithelium and the endothelium of all compartments).[17-21] Increased expression of HLA class II antigens provides a larger target for donor-specific antibodies (DSAs) and subsequent disorder.[17,24-26]

There are 2 types of rejection in organ transplant patients: TCMR and antibody-mediated rejection (AMR). TCMR is predominantly caused by CD4-positive and CD8-positive T cells, and leads to portal inflammation, endotheliitis, and bile duct injury. These features are graded on the Banff classification system using the grading criteria for a global assessment (indeterminate, mild, moderate, and severe) along with a quantitative scoring system known as the Rejection Activity Index. Six months is often used as a time marker for classification of early versus late TCMR even though the histologic features occur along a spectrum rather than in clear, time-defined categories. Both early and late TCMR show the classic histologic features described earlier but the latter also shows central perivenulitis with associated necrosis, less bile duct injury, and a more homogeneous inflammatory infiltrate of histiocytes, lymphocytes, and plasma cells with mild interface activity.[17,24]

AMR is caused by preformed antidonor antibodies, ABO incompatibilities, or de-novo antibodies that develop after transplant.[27-31] Preformed antidonor antibodies either bind to ABO antigens or to HLA class I and class II antigens expressed on endothelial cells. DSAs bind to endothelial cells and initiate a cascade of events complement fixation, activation, and C4d deposition, which stimulate endothelial pro-coagulant and chemotactic factors and culminates in cytotoxicity mediated by macrophages, NK cells, and neutrophils.[17,32-34] Endothelial cell damage causes margination of leukocytes and the histologic manifestations of fibrin micro-thrombi,[17,35-38] and capillary dilatation with subsequent repair and healing by myofibroblasts. This fibrosis and architectural remodeling causes shunting of blood flow, hypoxia, and impaired function.[39-41]

CLINICAL FEATURES

The incidence of AMR is low because of innate liver resistance, immunologic screening pretransplant, improved immunosuppressant therapies, and plasmapheresis.[42-44] The exact incidence of AMR is unknown because the diagnosis is difficult to establish, which has likely contributed to skepticism about whether AMR occurs in the post–liver transplant setting. Studies over the last 2 decades show that

ABO-incompatible grafts and DSAs are responsible for AMR.[45,46] The development of AMR varies from hours to days to months depending on the offending antibody, and the clinical features include an increase in serum liver enzyme levels, prothrombin time, and decreasing platelet counts.[16]

HISTOLOGIC FEATURES OF ACUTE ANTIBODY-MEDIATED REJECTION

The liver biopsy plays a crucial role during the management of liver transplant patients. Although each institution has its own customized protocol, a biopsy of the donor liver is often taken immediately after successful transplant and reperfusion. This biopsy is referred to as a time zero biopsy and serves as a baseline and reference to establish preexisting liver disease and the effects of organ preservation and reperfusion. Subsequent biopsies are performed on a routinely scheduled basis or when biochemical laboratory abnormalities arise because protocols vary by institution. Histopathology is important for establishing the diagnosis of cellular rejection, recurrent disease and progression (ie, necroinflammatory activity and fibrosis in hepatitis C), and vascular or biliary complications.[16]

The histologic features of acute AMR are not entirely specific. Obstructive cholangiopathy and reperfusion injury can show overlapping histologic features (**Figs. 1** and **2**). Therefore, a definitive diagnosis of acute AMR requires strict criteria. First, the liver biopsy shows endothelial cell injury within the vasculature of the portal tracts. Features of endothelial injury include endothelial cell hypertrophy (endothelial hobnailing and eosinophilic cytoplasm), and endotheliitis (**Figs. 3** and **4**) with intraepithelial and marginating eosinophils, macrophages, lymphocytes, and neutrophils.[47,48] Recognizing endotheliitis in the portal capillaries can be challenging because portal tracts may be obscured by an inflammatory infiltrate.[49] Immunohistochemical stains for CD31 and CD34 may be helpful in highlighting the vessels. Other features include a bile ductular proliferation, scattered apoptotic bodies within the lobules, centrizonal swelling of hepatocytes, and canalicular cholestasis.[50] Second, other causes with a similar injury pattern must be excluded. Third, serum donor-specific antibody levels should be consistent with AMR. In addition, there should be C4d deposition in the portal veins, capillaries, and periportal sinusoidal endothelium involving most of the portal

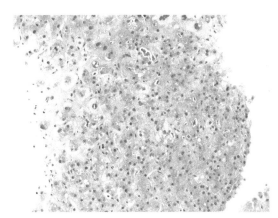

Fig. 1. Low-power magnification of liver tissue with dilated canaliculi and bile; this is one of the histologic features that can be seen in acute AMR that may be mistaken for biliary obstruction. Scattered swollen hepatocytes are present in the background (hematoxylin-eosin, original magnification ×200). (*Courtesy of* Alton Brad Farris, MD, Atlanta, GA.)

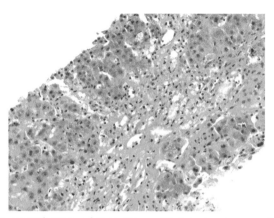

Fig. 2. Low-power magnification of liver tissue with hepatocyte necrosis and dropout as seen by areas of clear spaces with smudgy, pink eosinophilic material (hematoxylin-eosin, original magnification ×200). (*Courtesy of* Alton Brad Farris, MD, Atlanta, GA.)

tracts in a strong and diffuse fashion. According to the 2016 Banff Working Group on Liver Allograft Pathology, the histopathologic features for acute AMR are assigned a score of 1, 2, or 3 based on the degree of endotheliitis, an inflammatory infiltrate composed of lymphocytes, neutrophils, or eosinophils causing endothelial cell lifting/hobnailing and endothelial enlargement/hypertrophy with dilatation and edema within the portal veins, capillaries, and inlet venules.[24]

Hyperacute AMR is a severe example of AMR that presents with early graft failure. Biopsies taken within hours of transplant show endothelial injury, fibrin deposition, congestion, diffuse hepatocyte necrosis, hemorrhage, and a paucity of inflammation. On gross examination, the liver is markedly congested, indicating hemorrhagic necrosis.[16,45] The clinical and histologic features of hyperacute rejection are not entirely specific. There have been examples of early graft failure with hemorrhagic necrosis in which further examination did not detect an antibody-mediated cause.[51–53] Other diagnostic considerations are ischemia; infections by adenovirus, herpes simplex, zoster, enterovirus; and gram-negative sepsis.[16]

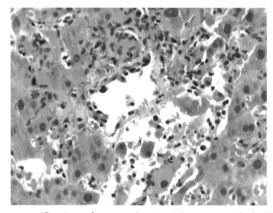

Fig. 3. High-power magnification of a central vein with severe endotheliitis. Intraepithelial lymphocytes lift the endothelial cells, causing hobnailing and hypertrophy (hematoxylin-eosin, original magnification ×400). (*Courtesy of* Alton Brad Farris, MD, Atlanta, GA.)

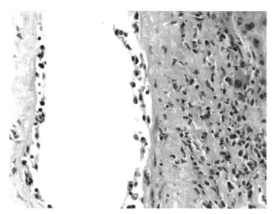

Fig. 4. Medium-power magnification of a vessel wall with a significant inflammatory infiltrate predominantly composed of lymphocytes with severe endotheliitis and endothelial lifting (hematoxylin-eosin, original magnification ×400). (*Courtesy of* Alton Brad Farris, MD, Atlanta, GA.)

COMPLEMENT 4D STAINING

There are 2 main methods to stain for C4d deposition: immunohistochemistry on formalin-fixed, paraffin-embedded tissue or immunofluorescence (IF) on frozen tissue. There are no significant studies directly comparing the 2 methods in liver allografts; however, according to anecdotal experience, IF is thought to be more sensitive than immunohistochemistry but more challenging to evaluate because of extensive nonspecific background staining. It is also harder to observe and evaluate the portal vasculature by IF.[17,54,55] Most institutions use immunohistochemistry staining of formalin-fixed, paraffin-embedded tissue by rabbit polyclonal or monoclonal anti-C4d antibodies instead of IF because of available laboratory resources. At present, there is no consensus on the most effective primary antibody. Positive control tissues from the liver, heart, and kidney are adequate.[24]

Normal liver allografts are usually C4d negative; however, nonspecific background staining can be seen in the elastic fibers of the portal tract and central vein, arterial elastic lamina, within necrotic or steatotic hepatocytes, and within sinusoidal fibrosis.[17] C4d positivity in the portal veins, capillaries, and central veins has also been seen in patients without rejection but with underlying hepatitis B, hepatitis C, autoimmune hepatitis, biliary obstruction, and other liver diseases.[54,56–58]

The ideal liver biopsy should contain 12 or more portal tracts for evaluation.[59] On further examination of the portal tracts, positive C4d staining is defined as linear or granular microvascular endothelial staining (**Figs. 5** and **6**).[32,60,61] The proposed Banff scoring system for C4d assigns a score of 0, 1, 2, or 3 based on the degree of C4d deposition in greater than 50% of the circumference of portal veins, portal capillaries, inlet venules, and periportal sinusoids. The higher the percentage of portal tracts with greater than 50% C4d staining in the portal tract endothelia, the higher the score.[24]

The portal vein, portal artery, portal capillaries, and sinusoidal and central vein endothelial cells that show C4d positivity show strong associations with DSA-positive recipients and acute AMR.[55,62,63] Portal vein and sinusoidal C4d staining is most specific for acute AMR,[47,48,63,64] whereas portal stroma staining is more often associated with TCMR, chronic rejection, and ABO-incompatible acute

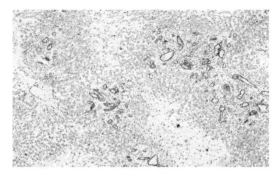

Fig. 5. Low-power view of C4d immunohistochemistry showing positive portal microvasculature staining within the portal veins, capillaries, and inlet venules (C4d immunohistochemical, original magnification ×100). (*Courtesy of* Alton Brad Farris, MD, Atlanta, GA.)

AMR.[26,31,43,55,65] Studies have shown that patients with a higher Banff grade TCMR episode also showed a directly proportional relationship with C4d positivity, suggesting that severe cellular rejection may represent a mixed TCMR/AMR picture.[30,43,54–56,66,67] It is thought that central perivenulitis leads to upregulation of HLA class II antigens and increases C4d-positive staining in the central vein endothelium.[24,26]

There are 4 criteria for establishing a diagnosis of acute AMR in liver allografts: positive serum DSA tests, histopathologic findings consistent with AMR, C4d staining, and clinical correlation to exclude other entities. These criteria are further outlined and scored by the Banff Working Group on Liver Allograft Pathology to stratify cases into 3 categories: indeterminate, suspicious, and definite acute AMR based on these criteria.[24]

CHRONIC ANTIBODY-MEDIATED REJECTION

Chronic AMR is a more difficult and challenging diagnosis to make because of the lack of specific clinical or histologic features. Because of these limitations, the exact percentage of liver transplant recipients who develop chronic AMR is unknown. It has been proved that alloantibodies can cause acute AMR; however, concomitant immunosuppression therapy, longer duration for clinical or histologic symptoms to develop, and overlap with other pathologic conditions continue to make chronic AMR a challenging diagnosis.[24]

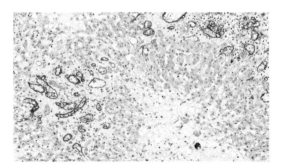

Fig. 6. High-power view of C4d immunohistochemistry stain (C4d immunohistochemical, original magnification ×200). (*Courtesy of* Alton Brad Farris, MD, Atlanta, GA.)

There are few studies that have prospectively examined liver allografts in nonhuman animal models over an extended period of time.[26,68,69] However, clinicians are learning more about chronic AMR histopathology from long-term follow-up of pediatric patients,[24,70–73] suboptimally immunosuppressed patients,[25,70,73,74] immunosuppression weaning,[70,75,76] and protocol biopsies along with serum samples.[25,47,48,77] Pediatric transplant patients are particularly revealing because the patients' original diseases are unlikely to recur, which makes chronic AMR easier to identify and often unrelated to viral hepatitis, TCMR, and vascular or biliary diseases that show histologic features that overlap with chronic AMR.[26,32,33,36,38,78,79]

The histopathologic features of chronic AMR that are strongly associated with a persistent DSA include portal, periportal, and central perivenular inflammation predominantly composed of lymphocytes and plasma cells; interface activity; central perivenular inflammation and necrosis; and variable degrees of fibrosis (portal, periportal, sinusoidal, and perivenular). Features that are less likely to be seen in chronic AMR include endotheliitis with endothelial cell hypertrophy, capillary dilatation, and marginated leukocytes. If these features are present, it may represent a mixed TCMR/chronic AMR picture.[24] Whether biliary strictures,[50,80,81] obliterative arteriopathy, and nodular regenerative hyperplasia are also caused by chronic AMR is unclear but this association has been suspected.[17,25,26] The histologic features of chronic AMR have not been well characterized because of the challenges discussed earlier.[24]

TREATMENT OF ANTIBODY-MEDIATED REJECTION

The treatment of AMR is a developing field in its early stages and many of the lessons learned from renal transplant disorders are applied to liver transplants. The most clinically effective and cost-effective method for treating AMR is prevention. Decreasing the patient's exposure to transfused blood products before liver transplant is essential because each transfusion can introduce various antigens and increases the risk of sensitization. This method is challenging because cirrhotic patients do not appropriately produce clotting factors and often need blood products, but using thromboelastography to assess coagulation function rather than platelet counts and International Normalized Ratio may be helpful.[82–85]

The options for treating AMR involve some combination of steroids, thymoglobulin, tacrolimus, rituximab, proteasome inhibitors (bortezomib), intravenous immunoglobulin (IVIg), and plasmapheresis. Mild AMR is usually treated with steroids with or without thymoglobulin and tacrolimus. Tacrolimus and thymoglobulin interfere with either or both T-cell and B-cell interactions to reduce immune competence.[82,86] There is no established protocol for treatment of moderate to severe acute AMR but some combination of rituximab, proteasome inhibitors, IVIg, and plasmapheresis is commonly used. Some physicians hypothesize that early, acute AMR is memory B cell predominant with fewer plasma cells and vice versa. Therefore, the timing of an AMR episode dictates which treatment a patient receives, with rituximab for early acute AMR because it targets B cells and proteasome inhibition to target longer-living plasma cells in late acute AMR.[82]

When chronic AMR is diagnosed, the most important intervention is compliance with an immunosuppressive regimen. Noncompliance is the most common cause of de-novo DSA formation. Tacrolimus has been shown to decrease de-novo DSA formation and could be used as the first therapeutic agent.[87,88] Steroids have also been shown to effectively decrease the likelihood of de-novo DSA and a combination of tacrolimus and steroids may be effective.[82,89,90]

SUMMARY

AMR in liver transplants is an area of study in its infancy compared with its allograft cohorts of the kidney and lung. It requires clinical and pathologic correlation and ongoing research has shown that DSAs, histopathologic findings on liver biopsy, and C4d deposition via immunohistochemistry or IF play important roles in determining AMR. Acute AMR can be diagnosed on a more consistent basis from specific histopathologic and clinical criteria established by the Banff Liver Allograft Working Group. What is a practical algorithm for diagnosing AMR? If a patient has an episode of rejection that is unresponsive to steroids or if clear histopathologic features of acute AMR are seen on biopsy before treatment, serum DSA testing, C4d tissue staining, and exclusion of other causes should be performed. In contrast, the histologic features of chronic AMR are not as specific and this is a more challenging diagnosis to make. Treatment regimens for both acute and chronic AMR should focus on prevention by decreasing exposure to blood products and encouraging compliance with immunosuppressive regimens. Subsequent episodes of acute and chronic AMR require some combination of steroids, immune-modulating agents, IVIg, plasmapheresis, and proteasome inhibitors. Despite the considerable progress made in liver allograft AMR, there is still much to learn about the pathobiology, the spectrum of histologic manifestations, and the interplay between TCMR and AMR with ongoing research.

REFERENCES

1. Starzl TE, Groth CG, Brettschneider L, et al. Orthotopic homotransplantation of the human liver. Ann Surg 1968;168(3):392–415.
2. Starzl TE, Koep LJ, Halgrimson CG, et al. Fifteen years of clinical liver transplantation. Gastroenterology 1979;77(2):375–88.
3. Starzl TE, Iwatsuki S, Van Thiel DH, et al. Evolution of liver transplantation. Hepatology 1982;2(5):614–36.
4. Hurst J. A modern Cosmas and Damian: Sir Roy Calne and Thomas Starzl receive the 2012 Lasker~Debakey Clinical Medical Research Award. J Clin Invest 2012; 122(10):3378–82.
5. Barber K, Blackwell J, Collett D, et al. Life expectancy of adult liver allograft recipients in the UK. Gut 2007;56(2):279–82.
6. Dawwas MF, Gimson AE, Lewsey JD, et al. Survival after liver transplantation in the United Kingdom and Ireland compared with the United States. Gut 2007; 56(11):1606–13.
7. Pomfret EA, Fryer JP, Sima CS, et al. Liver and intestine transplantation in the United States, 1996-2005. Am J Transplant 2007;7(5 Pt 2):1376–89.
8. Shimazono Y. The state of the international organ trade: a provisional picture based on integration of available information. Bull World Health Organ 2007; 85(12):955–62.
9. Durand F, Renz JF, Alkofer B, et al. Report of the Paris consensus meeting on expanded criteria donors in liver transplantation. Liver Transpl 2008;14(12): 1694–707.
10. Adam R, Hoti E. Liver transplantation: the current situation. Semin Liver Dis 2009; 29(1):3–18.
11. Clouston AD, Jonsson JR, Balderson GA, et al. Lymphocyte apoptosis and cell replacement in human liver allografts. Transplantation 2002;73(11): 1828–34.

12. Gouw AS, Houthoff HJ, Huitema S, et al. Expression of major histocompatibility complex antigens and replacement of donor cells by recipient ones in human liver grafts. Transplantation 1987;43(2):291–6.

13. Grassi A, Susca M, Ravaioli M, et al. Detection of recipient's cells in liver graft using antibodies to mismatched HLA class I antigens. Liver Transpl 2004;10(11): 1406–14.

14. Ng IO-L, Chan K-L, Shek W-H, et al. High frequency of chimerism in transplanted livers. Hepatology 2003;38(4):989–98.

15. Afzali B, Lechler RI, Hernandez-Fuentes MP. Allorecognition and the alloresponse: clinical implications. Tissue Antigens 2007;69(6):545–56.

16. Hubscher SG, Clouston AD. MacSween's pathology of the liver - transplantation pathology. 6th edition. London: Elsevier; 2012. p. 873–6.

17. Demetris AJ, Zeevi A, O'Leary JG. ABO-compatible liver allograft antibody-mediated rejection: an update. Curr Opin Organ Transplant 2015;20(3):314–24.

18. Daar AS, Fuggle SV, Fabre JW, et al. The detailed distribution of HLA-A, B, C antigens in normal human organs. Transplantation 1984;38(3):287–92.

19. Lautenschlager I, Taskinen E, Inkinen K, et al. Distribution of the major histocompatibility complex antigens on different cellular components of human liver. Cell Immunol 1984;85(1):191–200.

20. Ballardini G, Bianchi FB, Mirakian R, et al. HLA-A, B,C, HLA-D/DR and HLA-D/DQ expression on unfixed liver biopsy sections from patients with chronic liver disease. Clin Exp Immunol 1987;70(1):35–46.

21. Terada T, Nakanuma Y, Obata H. HLA-DR expression on the microvasculature of portal tracts in idiopathic portal hypertension. Immunohistochemical characteristics and relation to portal phlebosclerosis. Arch Pathol Lab Med 1991;115(10): 993–7.

22. Devaiah BN, Singer DS. CIITA and its dual roles in MHC gene transcription. Front Immunol 2013;4:476.

23. Pisapia L, Pozzo GD, Barba P, et al. Contrasting effects of IFNα on MHC class II expression in professional vs. nonprofessional APCs: role of CIITA type IV promoter. Results Immunol 2012;2:174–83.

24. Demetris AJ, Bellamy C, Hübscher SG, et al. 2016 Comprehensive update of the Banff Working Group on liver allograft pathology: introduction of antibody-mediated rejection. Am J Transplant 2016. http://dx.doi.org/10.1111/ajt.13909.

25. O'Leary JG, Demetris AJ, Friedman LS, et al. The role of donor-specific HLA alloantibodies in liver transplantation. Am J Transplant 2014;14(4):779–87.

26. O'Leary JG, Cai J, Freeman R, et al. Proposed diagnostic criteria for chronic antibody-mediated rejection in liver allografts. Am J Transplant 2016;16(2): 603–14.

27. Terminology for hepatic allograft rejection. International Working Party. Hepatology 1995;22(2):648–54.

28. Demetris AJ, Murase N, Nakamura K, et al. Immunopathology of antibodies as effectors of orthotopic liver allograft rejection. Semin Liver Dis 1992;12(1):51–9.

29. Ge X, Ericzon B-G, Nowak G, et al. Are preformed antibodies to biliary epithelial cells of clinical importance in liver transplantation? Liver Transpl 2003;9(11): 1191–8.

30. Krukemeyer MG, Moeller J, Morawietz L, et al. Description of B lymphocytes and plasma cells, complement, and chemokines/receptors in acute liver allograft rejection. Transplantation 2004;78(1):65–70.

31. Martelius T, Halme L, Arola J, et al. Vascular deposition of complement C4d is increased in liver allografts with chronic rejection. Transpl Immunol 2009;21(4): 244–6.

32. Valenzuela NM, McNamara JT, Reed EF. Antibody-mediated graft injury: complement-dependent and complement-independent mechanisms. Curr Opin Organ Transplant 2014;19(1):33–40.

33. Valenzuela NM, Reed EF. Antibodies in transplantation: the effects of HLA and non-HLA antibody binding and mechanisms of injury. Methods Mol Biol 2013; 1034:41–70.

34. Valenzuela NM, Mulder A, Reed EF. HLA class I antibodies trigger increased adherence of monocytes to endothelial cells by eliciting an increase in endothelial P-selectin and, depending on subclass, by engaging FcγRs. J Immunol 2013; 190(12):6635–50.

35. Adair A, Mitchell DR, Kipari T, et al. Peritubular capillary rarefaction and lymphangiogenesis in chronic allograft failure. Transplantation 2007;83(12):1542–50.

36. Escaned J, Flores A, García-Pavía P, et al. Assessment of microcirculatory remodeling with intracoronary flow velocity and pressure measurements: validation with endomyocardial sampling in cardiac allografts. Circulation 2009;120(16): 1561–8.

37. Greene AS, Tonellato PJ, Zhang Z, et al. Effect of microvascular rarefaction on tissue oxygen delivery in hypertension. Am J Physiol 1992;262(5 Pt 2): H1486–93.

38. Li X, Sun Q, Zhang M, et al. Capillary dilation and rarefaction are correlated with intracapillary inflammation in antibody-mediated rejection. J Immunol Res 2014; 2014:582902.

39. Shimizu A, Yamada K, Sachs DH, et al. Persistent rejection of peritubular capillaries and tubules is associated with progressive interstitial fibrosis. Kidney Int 2002;61(5):1867–79.

40. Dormond O, Dufour M, Seto T, et al. Targeting the intragraft microenvironment and the development of chronic allograft rejection. Hum Immunol 2012;73(12): 1261–8.

41. Bruneau S, Woda CB, Daly KP, et al. Key features of the intragraft microenvironment that determine long-term survival following transplantation. Front Immunol 2012;3:54.

42. Usuda M, Fujimori K, Koyamada N, et al. Successful use of anti-CD20 monoclonal antibody (rituximab) for ABO-incompatible living-related liver transplantation. Transplantation 2005;79(1):12–6.

43. Haga H, Egawa H, Fujimoto Y, et al. Acute humoral rejection and C4d immunostaining in ABO blood type-incompatible liver transplantation. Liver Transpl 2006;12(3):457–64.

44. Egawa H, Teramukai S, Haga H, et al. Present status of ABO-incompatible living donor liver transplantation in Japan. Hepatology 2008;47(1):143–52.

45. Demetris AJ, Jaffe R, Tzakis A, et al. Antibody mediated rejection of human liver allografts: transplantation across ABO blood group barriers. Transplant Proc 1989;21(1 Pt 2):2217–20.

46. Gugenheim J, Samuel D, Reynes M, et al. Liver transplantation across ABO blood group barriers. Lancet 1990;336(8714):519–23.

47. O'Leary JG, Kaneku H, Demetris AJ, et al. Antibody-mediated rejection as a contributor to previously unexplained early liver allograft loss. Liver Transpl 2014;20(2):218–27.

48. O'Leary JG, Michelle Shiller S, Bellamy C, et al. Acute liver allograft antibody-mediated rejection: an inter-institutional study of significant histopathological features. Liver Transpl 2014;20(10):1244–55.
49. Matsunaga Y, Terada T. Peribiliary capillary plexus around interlobular bile ducts in various chronic liver diseases: An immunohistochemical and morphometric study. Pathol Int 1999;49(10):869–73.
50. Demetris AJ, Nakamura K, Yagihashi A, et al. A clinicopathological study of human liver allograft recipients harboring preformed IgG lymphocytotoxic antibodies. Hepatology 1992;16(3):671–81.
51. Hübscher SG, Adams DH, Buckels JA, et al. Massive haemorrhagic necrosis of the liver after liver transplantation. J Clin Pathol 1989;42(4):360–70.
52. McCaughan GW, Huynh JC, Feller R, et al. Fulminant hepatic failure post liver transplantation: clinical syndromes, correlations and outcomes. Transpl Int 1995;8(1):20–6.
53. Zimmermann A, Lerut J. Early fulminant graft failure in orthotopic liver transplantation with massive haemorrhagic necrosis. Ital J Gastroenterol 1995;27(9):501–5.
54. Bu X, Zheng Z, Yu Y, et al. Significance of C4d deposition in the diagnosis of rejection after liver transplantation. Transplant Proc 2006;38(5):1418–21.
55. Sakashita H, Haga H, Ashihara E, et al. Significance of C4d staining in ABO-identical/compatible liver transplantation. Mod Pathol 2007;20(6):676–84.
56. Jain A, Ryan C, Mohanka R, et al. Characterization of CD4, CD8, CD56 positive lymphocytes and C4d deposits to distinguish acute cellular rejection from recurrent hepatitis C in post-liver transplant biopsies. Clin Transplant 2006;20(5): 624–33.
57. Bouron-Dal Soglio D, Rougemont A-L, Herzog D, et al. An immunohistochemical evaluation of C4d deposition in pediatric inflammatory liver diseases. Hum Pathol 2008;39(7):1103–10.
58. Aguilera I, Sousa JM, Gavilan F, et al. Complement component 4d immunostaining in liver allografts of patients with de novo immune hepatitis. Liver Transpl 2011;17(7):779–88.
59. Rockey DC, Caldwell SH, Goodman ZD, et al. American Association for the Study of Liver Diseases. Liver biopsy. Hepatology 2009;49(3):1017–44.
60. Cohen D, Colvin RB, Daha MR, et al. Pros and cons for C4d as a biomarker. Kidney Int 2012;81(7):628–39.
61. Sapir-Pichhadze R, Curran SP, John R, et al. A systematic review of the role of C4d in the diagnosis of acute antibody-mediated rejection. Kidney Int 2015; 87(1):182–94.
62. Troxell ML, Higgins JP, Kambham N. Evaluation of C4d staining in liver and small intestine allografts. Arch Pathol Lab Med 2006;130(10):1489–96.
63. Kozlowski T, Rubinas T, Nickeleit V, et al. Liver allograft antibody-mediated rejection with demonstration of sinusoidal C4d staining and circulating donor-specific antibodies. Liver Transpl 2011;17(4):357–68.
64. Salah A, Fujimoto M, Yoshizawa A, et al. Application of complement component 4d immunohistochemistry to ABO-compatible and ABO-incompatible liver transplantation. Liver Transpl 2014;20(2):200–9.
65. Musat AI, Agni RM, Wai PY, et al. The significance of donor-specific HLA antibodies in rejection and ductopenia development in ABO compatible liver transplantation. Am J Transplant 2011;11(3):500–10.
66. Bellamy COC, Herriot MM, Harrison DJ, et al. C4d immunopositivity is uncommon in ABO-compatible liver allografts, but correlates partially with lymphocytotoxic antibody status. Histopathology 2007;50(6):739–49.

67. Dankof A, Schmeding M, Morawietz L, et al. Portal capillary C4d deposits and increased infiltration by macrophages indicate humorally mediated mechanisms in acute cellular liver allograft rejection. Virchows Arch 2005;447(1):87–93.
68. Wan R, Ying W, Zeng L, et al. Antibody-mediated response in rat liver chronic rejection. Transplant Proc 2011;43(5):1976–9.
69. Shimizu A, Ishii E, Kuwahara N, et al. Chronic antibody-mediated responses may mediate chronic rejection in rat orthotopic liver transplantation. Transplant Proc 2013;45(5):1743–7.
70. Miyagawa-Hayashino A, Yoshizawa A, Uchida Y, et al. Progressive graft fibrosis and donor-specific human leukocyte antigen antibodies in pediatric late liver allografts. Liver Transpl 2012;18(11):1333–42.
71. Grabhorn E, Binder TMC, Obrecht D, et al. Long-term clinical relevance of de novo donor-specific antibodies after pediatric liver transplantation. Transplantation 2015;99(9):1876–81.
72. Markiewicz-Kijewska M, Kaliciński P, Kluge P, et al. Immunological factors and liver fibrosis in pediatric liver transplant recipients. Ann Transplant 2015;20:279–84.
73. Kosola S, Lampela H, Jalanko H, et al. Low-dose steroids associated with milder histological changes after pediatric liver transplantation. Liver Transpl 2013;19(2):145–54.
74. Wozniak LJ, Hickey MJ, Venick RS, et al. Donor-specific HLA antibodies are associated with late allograft dysfunction after pediatric liver transplantation. Transplantation 2015;99(7):1416–22.
75. Yoshitomi M, Koshiba T, Haga H, et al. Requirement of protocol biopsy before and after complete cessation of immunosuppression after liver transplantation. Transplantation 2009;87(4):606–14.
76. Koshiba T, Li Y, Takemura M, et al. Clinical, immunological, and pathological aspects of operational tolerance after pediatric living-donor liver transplantation. Transpl Immunol 2007;17(2):94–7.
77. O'Leary JG, Kaneku H, Jennings L, et al. Donor-specific alloantibodies are associated with fibrosis progression after liver transplantation in hepatitis C virus-infected patients. Liver Transpl 2014;20(6):655–63.
78. Colvin RB. Dimensions of antibody-mediated rejection. Am J Transplant 2010;10(7):1509–10.
79. Mauiyyedi S, Pelle PD, Saidman S, et al. Chronic humoral rejection: identification of antibody-mediated chronic renal allograft rejection by C4d deposits in peritubular capillaries. J Am Soc Nephrol 2001;12(3):574–82.
80. Song SH, Kim MS, Lee JJ, et al. Effect of donor-specific antibodies and panel reactive antibodies in living donor liver transplant recipients. Ann Surg Treat Res 2015;88(2):100–5.
81. Iacob S, Cicinnati VR, Dechêne A, et al. Genetic, immunological and clinical risk factors for biliary strictures following liver transplantation. Liver Int 2012;32(8):1253–61.
82. Kim PTW, Demetris AJ, O'Leary JG. Prevention and treatment of liver allograft antibody-mediated rejection and the role of the "two-hit hypothesis." Curr Opin Organ Transplant 2016;21(2):209–18.
83. Villanueva C, Colomo A, Bosch A, et al. Transfusion strategies for acute upper gastrointestinal bleeding. N Engl J Med 2013;368(1):11–21.
84. De Pietri L, Bianchini M, Montalti R, et al. Thrombelastography-guided blood product use before invasive procedures in cirrhosis with severe coagulopathy: a randomized, controlled trial. Hepatology 2016;63(2):566–73.

85. Rahimi RS, O'Leary JG. Transfusing common sense instead of blood products into coagulation testing in patients with cirrhosis: overtreatment ≠ safety. Hepatology 2016;63(2):368–70.

86. Woodle ES, Perdrizet GA, So SK, et al. FK 506 rescue therapy for hepatic allograft rejection: experience with an aggressive approach. Clin Transplant 1995;9(1): 45–52.

87. Sher LS, Cosenza CA, Michel J, et al. Efficacy of tacrolimus as rescue therapy for chronic rejection in orthotopic liver transplantation: a report of the U.S. Multicenter Liver Study Group. Transplantation 1997;64(2):258–63.

88. Kaneku H, O'Leary JG, Banuelos N, et al. De novo donor-specific HLA antibodies decrease patient and graft survival in liver transplant recipients. Am J Transplant 2013;13(6):1541–8.

89. Del Bello A, Congy-Jolivet N, Muscari F, et al. Prevalence, incidence and risk factors for donor-specific anti-HLA antibodies in maintenance liver transplant patients. Am J Transplant 2014;14(4):867–75.

90. Krishnamoorthy TL, Miezynska-Kurtycz J, Hodson J, et al. Longterm corticosteroid use after liver transplantation for autoimmune hepatitis is safe and associated with a lower incidence of recurrent disease. Liver Transpl 2016;22(1):34–41.

Immunohistochemistry in the Diagnosis of Hepatocellular Carcinoma

Won-Tak Choi, MD, PhD[a],*, Sanjay Kakar, MD[b]

KEYWORDS

- Hepatocellular carcinoma • Hepatocellular adenoma • Focal nodular hyperplasia
- Well-differentiated hepatocellular lesion • Immunohistochemistry

KEY POINTS

- In most situations, hepatocellular carcinoma (HCC) can be distinguished from metastatic tumor by using a panel of 2 hepatocellular (arginase-1, with Hep Par-1 or glypican-3) and 2 markers more commonly positive in adenocarcinoma (CK19 and MOC-31).
- A 2-stain approach using arginase-1 and CK19 can be a useful starting point if limited tissue is available.
- Use of less sensitive hepatocellular markers like polyclonal CEA and alpha-fetoprotein should be avoided for routine use and should be reserved for challenging cases. Similarly, use of large reflex panels of site-specific markers should be avoided.
- A panel of glutamine synthetase, β-catenin, and reticulin stains can help in differentiation of benign hepatocellular lesions from well-differentiated HCC. Additional stains like serum amyloid A, C-reactive protein, and liver-fatty acid binding protein can be obtained to subclassify hepatocellular adenoma.

INTRODUCTION

The morphologic features of hepatocellular carcinoma (HCC) often overlap with those of metastatic tumors and intrahepatic cholangiocarcinoma on the one hand, and with those of benign or borderline entities like focal nodular hyperplasia (FNH), hepatocellular adenoma (HCA), and high-grade dysplastic nodule (HGDN) on the other. In most instances, a panel of immunohistochemical stains is necessary to establish the diagnosis. This review summarizes recommendations for appropriate use of immunohistochemical markers in different settings and focuses on common pitfalls in diagnosis.

Disclosure Statement: The authors have nothing to disclose.
[a] Department of Pathology, University of California at San Francisco, 505 Parnassus Avenue, M552, Box 0102, San Francisco, CA 94143, USA; [b] Department of Pathology, University of California at San Francisco, 505 Parnassus Avenue, M543, Box 0102, San Francisco, CA 94143, USA
* Corresponding author.
E-mail address: Won-Tak.Choi@ucsf.edu

Gastroenterol Clin N Am 46 (2017) 311–325
http://dx.doi.org/10.1016/j.gtc.2017.01.006
0889-8553/17/© 2017 Elsevier Inc. All rights reserved.

gastro.theclinics.com

MOST USEFUL HEPATOCELLULAR MARKERS
Arginase-1

Arginase-1 (Arg-1) is the most sensitive and specific marker (greater than 90%, respectively) of hepatocellular differentiation and should be the first-line marker of HCC versus other tumors. It displays diffuse nuclear and cytoplasmic staining (**Fig. 1**A).[1] Arg-1 also shows higher sensitivities (85% and 85%, respectively) than Hep Par-1 (64% and 26%, respectively) for poorly differentiated HCC and scirrhous HCC.[1,2] Although Arg-1 is negative for most other tumors,[3] rare cases of adenocarcinoma (including colorectal, pancreatic, breast, and prostatic primaries), intrahepatic cholangiocarcinoma, and hepatoid carcinoma may show focal or weak Arg-1 positivity.[4–6]

Hepatocyte Paraffin-1

Hepatocyte paraffin-1 (Hep Par-1) has both sensitivity and specificity greater than 80% for HCC,[1,7–11] and it shows a diffuse cytoplasmic granular staining pattern (**Fig. 1**B). Although most adenocarcinomas and other HCC mimics (including neuroendocrine tumor [NET], renal cell carcinoma [RCC], adrenocortical carcinoma [ACC], melanoma, and epithelioid angiomyolipoma [AML]) do not express Hep Par-1, they may show focal positivity.[12] Also strong Hep Par-1 expression has been observed

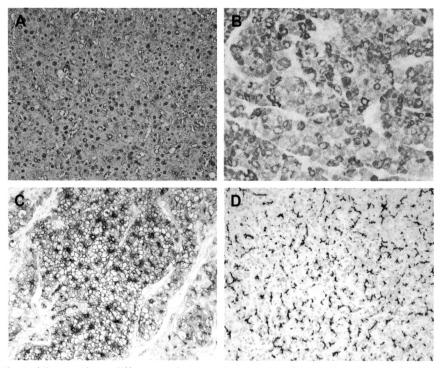

Fig. 1. (*A*) Arg-1 shows diffuse cytoplasmic and nuclear staining, and it is the most sensitive and specific marker of HCC (original magnification ×200). (*B*) Hep Par-1 demonstrates a diffuse cytoplasmic granular staining pattern (original magnification ×200). (*C*) GPC-3 has high sensitivities for poorly differentiated HCC and scirrhous HCC, and it shows a diffuse cytoplasmic, membranous, or Golgi expression pattern (original magnification ×200). (*D*) HCC shows a distinct canalicular staining pattern with pCEA (original magnification ×200).

in a subset of intrahepatic cholangiocarcinomas and metastatic adenocarcinomas (including esophageal, gastric, and pulmonary).[10–12] In addition, hepatoid carcinomas of various sites are positive for hepatocellular markers, including Hep Par-1.[2,6,12]

Glypican-3

Normal liver or benign hepatocellular lesion (including FNH and HCA) does not express glypican-3 (GPC-3),[13–18] which makes it an excellent marker of HCC if positive on small biopsies. It shows a diffuse cytoplasmic, membranous, or Golgi staining pattern in HCC (**Fig. 1**C). Although it has modest sensitivities for well-differentiated (56%–62%) and moderately differentiated (80%–83%) HCCs,[1,15] it has high sensitivities for poorly differentiated HCC (85%–89%) and scirrhous HCC (79%).[1,2,15] Its combined use with Arg-1 can identify most cases of poorly differentiated and scirrhous HCCs.[1] However, GPC-3 is not a specific hepatocellular marker and can be expressed in a wide variety of other tumors, including metastatic adenocarcinomas from various sites, intrahepatic cholangiocarcinoma (5%), melanoma (5%), nonseminomatous germ cell tumors (including yolk sac tumor and choriocarcinoma), and squamous cell carcinoma.[2,13]

Polyclonal Carcinoembryonic Antigen

Polyclonal carcinoembryonic antigen (pCEA) shows a distinct canalicular staining pattern in HCC (**Fig. 1**D), whereas most adenocarcinomas show diffuse membranous, luminal, and/or cytoplasmic positivity.[1,9,19,20] Although pCEA has high sensitivities for well-differentiated (92%) and moderately differentiated (88%) HCC,[1] it has poor sensitivities for poorly differentiated HCC (54%) and scirrhous HCC (37%).[1,2] Also, diffuse cytoplasmic pCEA expression, a common staining pattern in adenocarcinoma, can be present in up to 50% of HCCs.[12] Similarly, luminal or membranous staining in adenocarcinoma can be mistaken for the canalicular staining pattern of HCC.

LESS USEFUL HEPATOCELLULAR MARKERS
Other HCC Markers with Canalicular Staining Pattern

In addition to pCEA, a distinct canalicular staining pattern is seen with CD10 and villin.[9,19] However, these markers have low sensitivities for HCC (50% and 31%, respectively).[21] Bile salt export protein and multidrug-resistance protein 3 also show canalicular staining but have lower sensitivities than Arg-1 for poorly differentiated and scirrhous HCC.[6]

Alpha-Fetoprotein

Alpha-fetoprotein (AFP) has a low sensitivity for HCC (30%–50%), and germ cell tumors, including yolk sac tumor, can express AFP.[12] It tends to show patchy positivity with high background staining,[8,11,19,21] limiting its use as an HCC marker.

CD34

CD34 can be useful in identifying a hepatocellular lesion from the background liver parenchyma, as both malignant and benign hepatocellular (including FNH and HCA) lesions show increased CD34 sinusoidal staining (**Fig. 2**A, B).[22,23] Staining is confined to periportal sinusoids in normal liver (**Fig. 2**C); however, CD34 does not reliably distinguish HCC from benign hepatocellular lesions or metastatic tumors.

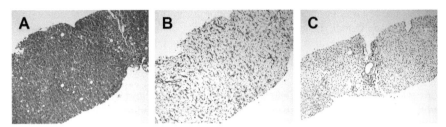

Fig. 2. (*A*) Well-differentiated HCC can be difficult to distinguish from benign hepatocellular lesions or normal background liver parenchyma on histologic ground. (*B*) CD34 sinusoidal positivity is increased in both HCC and benign hepatocellular lesions. (*C*) The background normal liver parenchyma does not show increased CD34 staining.

DIAGNOSTIC WORKUP OF MALIGNANT LIVER NEOPLASM

Because of overlap in staining patterns, a panel of 2 hepatocellular (Arg-1, with Hep Par-1 or GPC-3) and 2 adenocarcinoma (CK19 and MOC-31) markers is recommended to distinguish HCC from metastatic tumors. If limited tissue is available, an initial 2-stain approach with Arg-1 and CK19 help in providing direction for further diagnostic workup (**Table 1**). It should be noted that markers commonly associated with adenocarcinoma, such as CK7, CK19, and MOC-31, are positive in 10% to 20% of HCCs.[9,24–27] In addition to being positive in approximately 90% of metastatic adenocarcinomas, these markers also can be positive in NETs and RCCs.[9,26–29]

Group 1: Arg-1 Positive, CK19 Negative

This expression pattern supports the diagnosis of HCC in most cases (see **Table 1**). However, if Arg-1 expression is only focal or weak or if morphologic and/or imaging features are not typical of HCC, additional hepatocellular markers (Hep Par-1 and/or GPC-3) should be pursued before making the diagnosis of HCC.

Group 2: Arg-1 Negative, CK19 Positive

The likely diagnoses include metastatic adenocarcinoma, intrahepatic cholangiocarcinoma, and polygonal cell tumors (including NET and RCC). CK19-positive and Arg-1–negative HCC is possible, but is uncommon. Additional site-specific markers should be pursued based on morphology and clinical setting (see **Table 1**).

Group 3: Arg-1 Positive, CK19 Positive

This expression pattern most likely represents HCC with aberrant CK19 expression, which is thought to be an adverse prognostic factor.[24] Hepatoid carcinomas can show the same expression pattern. If morphologically distinct areas of the tumor show positivity for Arg-1 and CK19, the possibility of combined HCC-cholangiocarcinoma should be considered (see **Table 1**). Rarely, aberrant Arg-1 staining can be seen in metastatic adenocarcinoma or intrahepatic cholangiocarcinoma, but it is usually weak or focal.[4–6] Further staining with hepatocellular markers (Hep Par-1, GPC-3), cytokeratins (CK7, CK20), and/or site-specific markers can be considered based on the clinical setting.

Group 4: Arg-1 Negative, CK19 Negative

Pancytokeratin can help in narrowing the differential diagnosis when this pattern is observed. Pancytokeratin-positive tumors in this category include Arg-1-negative HCC, CK19-negative adenocarcinoma, NET, and RCC, whereas pancytokeratin-

Table 1
Two-stain approach for malignant hepatocellular neoplasms

Pattern	Likely Diagnosis	Other Differential Diagnoses
Arg-1+, CK19−	HCC → Hep Par-1 and/or GPC-3 can be considered to confirm the diagnosis of HCC	*If Arg-1 is weakly or focally positive*, adenocarcinomas (including cholangiocarcinoma, pancreas, colorectum, breast, and prostate)
Arg-1−, CK19+	*Pancreaticobiliary (including cholangiocarcinoma)* → CK7+, CK19+, pCEA+ (cytoplasmic) *Metastatic adenocarcinoma:* Upper GI → CK7+, CK19+ Colorectal → CK20+, CDX2+ Lung → CK7+, TTF-1+, Napsin+ Thyroid → CK7+, TTF-1+, Thyroglobulin+ Breast → ER+, Mammaglobin+, GATA+, GCDFP+ Ovary → CK7+, ER+, WT-1+ Prostate → PSA+, PAP+ *Polygonal cell tumor:* NET → Chromogranin+, Synaptophysin+ RCC → PAX-2+, PAX-8+, RCC+	HCC with aberrant CK19 positivity → Hep Par-1 and/or GPC-3 to rule out HCC
Arg-1+, CK19+	HCC with aberrant CK19 positivity → Hep Par-1 and/or GPC-3 should be performed Adenocarcinoma with aberrant Arg-1 positivity (rare) Combined HCC-cholangiocarcinoma Hepatoid carcinoma	
Arg-1−, CK19−	*If pancytokeratin is positive:* HCC → Hep Par-1 and/or GPC-3 to rule out HCC CK19-negative adenocarcinoma Polygonal cell tumor: NET, RCC Other carcinomas: SCC, urothelial carcinoma	*If pancytokeratin is negative:* ACC → Inhibin+, Melan-A+ Melanoma → SOX-10+, S100+, Melan-A+, HMB-45+ AML → SMA+, HMB-45+, Melan-A+ Epithelioid GIST → KIT+, DOG-1+ Sarcomas with epithelioid morphology

Abbreviations: ACC, adrenocortical carcinoma; AML, angiomyolipoma; Arg-1, arginine-1; GI, gastrointestinal; GIST, gastrointestinal stromal tumor; GPC-3, glypican-3; HCC, hepatocellular carcinoma; Hep Par-1, hepatocyte paraffin-1; NET, neuroendocrine tumor; PAP, prostate acid phosphatase; pCEA, polyclonal carcinoembryonic antigen; PSA, prostate-specific antigen; RCC, renal cell carcinoma; SCC, squamous cell carcinoma.

negative staining raises consideration for ACC, melanoma, AML, epithelioid gastroin-testinal stromal tumor (GIST), or sarcomas with epithelioid morphology (see **Table 1**). Additional hepatocellular markers (Hep Par-1, GPC-3) are necessary if the morpho-logic features suggest HCC. Site-specific markers can be obtained depending on the clinical scenario:

- *HCC versus metastatic NET*: Primary hepatic NET is extremely rare,[30] and strong cytoplasmic staining for chromogranin and/or synaptophysin usually supports NET. Some HCCs express CD56,[12] and this is not a reliable marker for this distinction.
- *Clear-cell HCC versus metastatic clear-cell RCC*: PAX-2 and PAX-8 are positive in 70% to 80% of clear-cell RCC, but negative in HCC.[31,32] Hepatocellular markers are typically negative in RCC.
- *HCC versus metastatic melanoma*: Positive staining for SOX-10, S-100, HMB-45, and/or Melan-A usually establishes the diagnosis of melanoma. Hepatocellular markers and cytokeratin are negative in melanoma.
- *HCC versus metastatic ACC*: Most ACCs are positive for inhibin (75%–86%) and Melan-A (50%–96%).[33,34] Although HCC is negative for Melan-A, rare positive staining for inhibin has been reported in HCC with high-grade pleomorphic morphology.[33]
- *HCC versus AML*: The lack of lipomatous and angiomatous components in monotypic epithelioid AML often makes it difficult to distinguish from HCC. How-ever, coexpression of melanocytic markers (HMB-45 and Melan-A) and smooth muscle actin usually establishes the diagnosis of AML, which is negative for he-patocellular markers and S100.[35]

HEPATOCELLULAR CARCINOMA WITH VARIANT HISTOLOGIC FEATURES
Early Hepatocellular Carcinoma Versus High-Grade Dysplastic Nodule

Diagnostic features of early HCC, especially vascular and/or stromal invasion, may not be evident on small biopsies, making it difficult to differentiate from HGDN.[36] In this regard, positive staining for at least 2 markers in a panel of heat shock protein (HSP)-70, GPC-3, and glutamine synthetase (GS) support the diagnosis of early HCC with the sensitivity of 60% to 78% (**Fig. 3**), whereas HGDN does not express more than 1 marker.[37] CK7 and CD34 stains may further help to distinguish early HCC from HGDN. HCC typically shows more diffuse CD34 staining without significant CK7-positive ductular reaction at the nodular interface, whereas HGDN shows focal CD34 staining at the periphery of the nodule but significant CK7 ductular staining at the nodular interface.[38,39]

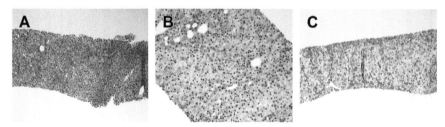

Fig. 3. (*A*) Early HCC and HGDN may have overlapping histologic features on small core bi-opsies. (*B, C*) Positive nuclear staining with HSP-70 (*B*) and diffuse GS (*C*) expression support the diagnosis of HCC.

Combined Hepatocellular Carcinoma–Cholangiocarcinoma

The diagnosis of mixed tumor requires both morphologic and immunohistochemical features of HCC and cholangiocarcinoma (CC) components. The presence of discrete glands (with or without mucin) indicates CC component, which should be confirmed by positive CK7, CK19, and/or MOC-31 stains.[2] HCC component should be confirmed using a combination of hepatocellular makers, which must include Arg-1.[2]

Scirrhous Hepatocellular Carcinoma

Scirrhous HCC is characterized by dense stromal fibrosis (**Fig. 4**A), and it often lacks positive staining for Hep Par-1 (26%) and pCEA (37%) (**Fig. 4**B).[2] Instead, up to 45% of scirrhous HCCs express 2 or more adenocarcinoma markers, including CK7 (53%), CK19 (26%), and MOC-31 (63%) (**Fig. 4**C, D), often leading to a mistaken diagnosis of metastatic adenocarcinoma or intrahepatic cholangiocarcinoma.[2] If scirrhous HCC is a diagnostic consideration, it is important to perform Arg-1 and GPC-3, as they have higher sensitivities for scirrhous HCC (85% and 79%, respectively).[2]

Fibrolamellar Carcinoma

This variant is characterized by lamellar pattern of fibrosis[40] and frequently expresses CK7 (80%–100%).[40,41] Hepatocellular markers, including Arg-1, Hep Par-1, and pCEA, are usually positive, whereas GPC-3 has a lower sensitivity (64%).[15,40] Nearly

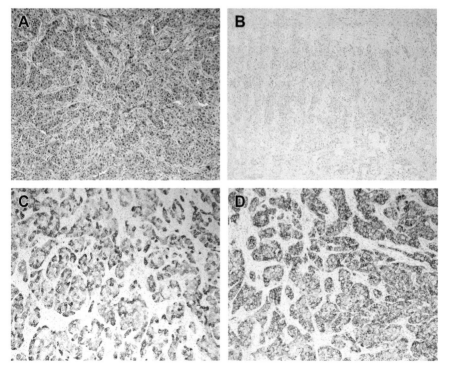

Fig. 4. (*A*) Scirrhous HCC is characterized by dense stromal fibrosis. (*B*) Scirrhous HCC is often negative for Hep Par-1. (*C*, *D*) Instead, adenocarcinoma markers, including CK19 (*C*) and MOC-31 (*D*), are often positive in scirrhous HCC.

all fibrolamellar carcinomas show a distinctive granular cytoplasmic staining pattern with CD68, compared with 25% of classic HCCs.[40,42] Hence, absence of CK7 and CD68 raises a doubt about this diagnosis, but positive staining does not confirm the diagnosis. More recently, *DNAJB1-PRKACA* fusion has been reported in 80% of fibrolamellar carcinomas.[43] The fusion can be detected by reverse transcription polymerase chain reaction or fluorescence in situ hybridization.[44]

WELL-DIFFERENTIATED HEPATOCELLULAR CARCINOMA: DISTINCTION FROM FOCAL NODULAR HYPERPLASIA AND HEPATOCELLULAR ADENOMA

Well-differentiated HCC can have overlapping histologic features with FNH and HCA, including focally thickened cell plates, pseudoacinar architecture, and mild cytologic atypia. However, HCC usually demonstrates loss of reticulin framework on reticulin stain, whereas FNH and HCA maintain an intact reticulin network.[36,45,46] In unequivocal cases, positive GPC-3 and/or diffuse nuclear HSP-70 staining favors well-differentiated HCC with the specificity of 100%, respectively, although they have modest sensitivities of 43% and 46%, respectively, for well-differentiated HCC.[47] FNH is a benign hepatocellular lesion resulting from blood flow abnormalities causing altered growth response.[36,48,49] HCA has 4 main subtypes (as described later in this article) based on the recent molecular-pathologic classification[50,51] and can be subclassified using immunohistochemistry (**Table 2**).[51]

Focal Nodular Hyperplasia

FNH is characterized by nodular architecture, thick fibrous septa, thick-walled blood vessels, and ductular reaction with or without central scar (**Fig. 5A**).[46] It demonstrates a moderate to strong "maplike" GS staining pattern interconnecting large groups of hepatocytes, while sparing small groups of hepatocytes adjacent to fibrous septa (**Fig. 5B**, see **Table 2**).[15,52] By contrast, normal liver shows staining of a few rims of hepatocytes around central veins.[15] Patchy weak staining with serum amyloid A (SAA) can be seen in up to 17% of FNHs.[52] β-catenin mutation/staining is not observed in FNH.[53]

Inflammatory Hepatocellular Adenoma

Although this subtype typically demonstrates sinusoidal dilatation/hemorrhage, patchy inflammation, and mild steatosis (**Fig. 6A**),[46,51] the same histologic features can be seen in FNH.[52] Granular cytoplasmic staining pattern of SAA can be helpful in establishing the diagnosis of inflammatory HCA (**Fig. 6B**, see **Table 2**), as it is positive in more than 90% of cases.[51,52] FNH can show positive staining for C-reactive protein (CRP), usually in periseptal location, with diffuse expression in up to 15% of FNHs.[52] Diffuse CRP expression favors the diagnosis of inflammatory HCA, as long as there is no "maplike" GS staining. β-catenin activation is present in 10% of inflammatory HCAs and can be associated with diffuse GS staining with or without nuclear β-catenin staining.[51,54]

Hepatocyte Nuclear Factor-1α-Inactivated Hepatocellular Adenoma

Hepatocyte nuclear factor (HNF)-1α-inactivated HCA shows prominent steatosis and lacks liver-fatty acid binding protein (LFABP) expression (see **Table 2**),[46,50,51] whereas normal liver and other variants of HCA maintain LFABP expression.[51] SAA, CRP, nuclear β-catenin are usually negative, and GS does not show "maplike" or diffuse pattern of staining in this variant.[46]

Table 2
Typical staining patterns in well-differentiated hepatocellular lesions

Stain	FNH	Inflammatory HCA	HNF-1α-Inactivated HCA	β-Catenin-Activated HCA	Unclassified HCA
GS	Maplike	Patchy (<50%) with perivascular accentuation	Patchy (<50%) with perivascular accentuation	Diffuse	Patchy (<50%) with perivascular accentuation
β-catenin	Membranous	Membranous (nuclear if β-catenin-activated)	Membranous	Nuclear (subset)	Membranous
SAA	Patchy + or −	Diffuse or patchy	−	−	−
CRP	Periseptal	Diffuse or patchy	−	−	−
LFABP	+	+	−	+	+
Reticulin	Intact	Intact	Intact	Intact	Intact

Abbreviations: −, negative staining; +, positive staining; CRP, C-reactive protein; FNH, focal nodular hyperplasia; GS, glutamine synthetase; HCA, hepatocellular adenoma; LFABP, liver-fatty acid binding protein; SAA, serum amyloid A.

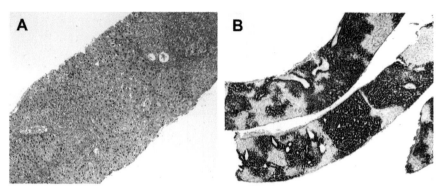

Fig. 5. (A) FNH shows nodular architecture, thick fibrous septa, thick-walled blood vessels, and ductular reaction (original magnification ×200). (B) A characteristic "maplike" GS staining pattern is diagnostic of FNH (original magnification ×100).

β-Catenin-Activated Hepatocellular Adenoma

This variant shows more prominent cytologic atypia and pseudoacinar formation (**Fig. 7**A) compared with other HCA subtypes.[46] Although a mutation in *CTNNB1* gene (β-catenin) or other components of the *Wnt* singling pathway leads to nuclear translocation of β-catenin and its aberrant nuclear expression (**Fig. 7**B, see **Table 2**),[36,51] this staining is usually restricted to a few isolated cells or may not be present. Diffuse GS overexpression is a more reliable marker of β-catenin activation and can show 2 patterns: diffuse GS staining involving more than 90% ("diffuse homogeneous," **Fig. 7**C) and diffuse GS staining involving 50% to 90% of tumor cells ("diffuse heterogeneous," **Fig. 7**D). Diffuse homogeneous pattern is strongly correlated with β-catenin activation due to mutation or deletion in exon 3 of *CTNNB1* (β-catenin) or other *Wnt* singling pathway genes, and is considered a high-risk feature for concurrent or subsequent HCC. Diffuse heterogeneous GS has a lower association with β-catenin activation, and the precise risk for HCC with this pattern remains to be determined and is likely related to the type of mutation involved.[36,55–57] For tumors with borderline or high-risk features that are insufficient for definite diagnosis of HCC, the term "atypical

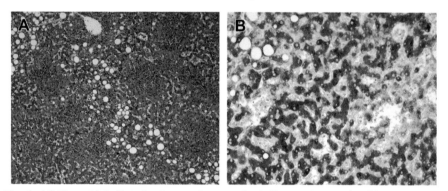

Fig. 6. (A) Sinusoidal dilatation/congestion, patchy inflammation, and mild steatosis are frequently present in inflammatory HCA (original magnification ×200). (B) SAA is the most specific marker for inflammatory HCA, and it shows strong and diffuse granular cytoplasmic staining (original magnification ×200).

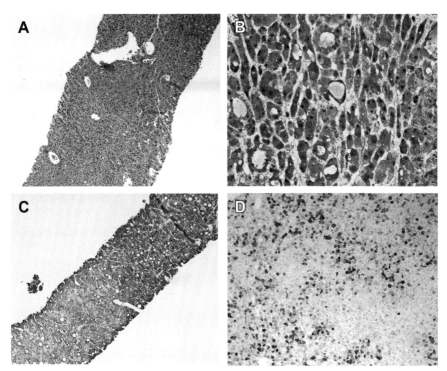

Fig. 7. (*A*) β-catenin-activated HCA is characterized by more prominent pseudoacinar formation and cytologic atypia compared with other HCA variants (original magnification ×200). (*B*) If present, aberrant β-catenin nuclear expression establishes the diagnosis of β-catenin-activated HCA (original magnification ×400). (*C, D*) β-catenin-activated HCA may show diffuse GS staining involving more than 90% ("diffuse homogenous" [*C*, original magnification ×200]) or 50% to 90% of tumor cells ("diffuse heterogeneous," [*D*, original magnification ×400]).

hepatocellular neoplasm" or "hepatocellular neoplasm with uncertain malignant potential" has been suggested.[58–60] High-risk features include male gender, older age (>50 years), focally atypical morphologic features insufficient for the diagnosis of definite HCC (eg, pseudoacinar architecture, reticulin loss), and β-catenin activation (nuclear β-catenin or diffuse GS staining).

Unclassified Hepatocellular Adenoma

This subtype does not show morphologic or immunohistochemical features of the other recognized subtypes (see **Table 2**).[46] GS staining is restricted to areas around central veins without "maplike" staining characteristics of FNH. A minority of cases previously classified as "unclassified" may have mutations in exon 7 or 8 of *CTNNB1* (β-catenin).[61] These tumors do not show diffuse GS staining and are not associated with high HCC risk, like the tumors with exon 3 *CTNNB1* (β-catenin) mutation.[61]

REFERENCES

1. Nguyen T, Phillips D, Jain D, et al. Comparison of 5 immunohistochemical markers of hepatocellular differentiation for the diagnosis of hepatocellular carcinoma. Arch Pathol Lab Med 2015;139:1028–34.

2. Krings G, Ramachandran R, Jain D, et al. Immunohistochemical pitfalls and the importance of glypican 3 and arginase in the diagnosis of scirrhous hepatocellular carcinoma. Mod Pathol 2013;26:782–91.

3. Timek DT, Shi J, Liu H, et al. Arginase-1, HepPar-1, and Glypican-3 are the most effective panel of markers in distinguishing hepatocellular carcinoma from metastatic tumor on fine-needle aspiration specimens. Am J Clin Pathol 2012;138: 203–10.

4. Fujiwara M, Kwok S, Yano H, et al. Arginase-1 is a more sensitive marker of hepatic differentiation than HepPar-1 and glypican-3 in fine-needle aspiration biopsies. Cancer Cytopathol 2012;120:230–7.

5. Yan BC, Gong C, Song J, et al. Arginase-1: a new immunohistochemical marker of hepatocytes and hepatocellular neoplasms. Am J Surg Pathol 2010;34: 1147–54.

6. Fujikura K, Yamasaki T, Otani K, et al. BSEP and MDR3: useful immunohistochemical markers to discriminate hepatocellular carcinomas from intrahepatic cholangiocarcinomas and hepatoid carcinomas. Am J Surg Pathol 2016;40:689–96.

7. Wennerberg AE, Nalesnik MA, Coleman WB. Hepatocyte paraffin 1: a monoclonal antibody that reacts with hepatocytes and can be used for differential diagnosis of hepatic tumors. Am J Pathol 1993;143:1050–4.

8. Minervini MI, Demetris AJ, Lee RG, et al. Utilization of hepatocyte-specific antibody in the immunocytochemical evaluation of liver tumors. Mod Pathol 1997; 10:686–92.

9. Morrison C, Marsh WJ, Frankel W. A comparison of CD10 to pCEA, MOC-31, and hepatocyte for the distinction of malignant tumors in the liver. Mod Pathol 2002; 15:1279–87.

10. Fan Z, van de Rijn M, Montgomery K, et al. Hep par 1 antibody stain for the differential diagnosis of hepatocellular carcinoma: 676 tumors tested using tissue microarrays and conventional tissue sections. Mod Pathol 2003;16:137–44.

11. Kakar S, Muir T, Murphy LM, et al. Immunoreactivity of Hep Par 1 in hepatic and extrahepatic tumors and its correlation with albumin in situ hybridization in hepatocellular carcinoma. Am J Clin Pathol 2003;119:361–6.

12. Kakar S, Gown AM, Goodman ZD, et al. Best practices in diagnostic immunohistochemistry: hepatocellular carcinoma versus metastatic neoplasms. Arch Pathol Lab Med 2007;131:1648–54.

13. Baumhoer D, Tornillo L, Stadlmann S, et al. Glypican 3 expression in human nonneoplastic, preoplastic, and neoplastic tissues: a tissue microarray analysis of 4,387 tissue samples. Am J Clin Pathol 2008;129:899–906.

14. Libbrecht L, Severi T, Cassiman D, et al. Glypican-3 expression distinguishes small hepatocellular carcinomas from cirrhosis, dysplastic nodules, and focal nodular hyperplasia-like nodules. Am J Surg Pathol 2006;30:1405–11.

15. Shafizadeh N, Ferrell LD, Kakar S. Utility and limitations of glypican-3 expression for the diagnosis of hepatocellular carcinoma at both ends of the differentiation spectrum. Mod Pathol 2008;21:1011–8.

16. Shirakawa H, Kuronuma T, Nishimura Y, et al. Glypican-3 is a useful diagnostic marker for a component of hepatocellular carcinoma in human liver cancer. Int J Oncol 2009;34:649–56.

17. Wang XY, Degos F, Dubois S, et al. Glypican-3 expression in hepatocellular tumors: diagnostic value for preoplastic lesions and hepatocellular carcinomas. Hum Pathol 2006;37:1435–41.

18. Yamauchi N, Watanabe A, Hishinuma M, et al. The glypican 3 oncofetal protein is a promising diagnostic marker for hepatocellular carcinoma. Mod Pathol 2005; 18:1591–8.
19. Lau SK, Prakash S, Geller SA, et al. Comparative immunohistochemical profile of hepatocellular carcinoma, cholangiocarcinoma, and metastatic adenocarcinoma. Hum Pathol 2002;33:1175–81.
20. Ma CK, Zarbo RJ, Frierson HFJ, et al. Comparative immunohistochemical study of primary and metastatic carcinomas of the liver. Am J Clin Pathol 1993;99: 551–7.
21. Chu PG, Ishizawa S, Wu E, et al. Hepatocyte antigen as a marker of hepatocellular carcinoma: an immunohistochemical comparison to carcinoembryonic antigen, CD10, and alpha-fetoprotein. Am J Surg Pathol 2002;26:978–88.
22. Kong CS, Appenzeller M, Ferrell LD. Utility of CD34 reactivity in evaluating focal nodular hepatocellular lesions sampled by fine needle aspiration biopsy. Acta Cytol 2000;44:218–22.
23. Kimura H, Nakajima T, Kagawa K, et al. Angiogenesis in hepatocellular carcinoma as evaluated by CD34 immunohistochemistry. Liver 1998;18:14–9.
24. Durnez A, Verslype C, Nevens F, et al. The clinicopathological and prognostic relevance of cytokeratin 7 and 19 expression in hepatocellular carcinoma. A possible progenitor cell origin. Histopathology 2006;49:138–51.
25. Maeda T, Kajiyama K, Adachi E, et al. The expression of cytokeratins 7, 19, and 20 in primary and metastatic carcinomas of the liver. Mod Pathol 1996;9:901–9.
26. Niemann TH, Hughes JH, Young De, et al. MOC-31 aids in the differentiation of metastatic adenocarcinoma from hepatocellular carcinoma. Cancer 1999;87: 295–8.
27. Proca DM, Niemann TH, Porcell AI, et al. MOC31 immunoreactivity in primary and metastatic carcinoma of the liver. Report of findings and review of other utilized markers. Appl Immunohistochem Mol Morphol 2000;8:120–5.
28. Ordóñez NG. The diagnostic utility of immunohistochemistry in distinguishing between mesothelioma and renal cell carcinoma: a comparative study. Hum Pathol 2004;35:697–710.
29. Ordóñez NG. Value of the MOC-31 monoclonal antibody in differentiating epithelial pleural mesothelioma from lung adenocarcinoma. Hum Pathol 1998;29:166–9.
30. Sano K, Kosuge T, Yamamoto J, et al. Primary hepatic carcinoid tumors confirmed with long-term follow-up after resection. Hepatogastroenterology 1999;46:2547–50.
31. Mazal PR, Stichenwirth M, Koller A, et al. Expression of aquaporins and PAX-2 compared to CD10 and cytokeratin 7 in renal neoplasms: a tissue microarray study. Mod Pathol 2005;18:535–40.
32. Barr ML, Jilaveanu LB, Camp RL, et al. PAX-8 expression in renal tumours and distant sites: a useful marker of primary and metastatic renal cell carcinoma? J Clin Pathol 2015;68:12–7.
33. Renshaw AA, Granter SR. A comparison of A103 and inhibin reactivity in adrenal cortical tumors: distinction from hepatocellular carcinoma and renal tumors. Mod Pathol 1998;11:1160–4.
34. Ghorab Z, Jorda M, Ganjei P, et al. Melan A (A103) is expressed in adrenocortical neoplasms but not in renal cell and hepatocellular carcinomas. Appl Immunohistochem Mol Morphol 2003;11:330–3.
35. Tsui WM, Colombari R, Portmann BC, et al. Hepatic angiomyolipoma: a clinicopathologic study of 30 cases and delineation of unusual morphologic variants. Am J Surg Pathol 1999;23:34–48.

36. Shafizadeh N, Kakar S. Diagnosis of well-differentiated hepatocellular lesions: role of immunohistochemistry and other ancillary techniques. Adv Anat Pathol 2011;18:438–45.
37. Di Tommaso L, Destro A, Seok JY, et al. The application of markers (HSP70 GPC3 and GS) in liver biopsies is useful for detection of hepatocellular carcinoma. J Hepatol 2009;50:746–54.
38. Park YN, Kojiro M, Di Tommaso L, et al. Ductular reaction is helpful in defining early stromal invasion, small hepatocellular carcinomas, and dysplastic nodules. Cancer 2007;109:915–23.
39. Park YN, Yang CP, Fernandez GJ, et al. Neoangiogenesis and sinusoidal "capillarization" in dysplastic nodules of the liver. Am J Surg Pathol 1998;22:656–62.
40. Shafizadeh N, Kakar S. Hepatocellular carcinoma: histologic subtypes. Surg Pathol Clin 2013;6:367–84.
41. Górnicka B, Ziarkiewicz-Wróblewska B, Wróblewski T, et al. Carcinoma, a fibrolamellar variant–immunohistochemical analysis of 4 cases. Hepatogastroenterology 2005;52:519–23.
42. Ross HM, Daniel HD, Vivekanandan P, et al. Fibrolamellar carcinomas are positive for CD68. Mod Pathol 2011;24:390–5.
43. Honeyman JN, Simon EP, Robine N, et al. Detection of a recurrent DNAJB1-PRKACA chimeric transcript in fibrolamellar hepatocellular carcinoma. Science 2014;343:1010–4.
44. Graham RP, Jin L, Knutson DL, et al. DNAJB1-PRKACA is specific for fibrolamellar carcinoma. Mod Pathol 2015;28:822–9.
45. Ferrell LD, Crawford JM, Dhillon AP, et al. Proposal for standardized criteria for the diagnosis of benign, borderline, and malignant hepatocellular lesions arising in chronic advanced liver disease. Am J Surg Pathol 1993;17:1113–23.
46. Dhingra S, Fiel MI. Update on the new classification of hepatic adenomas: clinical, molecular, and pathologic characteristics. Arch Pathol Lab Med 2014;138:1090–7.
47. Lagana SM, Salomao M, Bao F, et al. Utility of an immunohistochemical panel consisting of glypican-3, heat-shock protein-70, and glutamine synthetase in the distinction of low-grade hepatocellular carcinoma from hepatocellular adenoma. Appl Immunohistochem Mol Morphol 2013;21:170–6.
48. Wanless IR, Mawdsley C, Adams R. On the pathogenesis of focal nodular hyperplasia of the liver. Hepatology 1985;5:1194–200.
49. Fukukura Y, Nakashima O, Kusaba A, et al. Angioarchitecture and blood circulation in focal nodular hyperplasia of the liver. J Hepatol 1998;29:470–5.
50. Zucman-Rossi J, Jeannot E, Nhieu JT, et al. Genotype-phenotype correlation in hepatocellular adenoma: new classification and relationship with HCC. Hepatology 2006;43:515–24.
51. Bioulac-Sage P, Rebouissou S, Thomas C, et al. Hepatocellular adenoma subtype classification using molecular markers and immunohistochemistry. Hepatology 2007;46:740–8.
52. Joseph NM, Ferrell LD, Jain D, et al. Diagnostic utility and limitations of glutamine synthetase and serum amyloid-associated protein immunohistochemistry in the distinction of focal nodular hyperplasia and inflammatory hepatocellular adenoma. Mod Pathol 2014;27:62–72.
53. Bioulac-Sage P, Laumonier H, Sa Cunha A, et al. Hepatocellular adenomas. Liver Int 2009;29:142.
54. Rebouissou S, Amessou M, Couchy G, et al. Frequent in-frame somatic deletions activate gp130 in inflammatory hepatocellular tumours. Nature 2009;457:200–4.

55. Bioulac-Sage P, Balabaud C, Bedossa P, et al. Pathological diagnosis of liver cell adenoma and focal nodular hyperplasia: bordeaux update. J Hepatol 2007;46: 521–7.
56. Hale G, Liu X, Hu J, et al. Correlation of exon 3 β-catenin mutations with glutamine synthetase staining patterns in hepatocellular adenoma and hepatocellular carcinoma. Mod Pathol 2016;29(11):1370–80.
57. Rebouissou S, Franconi A, Calderaro J, et al. Genotype-phenotype correlation of CTNNB1 mutations reveals different ß-catenin activity associated with liver tumor progression. Hepatology 2016;64(6):2047–61.
58. Evason KJ, Grenert JP, Ferrell LD, et al. Atypical hepatocellular adenoma-like neoplasms with β-catenin activation show cytogenetic alterations similar to well-differentiated hepatocellular carcinomas. Hum Pathol 2013;44:750–8.
59. Bedossa P, Burt AD, Brunt EM, et al. Well-differentiated hepatocellular neoplasm of uncertain malignant potential: proposal for a new diagnostic category. Hum Pathol 2014;45:658–60.
60. Kakar S, Evason KJ, Ferrell LD. Well-differentiated hepatocellular neoplasm of uncertain malignant potential: proposal for a new diagnostic category–reply. Hum Pathol 2014;45:660–1.
61. Pilati C, Letouzé E, Nault JC, et al. Genomic profiling of hepatocellular adenomas reveals recurrent FRK-activating mutations and the mechanisms of malignant transformation. Cancer Cell 2014;25:428–41.

Human Immunodeficiency Virus Infection, Antiretroviral Therapy, and Liver Pathology

CrossMark

Mark W. Sonderup, MBChB, FCP (SA), MMED (MED)[a],*,
Helen Cecilia Wainwright, MBChB, FFPath[b]

KEYWORDS

- HIV • Drug-induced liver injury • Coinfections • Obesity
- Low/high-income countries

KEY POINTS

- Antiretroviral therapy has resulted in a dramatic decrease in death in human immunodeficiency virus infection.
- Hepatitis B and C coinfection alters the natural history of viral hepatitis.
- Drug-induced liver injuries cause mortality and morbidity, so early diagnosis is crucial.

INTRODUCTION

The 25-year global human immunodeficiency virus (HIV)/AIDS pandemic has resulted in more than 35 million deaths and currently 37 million people living with HIV.[1] More than 70% live in sub-Saharan Africa with Southern Africa an epicenter with more than half of the global disease burden concentrated in this area.[2] Developments in antiretroviral therapy (ART) with sustained viral suppression has resulted in HIV infection becoming a treatable chronic lifelong disease with a life expectancy significantly prolonged.[3] Coinfections and coexistent diseases are now the target of therapy, as they are increasingly responsible for liver-related morbidity and mortality.[4]

Low-income and middle-income countries disproportionately carry the HIV/AIDS burden with South Africa, as an example, having 6.4 million people living with HIV representing an adult population prevalence of 12%.[5] Its public ART program now has 3.4

[a] Division of Hepatology, Department of Medicine, Groote Schuur Hospital, University of Cape Town, Observatory, Cape Town 7925, South Africa; [b] Department of Anatomical Pathology, National Health Laboratory Services, D7 Groote Schuur Hospital, University of Cape Town, Observatory, Cape Town 7925, South Africa
* Corresponding author.
E-mail address: msonderup@samedical.co.za

Gastroenterol Clin N Am 46 (2017) 327–343
http://dx.doi.org/10.1016/j.gtc.2017.01.007
0889-8553/17/© 2017 Elsevier Inc. All rights reserved.

million people receiving ART.[2,5] Apart from HIV, sub-Saharan Africa, Eastern Europe, and India shoulder a tuberculosis (TB) burden with the associated problem of drug-resistant TB.[6] In South Africa, TB-HIV coinfection is frequent, with up to 65% of new sputum-positive TB cases HIV positive.[7] Sub-Saharan Africa is endemic for hepatitis B (HBV), mostly acquired in childhood with HIV acquisition in adulthood.[8] This differs from high-income or developed countries where HBV and HIV are acquired through similar transmission routes, invariably in adulthood. Globally, HIV-HBV coinfection rates are between 5% and 20%, with approximately 4 to 6 million people HIV-HBV coinfected, rates being highest in Western and Southern Africa.[9] Hepatitis C (HCV) and HIV share similar transmission routes, with HIV adversely impacting the natural history of hepatitis C, with accelerated liver disease and elevated hepatocellular carcinoma risk.[10] Viral hepatitis coinfection significantly contributes to liver-related mortality in the ART era of HIV management, most notably with HIV-HBV coinfected patients in whom incident risk rate is doubled.[11]

With the obesity epidemic and the long-term metabolic consequences of ART, nonalcoholic fatty liver disease (NAFLD) is an additional burden in HIV. In a high HIV burden area, such as sub-Saharan Africa, obesity rates are increasing. In South Africa, 13.5% of men and 42.0% of women are obese.[12] Additional comorbidities include alcohol, drug use, and hepatotoxic traditional/herbal remedies.

Liver disease manifests though clinical symptoms, jaundice, hepatomegaly, abnormal liver function tests or imaging, and biopsy forms part of this assessment in HIV. With careful clinic-pathological assessment, biopsy has significant clinical value. Pathology findings have changed over the 3 decades of the HIV pandemic, and can appropriately be differentiated into the pre-ART and ART era of HIV/AIDS.

PRE-ANTIRETROVIRAL THERAPY

Most liver pathology data were published in the pre-ART era, with fewer data from the ART era. Findings on biopsy invariably differed between the developed and developing world and influenced by local prevalence of infectious diseases.

The largest series published was of 501 biopsies in HIV-infected patients from New York, biopsied for investigation of abnormal liver enzymes, persistent fever, or hepatomegaly.[13] Biopsy yielded a histologic diagnosis in 64%, whereas in 46% it was treatable. *Mycobacterium avium intracellulare* (MAC) was present in 17.6%, TB in 2.6%, and chronic viral hepatitis in 12%. Other opportunistic infection accounted for 2.8% and the commonest neoplasm was lymphoma in 2.6%. *Mycobacterium tuberculosis* (MTB) was an infrequent finding. Another series from Boston of 36 patients biopsied for unexplained fever (83%) and abnormal liver profiles (89%), provided a diagnosis in 75% with a low CD_4 as compared with 25% of those with more preserved immunity. Opportunistic infections included mycobacteria, cytomegalovirus (CMV), and schistosomiasis. Noninfective observations included granulomas of unknown etiology, cirrhosis, and "chronic persistent hepatitis."[14] An Irish study of 39 biopsies revealed pathologic change in 86% of cases. Findings included nonspecific changes, chronic viral hepatitis, acute hepatitis, and cirrhosis. Granulomatous change was an infrequent finding and liver biopsy in this study was deemed very useful in diagnosing hepatic pathology. In several instances, it provided the source of a "pyrexia of unknown origin" but was less useful for detecting opportunistic infection.[15] A 58-case Spanish study found liver biopsy to be diagnostic/suggestive of a specific diagnosis in 63% of cases. Here, MTB was present in 50% and Leishmaniasis in 20%.[16]

Data from low-income or middle-income countries include a 1999 Thai study of 46 liver biopsies in HIV-positive patients with abnormal liver profiles. This series included culture of a portion of the biopsy. TB was diagnosed in 32% and other opportunistic infections included histoplasmosis, cryptococcosis, and *Penicillium marneffei*. In 89%, opportunistic infections were detected, with dual infections in 3 patients **(Fig. 1)**.[17]

From Mumbai, India, a study of 74 patients with HIV, 34 who had a liver biopsy, revealed 30% HIV-HCV and 16% HIV-HBV coinfection. Overall, 14% had established cirrhosis and in 14% TB was diagnosed. Alcohol was a contributing factor in 45%.[18] Furthermore, a study from Mexico looking at 85 liver biopsies from a series of 161 HIV-infected patients between 1987 and 1996, demonstrated granulomatous inflammation in 29%, steatosis and granulomatous inflammation in 19.5%, and steatosis in 14.6%. Infections were cultured in 27.9%: 26.6% MTB, 20% histoplasmosis, 13.3% CMV, and MAC in 11%. Hepatitis B surface antigen was positive in 30%.[19]

A study from Cape Town, South Africa, clinicopathologically evaluated liver biopsies in 301 patients with the study covering the pre-ART/ART eras at which time 26,317 adults were receiving ART. Drug-induced liver injury (DILI) was the commonest finding in 42%, granulomatous inflammation in 29%, steatosis/steatohepatitis in 19%, hepatitis B in 19%, and hepatitis C in 3%. In 16%, more than 1 pathology was diagnosed.[20]

Liver pathology data in HIV-HBV coinfection in the pre-ART era is few and contradictory. Data from US cohorts of coinfected men who have sex with men (MSM) demonstrated significantly less severe necroinflammatory activity in coinfected patients, whereas studies from other US and French cohorts, including people who inject drugs, showed increased necroinflammatory activity.[21,22] With fibrosis, data in the pre-ART era from Europe and the United States showed no difference in fibrosis or cirrhosis scores, whereas 3 French cohort studies identified a more rapid progression toward cirrhosis in coinfected individuals.[23] Scant data from sub-Saharan Africa, an HBV endemic area, exists. A preliminary study from South Africa comparing HIV-HBV coinfected (median CD4 117, ART naive) and HBV monoinfected (pretreatment) patients, observed significantly higher histologic necroinflammatory and fibrosis scores (Ishak modified histologic activity index) in coinfected patients.[24]

Biliary system involvement occurs via opportunistic infections or as a direct consequence of HIV infection. HIV or AIDS cholangiopathy is often associated with CMV or

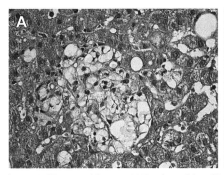 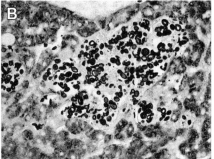

Fig. 1. A 33-year-old man, ART naive with a CD4 1 cell/mm³, presented with a cholestatic liver profile, mild jaundice, hepatomegaly, and fever. Liver biopsy was performed. (*A*) Aggregates of fungal yeasts are splaying the sinusoids (original magnification ×400). (*B*) Grocott stain demonstrates numerous fungal yeasts present, some of which are budding. Fungal culture of liver tissue confirmed *Cryptococcus neoformans* (original magnification ×400).

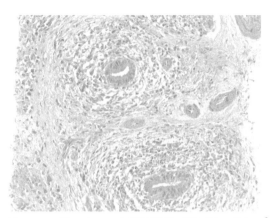

Fig. 2. A 45-year-old man with advanced HIV/AIDS, CD4 30 cells/mm^3, presented with cryptosporidium-related chronic diarrhea and a markedly cholestatic liver profile. Ultrasound of the liver excluded a dilated biliary system. Magnetic resonance pancreatography confirmed a cholangiopathic picture. Portal tract shows chronic inflammation targeting 2 bile ducts with periductal cuffing (hematoxylin-eosin, original magnification ×200).

cryptosporidium that promotes biliary tract inflammation and a secondary sclerosing cholangitis. The bile duct injury is not through HIV directly but possibly through HIV-1 tat protein, via a Fas ligand-dependent mechanism, that is able to increase cryptosporidium-induced apoptosis in cholangiocytes (**Fig. 2**).[25]

The small intrahepatic cholangioles can be the target of several drugs used in management and can produce a ductopenic or vanishing bile duct DILI.[26–29] Implicated drugs include cotrimoxazole and fluconazole.

Last, malignancies that frequently occur in HIV/AIDS, such as lymphomas and Kaposi sarcoma, may involve the liver and can be diagnosed on biopsy.

ANTIRETROVIRAL THERAPY ERA

ART now maintains long-term HIV viral suppression with immune restoration and markedly reduces opportunistic infection risk and HIV-related morbidity and mortality.[30,31] HIV-related mortality is declining and non-HIV–related causes of mortality are contributed by liver disease with 14% to 18% related to coinfections with HBV and HCV. Additional mortality is accounted for by cardiovascular disease, alcohol abuse, and NAFLD.[32]

The frequency of coinfection with hepatitis B or C, occasionally both, is due to shared risk factors. People who inject/use drugs account for up to 90% of HIV-HCV coinfection in high-income countries. Sexual transmission of HCV is infrequent and transmission risk is mostly in MSM.[33] HIV coinfection negatively alters the natural history of hepatitis C with reduced spontaneous clearance of virus following acute infection and higher RNA levels with chronicity. HCV-related liver fibrosis progression is accelerated with a more rapid progression to cirrhosis and decompensated liver disease.[34] Progression to cirrhosis is threefold higher and the relative risk of decompensated liver disease sixfold higher. Hepatocellular carcinoma (HCC) occurs earlier and may be more aggressive.[35] Treating hepatitis C in coinfected patients and achieving cure with a sustained virological response, notably in the era of direct-acting antiviral therapies for hepatitis C, significantly improves outcomes.[36]

HIV coinfection with HBV has an equally deleterious effect on its natural history. People living with HIV are 3 to 6 times more likely to develop chronic HBV compared with HIV-negative individuals following acute HBV infection. HBV replication is higher despite often normal alanine transaminase (ALT), HBV reactivation risk is elevated, and acute liver failure with acute HBV infection is greater as are rates of occult HBV. Fibrosis and cirrhosis progression rates are enhanced and similarly HCC risk is elevated. As with HIV-HCV coinfection, ART-related hepatotoxicity risk is elevated. Immune reconstitution hepatitis can occur after ART initiation. The pathologic staging of the liver biopsies with HIV/HBV can be problematic, as HIV can influence the degree of necroinflammation. Dual HBV-based ART, namely, lamivudine/tenofovir or emtricitabine/tenofovir, is the cornerstone of HBV management in HIV-HBV coinfection.[37] Tenofovir-based therapy has demonstrated long-term durability to HBV resistance[32] (**Fig. 3**).

Drug Toxicity in Human Immunodeficiency Virus Disease

Liver biopsy is the gold standard for assessing hepatotoxicity, but is limited by its invasiveness. It provides a means of assessing the pattern of liver injury and the specific type of inflammatory response, namely, immunoallergic, nonspecific hepatitis with apoptosis, biliary involvement with bile duct targeting or paucity of bile ducts,

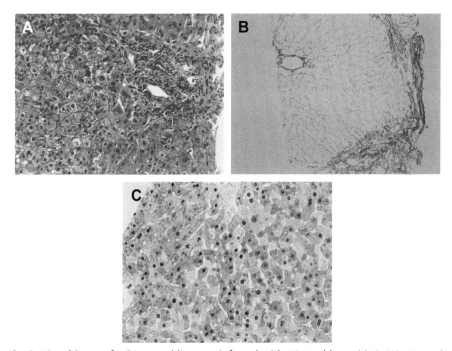

Fig. 3. Liver biopsy of a 31-year-old man coinfected with HIV and hepatitis B, HBeAg positive, ALT 141 U/L, and hepatitis B DNA viral load of $\log_{10}$ 9.3. Efavirenz/FTC/TDF was initiated and within 1 month, ALT rose sharply with no jaundice or coagulopathy. Patient biopsied. HBeAg remained positive and patient maintained on ART and carefully followed. ALT settled within 3 months. (*A*) Portal tract shows moderate inflammation, with mild interface hepatitis and zone 1 hepatocytes with ground-glass cytoplasm (hematoxylin-eosin, original magnification ×400). (*B*) Portal-portal bridging fibrosis and a normal central vein is seen indicating F3 fibrosis (original magnification ×200). (*C*). Extensive intranuclear positivity to hepatitis B core antigen (original magnification ×400).

cholestatic without inflammation or cholestatic with inflammation, granulomatous or steatohepatitis. It also may identify unexpected underlying pathology.

Non-antiretroviral drugs

Several drugs used for management of opportunistic infections in HIV/AIDS are potentially hepatotoxic. These include cotrimoxazole, pentamidine, antifungals, including ketoconazole and fluconazole, and antituberculous drugs, such as rifampicin, isoniazid, and pyrazinamide. Cotrimoxazole typically causes a mixed cholestatic-hepatitis or pure cholestatic injury, with the potential for a progressive ductopenic injury. A series of 38 patients in whom 29 developed drug toxicity, 19 with a severe reaction, was described in 1984.[38,39] A significantly lower rate of hepatotoxicity was reported with pentamidine[40] (**Fig. 4**).

Isoniazid (INH) produces a range of patterns of DILI from steatosis, focal necrosis, and chronic active hepatitis to massive hepatic necrosis, with 95% demonstrating focal hepatocyte necrosis with ballooning, apoptosis, and mild inflammation in portal tracts. Incidence is approximately 1%, rising to 2.3% in those older than 50. Massive hepatic necrosis is idiosyncratic, with an overall mortality of 10%. Rifampicin DILI is less frequent when used individually; however, with INH, the incidence rises to 5% to 8%.

The imidazole drugs have hepatotoxic potential with cholestatic injuries being the most frequent pattern. Ketoconazole, however, can produce a florid hepatocellular injury. Given the possibility of polypharmacy in HIV/AIDS management, clinicians must obtain a complete drug history when a liver biopsy is being assessed for hepatotoxicity (**Fig. 5**).

Antiretroviral drugs

There are 6 classes of antiretroviral drugs:

1. Nucleoside reverse transcriptase inhibitors (NRTIs), for example, didanosine (DDI), emtricitabine (FTC), lamivudine (3 TC), stavudine (D4T), tenofovir (TDF), abacavir (ABC), and zidovudine (AZT)

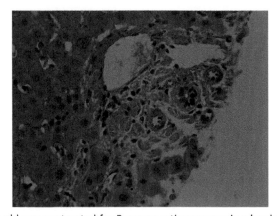

Fig. 4. A 32-year-old woman treated for Pneumocystis pneumonia who developed jaundice and a cholestatic liver injury in the last week of treatment. Despite cessation of therapy and treatment with ursodeoxycholic acid, cholestasis and jaundice were progressive. Portal tract demonstrates absent bile duct as seen in this vanishing bile duct syndrome. There is a residual bile duct with adjacent hepatic artery and 2 unpaired arteries. Lymphocytes are present within the biliary epithelial lining (hematoxylin-eosin, original magnification ×400).

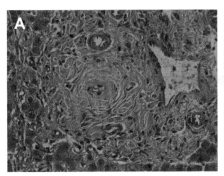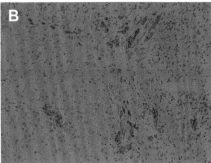

Fig. 5. A 28-year-old woman, CD4 cell count greater than 500 cells/mm³, ART naive, presented with cholestatic liver profile after using a supplement with African potato (*Hypoxis hemerocallidea*). (*A*) The portal tract has a portal vein and hepatic arteries. The bile duct is atrophic, surrounded by dense fibrosis and has no functional lumen. There is minimal inflammation portal inflammation (hematoxylin-eosin, original magnification ×400). (*B*) CK 19 immunostaining of a portal tract showing no residual bile ducts and a ductular reaction at the periphery (original magnification ×400).

2. Non-nucleoside reverse transcriptase inhibitors (NNRTIs), for example, efavirenz, nevirapine, etravirine, and rilpivirine
3. Protease inhibitors (PIs), for example, amprenavir, atazanavir, darunavir, fosamprenavir, indinavir, lopinavir/ritonavir, nelfinavir, ritonavir
4. Integrase inhibitors (INSTIs), for example, raltegravir, dolutegravir
5. Fusion inhibitors (FIs), for example, enfuvirtide
6. Chemokine receptor antagonists (CCR5 antagonists), for example, maraviroc

ART is based on the principle of combining different classes of drugs, acting at different stages in the HIV-host cell life cycle, to increase efficacy and reduce resistance. ART-related DILI is consequent to a range of potential mechanisms, including direct drug toxicity, hypersensitivity, mitochondrial toxicity, or immune reconstitution related.[32] The toxicity or DILI potential of each class of ART varies and is mostly unpredictable. However, in some instances, predictable risk can occur, as is seen with abacavir-induced steatosis and lactic acidosis in those with HLA-B*5701 phenotype.[41]

Nucleoside reverse transcriptase inhibitors

NRTI toxicity mechanisms include mitochondrial and hypersensitivity reactions. Late 1980s data suggested moderate to severe hepatotoxicity rates ranging from 7% with AZT, 9% to 13% with D4T, to 16% with DDI.[42] The newer FTC, TDF, 3 TC, and ABC are associated with a significantly lower risk. Mitochondrial toxicity is an infrequent but distinctive DILI pattern causing acute liver failure preceded by tender hepatomegaly (due to steatosis) and lactic acidosis.[43] In vitro, NRTIs inhibit mitochondrial γ-polymerase required for the maintenance of mitochondrial mass and function. Drug depletion of hepatic mitochondria can be demonstrated on Southern blot analysis.[44] Fatalities have been documented in medical personnel with needle-stick injuries given short courses and hence the use of older NRTIs as postexposure prophylaxis is discouraged.[45]

The various NRTIs differ widely in their propensity to induce mitochondrial toxicity. Those with greatest risk are zalcitabine, DDI, D4T, and AZT and lesser risk, ABC.[46] Combining certain agents, such as D4T and DDI, is additive and enhances risk.[47] The steatosis is usually mixed macro/microvesicular and is secondary to increased fatty acid synthesis with respiratory electron chain activation with simultaneous mitochondrial uncoupling. Myopathy also can occur. DDI use is now generally discouraged because of its toxicity potential. DDI liver toxicity producing portal fibrosis with nodular regenerative hyperplasia (NRH) has been documented.[48] DDI-related noncirrhotic portal hypertension secondary to NRH and obliterative portal venopathy are reported, albeit rarely.[49] Patients clinically manifest with portal hypertension features, including ascites and variceal hemorrhage with muscle wasting and weakness. Jaundice is infrequent and liver enzymes are modestly elevated. Mechanisms are thought to relate to DDI damaging endothelial cells producing thrombotic occlusion with secondary nodular hyperplasia. Potential contributing factors are acquired protein S deficiency, and direct HIV-related endothelial cell activation–related thrombosis (**Fig. 6**).[48,50,51]

Non-nucleoside reverse transcriptase inhibitors

Nevirapine Nevirapine, a potent inhibitor of HIV replication, is typically given in combination with 2 NRTIs. Nevirapine, first approved in the United States in 1996, causes elevations in ALT levels (>5 times upper limit of normal [ULN]) in 4% to 20% of patients and symptomatic elevation in 1% to 5% of patients. In 17 randomized trials, 10% of patients developed ALT/aspartate transaminase (AST) more than 5 times ULN, 6.3% symptomatic.[52] Risk factors included HCV or HBV coinfection, female gender, CD4 greater than 250/μL, and when used for postexposure prophylaxis.[53] Overall, the 1% frequency of nevirapine DILI is significant with an approximately 0.1% mortality.

There are 2 patterns of nevirapine DILI. The early being a drug hypersensitivity reaction/immune-mediated DILI in which patients present within the first 6 to 8 weeks of therapy with abdominal pain, fever, rash, and jaundice, collectively a DRESS-type phenomenon (drug reaction with eosinophilia and systemic symptoms). The rash can be severe and be a toxic epidermal necrosis or Stevens-Johnson syndrome. The second hepatotoxicity mechanism is a delayed onset occurring 4 to 5 months after initiation and is not immunoallergic/hypersensitivity in nature. Infrequently, bile duct targeting and loss of bile ducts resulting in a vanishing bile duct syndrome, has been documented.[29] It has never been associated with causing steatosis.[54]

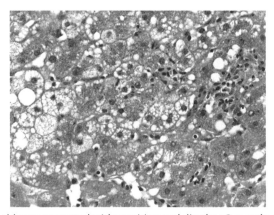

Fig. 6. A 28-year-old man presented with vomiting and diarrhea 3 months after starting ART with AZT, DDI, and lopinavir/ritonavir. Liver profile demonstrated a mild hepatocellular injury with jaundice. Liver core shows microvesicular steatosis, hepatocyte ballooning, and small necroinflammatory foci, which are in keeping with an NRTI injury (hematoxylin-eosin, original magnification ×400).

A 2002 study of 568 patients found the frequency of hepatotoxicity with nevirapine 15.6% and 8.5% with efavirenz. Coinfection with HCV and HBV were 43.0% and 7.7%, respectively, and presentation within the first 12 weeks occurred in 32.0% of the efavirenz and 50.0% of the nevirapine group. Liver injury was more severe with coinfection and PIs.[55] A 2005 South African study of 468 patients using either nevirapine or efavirenz as the NNRTI, showed a 17% hepatotoxicity rate with nevirapine and 2 deaths due to hepatic failure with high body mass index an identified risk factor.[56] Efavirenz was suggested as the preferred NNRTI option with perceived lower rates of hepatotoxicity (**Fig. 7**).[57]

Efavirenz Efavirenz, an NNRTI was first approved in 1998, and is similar to nevirapine in its mechanism of action but has no structural similarity. ALT/AST elevations greater than 5 times ULN have been reported in 1% to 8% with higher rates in HCV coinfection. DRESS phenomenon, although described, is less common than with nevirapine. Efavirenz can activate a nuclear receptor, constitutive androstane receptor (CAR), and induce *CYP2B6* mRNA expression.[58] Single nucleotide polymorphisms of CYP2B6 in a Thai study were demonstrated in patients with efavirenz hepatotoxicity risk.[59] Efavirenz has been shown to induce mitochondrial dysfunction stimulating mitochondria with abnormal morphology and increased mass leading to apoptosis.[60]

In pregnancy, nevirapine was the preferred NNRTI but 12 studies in pregnancy suggested no difference in the overall risks of congenital anomalies between the 2 drugs and is now used in pregnancy.[61] We have reported our experience with efavirenz DILI in 81 patients with liver biopsy in 73 and demonstrated 3 histologic patterns of injury: a nonspecific hepatitis with mild elevation of serum transaminases; a mixed cholestatic-hepatitis with mild to moderate jaundice and moderate elevation of transaminases, alkaline phosphatase (ALP) and gamma-glutamyl transferase (GGT); and an immune-allergic hypersensitivity DILI causing submassive necrosis with markedly elevated transaminases, severe jaundice, and coagulopathy. The patient profile was predominantly female, aged younger than 30 years, and more than half were pregnant at ART initiation. High baseline CD4 predicted for submassive necrosis and mortality was 17%.[62] Reported cases of efavirenz-associated liver failure and death within

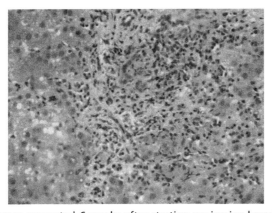

Fig. 7. Young woman presented 6 weeks after starting nevirapine-based ART with fever, marked generalized maculopapular rash, and severe hepatitis. An expanded portal tract is shown with a marked inflammatory reaction including eosinophils extending into the parenchyma. There is a ductular reaction and zone 1 steatosis (hematoxylin-eosin, original magnification ×400).

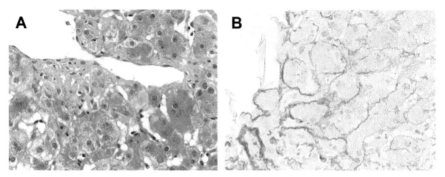

Fig. 8. A 43-year-old man presented with a mixed cholestatic-hepatitis liver profile and jaundice 5 months after initiating efavirenz-based ART with a baseline CD4 count of 180 cells/mm³. (*A*) Zone 3 hepatocytes show multinucleation and bilirubinostasis with a mild associated mononuclear infiltrate (hematoxylin-eosin, original magnification ×400). (*B*) Emerald green staining of the intracytoplasmic bile is seen and the pericellular fibrosis is highlighted with the bile Sirius red stain (original magnification ×400).

months of initiating ART may well be patients with the submassive necrosis type injury described (**Figs. 8** and **9**).[63,64]

In pooled data, rilpivirine, a newer NNRTI used in treatment-naive patients with low viral loads, demonstrated a twofold lower incidence of any grade 2 to 4 liver adverse events compared with efavirenz. With longer follow-up, the difference in incident hepatoxicity when compared with efavirenz was no longer observed.[65,66]

Protease Inhibitors

PIs were introduced in the mid to late 1990s as part of ART. As a group, rates of hepatotoxicity are seemingly lower. Elevations in serum ALT/AST (>5 times ULN) is reported in up to 15% and are more common in patients with HIV-HCV coinfection. However, with ritonavir, when the dose is lowered and used in "booster" doses, the frequency and severity of ALT/AST elevation decreases. Immuno-allergic features are rare. Atazanavir and indinavir increases unconjugated serum bilirubin due to the

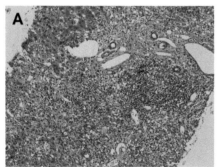
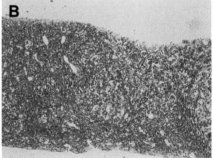

Fig. 9. A 25-year-old woman initiated efavirenz/FTC/TDF during pregnancy with a baseline CD4 count of 570 cells/mm³. She presented 3 months' postpartum with marked jaundice, hepatitis, and coagulopathy. (*A*) The liver core shows marked immune-allergic portal inflammation with lymphocytes, plasma cells, eosinophils, and neutrophils. There is panlobular extension of the inflammation to involve the zone 3 hepatocytes (hematoxylin-eosin, original magnification ×400). (*B*) Reticulin stain shows the collapsed framework in areas of submassive necrosis (original magnification ×200).

inhibition of UDP glucuronyl-transferase in a Gilbert syndrome–like fashion with jaundice not indicative of hepatic injury. Factors that contributing to PI-induced hepatotoxicity include age, CD4 count, viral hepatitis coinfection, alcohol, and drug-drug interactions, for example, anti-TB drugs.[67]

Integrase inhibitors, fusion inhibitors, and CCR5 antagonists

In 2005, aplaviroc development, a CCR5 antagonist, was halted because of severe hepatotoxicity.[68] In contrast, maraviroc and vicriviroc have safer hepatotoxicity profiles. Case reports of maraviroc DILI have been reported, although given the extensive range of other drugs used, causality is doubtful.[69,70] Enfuvirtide, the only approved FI, has demonstrated a consistent safety record, similarly with integrase inhibitors, although data are limited. A small prospective study in 8 patients on dolutegravir and Child-Pugh B cirrhosis noted no hepatotoxicity.[71]

Immune reconstitution inflammatory syndrome

Immune reconstitution inflammatory syndrome (IRIS), or immune restoration disease, is a disease-specific or pathogen-specific inflammatory response in HIV-infected patients after initiation/reinitiation of ART or a change to more active ART. It is accompanied by a rapid rise in CD4 count and/or a rapid decrease in HIV viremia. Most clinically apparent cases occur in patients with low CD4 counts and high viral loads. Presentation is usually within the first 4 to 8 weeks after ART initiation and inflammatory reactions to many pathogens are described, including mycobacterium, fungi, viruses, and bacteria.

In low-income and medium-income countries, given the high rates of TB-HIV coinfection, TB-IRIS is frequent. Two forms of TB-IRIS are recognized: *paradoxic*, in which IRIS occurs in those who start TB treatment before ART, and *unmasking*, which occurs in those with undiagnosed TB who start ART. Cohort studies have reported that 8% to 43% of patients starting ART while on TB treatment develop paradoxic TB-IRIS and a recent meta-analysis estimated the pooled cumulative incidence as 15.7%.[72,73] The largest systematic review and meta-analysis of early initiation of ART from 6 studies demonstrated mortality reduction and increased rate of TB-IRIS requiring proper management to avoid excess deaths.[74] A second review and meta-analysis of studies from 1996 to 2013 demonstrated the same. The case fatality rate was 8% to 14%.[75]

Hepatic TB-IRIS is probably more common than clinically appreciated. Hematogenous dissemination of TB is frequent in advanced HIV and with TB-IRIS, liver involvement is likely. In a case series of patients with hepatic TB-IRIS, presentations were characterized by hepatomegaly (56%) and an abnormal liver profile, with two-thirds having a fever. The pattern of liver enzyme abnormality was a mixed picture with moderate elevation of ALT/AST but a more significant elevation in GGT over ALP.[76] Histologic features observed in hepatic TB-IRIS include increased numbers of granulomas per liver core with abundant eosinophils palisading around these granulomas (**Fig. 10**).[20]

Causes of death on antiretroviral therapy

A South African 2012 postmortem biopsy series of 39 adults, 14 pre-ART; 15 early ART, and 10 on established ART, noted mycobacterial infection in 69% (MTB in 26/27), bacterial infection in 33%, fungal infection in 21%, and neoplasms in 26%. IRIS was implicated in 73%. In 49%, a previously undiagnosed cause of death was found with multiple pathologies in 62%.[77]

A 10-year French study covering 1995 to 2005 after ART introduction yielded an increase in deaths due to end-stage liver disease from 2% to 17%; 75% had HCV coinfection, 48% alcohol related and death due to HCC increased from 5% to 25%.[78] In

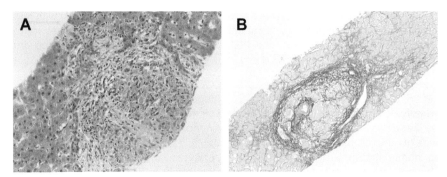

Fig. 10. A 46-year-old man presented with hepatomegaly, right upper quadrant pain, mild fever, and marked cholestasis and mild jaundice 1 month after initiating ART. Sputum cultured MTB. (*A*) There is an expanded portal tract with moderate inflammation and a large non-necrotizing granuloma. Ziehl Neelsen stain was negative (hematoxylin-eosin, original magnification ×400). (*B*) BSR stain showing periportal fibrosis extending into the parenchyma (original magnification ×200).

2006, the Data collection on Adverse effects of anti-HIV Drugs (D:A:D) study reported 1246 deaths (5.3%) in a 23,441-participant cohort with 14.5% liver related, 16.9% HBV coinfected, 66% HCV, and 71% tri-coinfected.[79] In 2010, D:A:D reported 2482 deaths in 33,308 participants with death rate decreasing from 16.9% in 1999/2000 to 9.6% in 2007/2008. There were 341 liver-related deaths due to HCV, HBV, and liver complications of the metabolic syndrome.[80]

SUMMARY

ART has had a huge impact on those living with HIV. HIV has become a treatable chronic disease with a reasonable life expectancy. Liver disease in this population has now shifted away from predominantly opportunistic infections to viral coinfection and the metabolic and potential DILI consequences of ART, although this is still influenced as to whether patients reside in low-income or high-income countries.

REFERENCES

1. UNAIDS Global Fact Sheet. Available at: http://www.unaids.org/sites/default/files/media_asset/UNAIDS_FactSheet_en.pdf. Accessed February 27, 2017.
2. UN AIDS Global AIDS update. 2016. Available at: http://www.unaids.org/sites/default/files/media_asset/global-AIDS-update-2016_en.pdf. Accessed February 27, 2017.
3. Teeraananchai S, Kerr SJ, Amin J, et al. Life expectancy of HIV-positive people after starting combination antiretroviral therapy: a meta-analysis. HIV Med 2016. [Epub ahead of print].
4. Smith CJ, Ryom L, Weber R, et al. Trends in underlying causes of death in people with HIV from 1999 to 2011 (D:A:D): a multicohort collaboration. Lancet 2014; 384(9939):241–8.
5. Shisana O, Rehle T, Simbayi LC, et al. South African national HIV prevalence, incidence and behaviour survey, 2012. Cape Town (South Africa): HSRC Press; 2014. Available at: http://www.hsrc.ac.za/uploads/pageContent/4565/SABSSM%20IV%20LEO%20final. Accessed February 27, 2017.
6. Zumla A, George A, Sharma V, et al. The WHO 2014 global tuberculosis report–further to go. Lancet Glob Health 2015;3(1):e10–2.

7. Wood R, Lawn SD, Caldwell J, et al. Burden of new and recurrent tuberculosis in a major South African city stratified by age and HIV-status. PLoS One 2011;6(10): e25098.

8. Matthews PC, Geretti AM, Goulder PJ, et al. Epidemiology and impact of HIV co-infection with hepatitis B and hepatitis C viruses in sub-Saharan Africa. J Clin Virol 2014;61(1):20–33.

9. Kourtis AP, Bulterys M, Hu DJ, et al. HIV-HBV coinfection–a global challenge. N Engl J Med 2012;366(19):1749–52.

10. Naggie S, Sulkowski MS. Management of patients coinfected with HCV and HIV: a close look at the role for direct-acting antivirals. Gastroenterology 2012;142(6): 1324–34.e1323.

11. Falade-Nwulia O, Seaberg EC, Rinaldo CR, et al. Comparative risk of liver-related mortality from chronic hepatitis B versus chronic hepatitis C virus infection. Clin Infect Dis 2012;55(4):507–13.

12. Ng M, Fleming T, Robinson M, et al. Global, regional, and national prevalence of overweight and obesity in children and adults during 1980-2013: a systematic analysis for the Global Burden of Disease Study 2013. Lancet 2014;384(9945): 766–81.

13. Poles MA, Dieterich DT, Schwarz ED, et al. Liver biopsy findings in 501 patients infected with human immunodeficiency virus (HIV). J Acquir Immune Defic Syndr Hum Retrovirol 1996;11(2):170–7.

14. Cappell MS, Schwartz MS, Biempica L. Clinical utility of liver biopsy in patients with serum antibodies to the human immunodeficiency virus. Am J Med 1990; 88(2):123–30.

15. Kennedy M, O'Reilly M, Bergin CJ, et al. Liver biopsy pathology in human immu-nodeficiency virus infection. Eur J Gastroenterol Hepatol 1998;10(3):255–8.

16. Garcia-Ordonez MA, Colmenero JD, Jimenez-Onate F, et al. Diagnostic useful-ness of percutaneous liver biopsy in HIV-infected patients with fever of unknown origin. J Infect 1999;38(2):94–8.

17. Piratvisuth T, Siripaitoon P, Sriplug H, et al. Findings and benefit of liver biopsies in 46 patients infected with human immunodeficiency virus. J Gastroenterol Hep-atol 1999;14(2):146–9.

18. Rathi PM, Amarapurkar DN, Borges NE, et al. Spectrum of liver diseases in HIV infection. Indian J Gastroenterol 1997;16(3):94–5.

19. Lizardi-Cervera J, Soto Ramirez LE, Poo JL, et al. Hepatobiliary diseases in pa-tients with human immunodeficiency virus (HIV) treated with non highly active anti-retroviral therapy: frequency and clinical manifestations. Ann Hepatol 2005; 4(3):188–91.

20. Sonderup MW, Wainwright H, Hall P, et al. A clinicopathological cohort study of liver pathology in 301 patients with human immunodeficiency virus/acquired im-mune deficiency syndrome. Hepatology 2015;61(5):1721–9.

21. Goldin RD, Fish DE, Hay A, et al. Histological and immunohistochemical study of hepatitis B virus in human immunodeficiency virus infection. J Clin Pathol 1990; 43(3):203–5.

22. Housset C, Pol S, Carnot F, et al. Interactions between human immunodeficiency virus-1, hepatitis delta virus and hepatitis B virus infections in 260 chronic carriers of hepatitis B virus. Hepatology 1992;15(4):578–83.

23. Colin JF, Cazals-Hatem D, Loriot MA, et al. Influence of human immunodeficiency virus infection on chronic hepatitis B in homosexual men. Hepatology 1999;29(4): 1306–10.

24. Sonderup MW, Wainwright H, Hairwadzi H, et al. A clinicopathological comparison of HIV/Hepatitis B co-infection and Hepatitis B mono-infection in Cape Town, South Africa. Hepatology 2008;48(4):1176A.

25. O'Hara SP, Small AJ, Nelson JB, et al. The human immunodeficiency virus type 1 tat protein enhances *Cryptosporidium parvum*-induced apoptosis in cholangiocytes via a Fas ligand-dependent mechanism. Infect Immun 2007;75(2):684–96.

26. Bonacini M. Hepatobiliary complications in patients with human immunodeficiency virus infection. Am J Med 1992;92(4):404–11.

27. Cappell MS. Hepatobiliary manifestations of the acquired immune deficiency syndrome. Am J Gastroenterol 1991;86(1):1–15.

28. Oppenheimer AP, Koh C, McLaughlin M, et al. Vanishing bile duct syndrome in human immunodeficiency virus infected adults: a report of two cases. World J Gastroenterol 2013;19(1):115–21.

29. Hindupur S, Yeung M, Shroff P, et al. Vanishing bile duct syndrome in a patient with advanced AIDS. HIV Med 2007;8(1):70–2.

30. Maartens G, Celum C, Lewin SR. HIV infection: epidemiology, pathogenesis, treatment, and prevention. Lancet 2014;384(9939):258–71.

31. Ford N, Shubber Z, Meintjes G, et al. Causes of hospital admission among people living with HIV worldwide: a systematic review and meta-analysis. Lancet HIV 2015;2(10):e438–44.

32. Price JC, Thio CL. Liver disease in the HIV-infected individual. Clin Gastroenterol Hepatol 2010;8(12):1002–12.

33. Chan DP, Sun HY, Wong HT, et al. Sexually acquired hepatitis C virus infection: a review. Int J Infect Dis 2016;49:47–58.

34. Ingiliz P, Rockstroh JK. Natural history of liver disease and effect of hepatitis C virus on HIV disease progression. Curr Opin HIV AIDS 2015;10(5):303–8.

35. Lewden C, May T, Rosenthal E, et al. Changes in causes of death among adults infected by HIV between 2000 and 2005: The "Mortalite 2000 and 2005" surveys (ANRS EN19 and Mortavic). J Acquir Immune Defic Syndr 2008;48(5):590–8.

36. Mandorfer M, Schwabl P, Steiner S, et al. Advances in the management of HIV/HCV coinfection. Hepatol Int 2016;10(3):424–35.

37. Nunez M, Mendes-Correa MC. Viral hepatitis and HIV: update and management. Antivir Ther 2013;18(3 Pt B):451–8.

38. Smilack JD. Trimethoprim-sulfamethoxazole. Mayo Clin Proc 1999;74(7):730–4.

39. Gordin FM, Simon GL, Wofsy CB, et al. Adverse reactions to trimethoprim-sulfamethoxazole in patients with the acquired immunodeficiency syndrome. Ann Intern Med 1984;100(4):495–9.

40. O'Brien JG, Dong BJ, Coleman RL, et al. A 5-year retrospective review of adverse drug reactions and their risk factors in human immunodeficiency virus-infected patients who were receiving intravenous pentamidine therapy for *Pneumocystis carinii* pneumonia. Clin Infect Dis 1997;24(5):854–9.

41. Sousa-Pinto B, Pinto-Ramos J, Correia C, et al. Pharmacogenetics of abacavir hypersensitivity: A systematic review and meta-analysis of the association with HLA-B*57:01. J Allergy Clin Immunol 2015;136(4):1092–4.e1093.

42. Ogedegbe AO, Sulkowski MS. Antiretroviral-associated liver injury. Clin Liver Dis 2003;7(2):475–99.

43. Brinkman K, ter Hofstede HJ, Burger DM, et al. Adverse effects of reverse transcriptase inhibitors: mitochondrial toxicity as common pathway. AIDS 1998;12(14):1735–44.

44. Chariot P, Drogou I, de Lacroix-Szmania I, et al. Zidovudine-induced mitochondrial disorder with massive liver steatosis, myopathy, lactic acidosis, and mitochondrial DNA depletion. J Hepatol 1999;30(1):156–60.
45. Nunez M. Clinical syndromes and consequences of antiretroviral-related hepatotoxicity. Hepatology 2010;52(3):1143–55.
46. Birkus G, Hitchcock MJ, Cihlar T. Assessment of mitochondrial toxicity in human cells treated with tenofovir: comparison with other nucleoside reverse transcriptase inhibitors. Antimicrob Agents Chemother 2002;46(3):716–23.
47. Walker UA, Setzer B, Venhoff N. Increased long-term mitochondrial toxicity in combinations of nucleoside analogue reverse-transcriptase inhibitors. AIDS 2002;16(16):2165–73.
48. Vispo E, Moreno A, Maida I, et al. Noncirrhotic portal hypertension in HIV-infected patients: unique clinical and pathological findings. AIDS 2010;24(8):1171–6.
49. Vispo E, Morello J, Rodriguez-Novoa S, et al. Noncirrhotic portal hypertension in HIV infection. Curr Opin Infect Dis 2011;24(1):12–8.
50. Mallet VO, Varthaman A, Lasne D, et al. Acquired protein S deficiency leads to obliterative portal venopathy and to compensatory nodular regenerative hyperplasia in HIV-infected patients. AIDS 2009;23(12):1511–8.
51. Schiano TD, Kotler DP, Ferran E, et al. Hepatoportal sclerosis as a cause of noncirrhotic portal hypertension in patients with HIV. Am J Gastroenterol 2007; 102(11):2536–40.
52. Dieterich DT, Robinson PA, Love J, et al. Drug-induced liver injury associated with the use of nonnucleoside reverse-transcriptase inhibitors. Clin Infect Dis 2004; 38(Suppl 2):S80–9.
53. Wooltorton E. HIV drug nevirapine (Viramune): risk of severe hepatotoxicity. CMAJ 2004;170(7):1091.
54. Terelius Y, Figler RA, Marukian S, et al. Transcriptional profiling suggests that Nevirapine and Ritonavir cause drug induced liver injury through distinct mechanisms in primary human hepatocytes. Chem Biol Interact 2016;255:31–44.
55. Sulkowski MS, Thomas DL, Mehta SH, et al. Hepatotoxicity associated with nevirapine or efavirenz-containing antiretroviral therapy: role of hepatitis C and B infections. Hepatology 2002;35(1):182–9.
56. Sanne I, Mommeja-Marin H, Hinkle J, et al. Severe hepatotoxicity associated with nevirapine use in HIV-infected subjects. J Infect Dis 2005;191(6):825–9.
57. Shubber Z, Calmy A, Andrieux-Meyer I, et al. Adverse events associated with nevirapine and efavirenz-based first-line antiretroviral therapy: a systematic review and meta-analysis. AIDS 2013;27(9):1403–12.
58. Meyer zu Schwabedissen HE, Oswald S, Bresser C, et al. Compartment-specific gene regulation of the CAR inducer efavirenz in vivo. Clin Pharmacol Ther 2012; 92(1):103–11.
59. Manosuthi W, Sukasem C, Lueangniyomkul A, et al. CYP2B6 haplotype and biological factors responsible for hepatotoxicity in HIV-infected patients receiving efavirenz-based antiretroviral therapy. Int J Antimicrob Agents 2014;43(3):292–6.
60. Apostolova N, Gomez-Sucerquia LJ, Gortat A, et al. Autophagy as a rescue mechanism in efavirenz-induced mitochondrial dysfunction: a lesson from hepatic cells. Autophagy 2011;7(11):1402–4.
61. Ford N, Mofenson L, Shubber Z, et al. Safety of efavirenz in the first trimester of pregnancy: an updated systematic review and meta-analysis. AIDS 2014; 28(Suppl 2):S123–31.

62. Sonderup MW, Maughan D, Gogela N, et al. Identification of a novel and severe pattern of efavirenz drug-induced liver injury in South Africa. AIDS 2016;30(9): 1483–5.

63. Qayyum S, Dong H, Kovacic D, et al. Combination therapy efavirenz/emtricitabine/tenofovir disoproxil fumarate associated with hepatic failure. Curr Drug Saf 2012;7(5):391–3.

64. Patil R, Ona MA, Papafragkakis H, et al. Acute liver toxicity due to efavirenz/emtricitabine/tenofovir. Case Reports Hepatol 2015;2015:280353.

65. Cohen CJ, Molina JM, Cahn P, et al. Efficacy and safety of rilpivirine (TMC278) versus efavirenz at 48 weeks in treatment-naive HIV-1-infected patients: pooled results from the phase 3 double-blind randomized ECHO and THRIVE trials. J Acquir Immune Defic Syndr 2012;60(1):33–42.

66. Pozniak AL, Morales-Ramirez J, Katabira E, et al. Efficacy and safety of TMC278 in antiretroviral-naive HIV-1 patients: week 96 results of a phase IIb randomized trial. AIDS 2010;24(1):55–65.

67. Sulkowski MS. Drug-induced liver injury associated with antiretroviral therapy that includes HIV-1 protease inhibitors. Clin Infect Dis 2004;38(Suppl 2):S90–7.

68. Crabb C. GlaxoSmithKline ends aplaviroc trials. AIDS 2006;20(5):641.

69. Abel S, Back DJ, Vourvahis M. Maraviroc: pharmacokinetics and drug interactions. Antivir Ther 2009;14(5):607–18.

70. Hardy WD, Gulick RM, Mayer H, et al. Two-year safety and virologic efficacy of maraviroc in treatment-experienced patients with CCR5-tropic HIV-1 infection: 96-week combined analysis of MOTIVATE 1 and 2. J Acquir Immune Defic Syndr 2010;55(5):558–64.

71. Song IH, Borland J, Savina PM, et al. Pharmacokinetics of single-dose dolutegravir in HIV-Seronegative subjects with moderate hepatic impairment compared to healthy matched controls. Clin Pharmacol Drug Dev 2013;2(4):342–8.

72. Meintjes G, Lawn SD, Scano F, et al. Tuberculosis-associated immune reconstitution inflammatory syndrome: case definitions for use in resource-limited settings. Lancet Infect Dis 2008;8(8):516–23.

73. Muller M, Wandel S, Colebunders R, et al. Immune reconstitution inflammatory syndrome in patients starting antiretroviral therapy for HIV infection: a systematic review and meta-analysis. Lancet Infect Dis 2010;10(4):251–61.

74. Abay SM, Deribe K, Reda AA, et al. The effect of early initiation of antiretroviral therapy in tb/hiv-coinfected patients: a systematic review and meta-analysis. J Int Assoc Provid AIDS Care 2015;14(6):560–70.

75. Odone A, Amadasi S, White RG, et al. The impact of antiretroviral therapy on mortality in HIV positive people during tuberculosis treatment: a systematic review and meta-analysis. PLoS One 2014;9(11):e112017.

76. Sonderup MW, Wainwright H, Spearman CW. Hepatic tuberculosis-associated immune reconstitution inflammatory syndrome compared to antiretroviral naive HIV positive patients with hepatic tuberculosis. Hepatology 2009;50(Suppl. 4): 1246A.

77. Wong EB, Omar T, Setlhako GJ, et al. Causes of death on antiretroviral therapy: a post-mortem study from South Africa. PLoS One 2012;7(10):e47542.

78. Rosenthal E, Salmon-Ceron D, Lewden C, et al. Liver-related deaths in HIV-infected patients between 1995 and 2005 in the French GERMIVIC Joint Study Group Network (Mortavic 2005 study in collaboration with the Mortalite 2005 survey, ANRS EN19). HIV Med 2009;10(5):282–9.

79. Weber R, Sabin CA, Friis-Moller N, et al. Liver-related deaths in persons infected with the human immunodeficiency virus: the D:A:D study. Arch Intern Med 2006; 166(15):1632–41.
80. Smith C, Sabin CA, Lundgren JD, et al. Factors associated with specific causes of death amongst HIV-positive individuals in the D:A:D Study. AIDS 2010;24(10): 1537–48.

Autoimmune Hepatitis Overlap Syndromes and Liver Pathology

Albert J. Czaja, MD[a],*, Herschel A. Carpenter, MD[b]

KEYWORDS

- Autoimmune hepatitis • Overlap • Variants • Cholestatic • Histologic findings

KEY POINTS

- Autoimmune hepatitis may have cholestatic laboratory and histologic features that resemble primary biliary cholangitis, primary sclerosing cholangitis, or a cholestatic syndrome.
- Histologic findings may include destructive and nondestructive cholangitis, portal edema, portal fibrosis, periductal fibrosis, and ductopenia.
- Serum alkaline phosphatase levels greater than 2-fold the upper limit of normal range, concurrent inflammatory bowel disease, antimitochondrial antibodies, and recalcitrance to corticosteroid therapy are key clinical manifestations.
- Evaluation should include histologic assessment and endoscopic retrograde or MR cholangiography.
- Treatment recommendations emphasize mainly combination therapy with prednisone or prednisolone, azathioprine, and ursodeoxycholic acid, and outcomes vary depending on the predominant disease component.

INTRODUCTION

Autoimmune hepatitis (AIH) is a chronic inflammatory liver disease that is characterized by the presence of autoantibodies, hypergammaglobulinemia (especially increased serum levels of immunoglobulin G), and histologic findings of interface hepatitis (**Fig. 1**).[1–3] Lymphocytic aggregates in the portal tracts typically accompany interface hepatitis and, in 66% of patients, portal plasma cells are prominent (**Fig. 2**).[4] None of the serologic, laboratory, or histologic features of AIH is disease specific, and the diagnosis requires the presence of a constellation of compatible findings

Disclosure Statement: The authors have nothing to disclose.
[a] Division of Gastroenterology and Hepatology, Mayo Clinic College of Medicine, 200 First Street Southwest, Rochester, MN 55905, USA; [b] Department of Laboratory Medicine and Pathology, Mayo Clinic College of Medicine, 200 First Street Southwest, Rochester, MN 55905, USA
* Corresponding author:
E-mail address: czaja.albert@mayo.edu

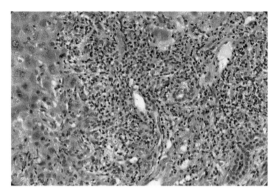

Fig. 1. Interface hepatitis associated with classical autoimmune hepatitis. Lymphoplasma-cytic infiltrates extend from the portal tract into the acinar tissue with disruption of the limiting plate. Original magnification ×200. Hematoxylin and eosin stain.

and the exclusion of virus-related, drug-induced, alcoholic, metabolic, and hereditary liver diseases.[3,5]

The diagnostic criteria for AIH have been codified by the International Autoimmune Hepatitis Group,[6] and a revised comprehensive scoring system and a simplified diagnostic scoring system have been promulgated to aid in the diagnosis of difficult cases.[6–8] All diagnostic algorithms have emphasized the inflammatory components of AIH and the absence of prominent cholestatic manifestations.[9,10] The presence of cholestatic features in a patient with otherwise classical AIH constitutes a phenotype that must be categorized separately and managed individually.[11–14] The variable response of such patients to conventional immunosuppressive therapy is the most compelling reason for their early recognition.[11,13,14]

Three major cholestatic phenotypes of AIH have been described, and they constitute the overlap syndromes (**Table 1**).[13,14]

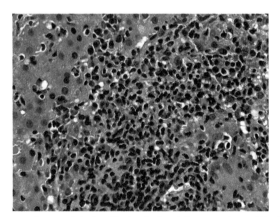

Fig. 2. Portal plasma cells associated with classical autoimmune hepatitis. Plasma cells characterized by cytoplasmic halo around the nucleus infiltrate the hepatic parenchyma. Original magnification ×400. Hematoxylin and eosin stain. (*From* Czaja AJ, Carpenter HA. Optimizing diagnosis from the medical liver biopsy. Clin Gastroenterol Hepatol 2007;5(8):899; with permission.)

Table 1
Diagnostic features of overlap syndromes of autoimmune hepatitis

Overlap Syndrome	Laboratory Features	Histologic Findings
AIH and PBC	ANA or SMA[11,17] Hypergammaglobulinemia[17] Serum IgG level increased[17] Marked serum AST/ALT abnormalities[17] AP or GGT level > ULN[11,24] AMA present[15,24]	Interface hepatitis[1,11] Lymphocytic portal infiltrate[1] Portal plasma cells[4] Destructive cholangitis[1,11,15,16]

AIH and PBC (Paris criteria)	AIH features (2 of 3)[15,36]
	    Serum ALT level ≥5-fold ULN
	    Serum IgG level ≥2-fold ULN or SMA present
	    Interface hepatitis
	PBC features (2 of 3)[15,36]
	    Serum AP level ≥2-fold ULN or GGT level ≥5-fold ULN
	    AMA present
	    Florid duct lesions
		Interface hepatitis (moderate to severe)[12,36]
		Destructive cholangitis[15,36]

AIH and PSC	ANA or SMA[11,32] Hypergammaglobulinemia[17] Serum IgG level increased[17] Marked serum AST/ALT abnormalities[17] Focal biliary strictures and dilations by ERC or MRC[20,32,43,44]	Lymphocytic portal infiltrate[19] Ductular proliferation[31] Periductular fibrosis[19,31,53] Portal edema[1,53] Cholate stasis[1,53] Fibrous obliterative cholangitis (rare)[19] Ductopenia[31,53] Increased stainable hepatic copper[53]
AIH and undefined cholestatic syndrome (possible AMA-negative PBC or small duct PSC)	ANA or SMA[11,32] Hypergammaglobulinemia[17] Serum IgG level increased[17] Marked serum AST/ALT abnormalities[17] AMA absent[11,13,14,21] ERC or MRC normal[11,14,17]	Interface hepatitis plus at least[1,14,21] Destructive cholangitis Periductular fibrosis Ductopenia Portal edema

Abbreviations: AIH, autoimmune hepatitis; ALT, alanine aminotransferase; AMA, antimitochondrial antibodies; ANA, antinuclear antibodies; AP, alkaline phosphatase; AST, aspartate aminotransferase; ERC, endoscopic retrograde cholangiography; GGT, gamma glutamyl transferase; IgG, immunoglobulin G; MRC, MR cholangiography; PBC, primary biliary cholangitis; PSC, primary sclerosing cholangitis; SMA, smooth muscle antibodies; ULN, upper limit of the normal range.

- Patients with AIH may have antimitochondrial antibodies (AMA) and histologic features of bile duct injury or loss.[1,11,15–17] Their resemblance to patients with primary biliary cholangitis (PBC) has justified the designation of an overlap syndrome between AIH and PBC.[13,14,17,18]
- Patients with AIH may have cholestatic laboratory changes, absence of AMA, histologic features of bile duct injury or loss, and cholangiographic changes that are suggestive of primary sclerosing cholangitis (PSC).[1,13,14,16,19,20] These patients have been designated as having an overlap syndrome between AIH and PSC, and they may or may not have concurrent inflammatory bowel disease.[11,12,17]

- Patients with AIH may also have a cholestatic laboratory profile, absent AMA, histologic features of bile duct injury or loss, and normal cholangiography.[1,13,14,21] These patients have AIH and a cholestatic syndrome. This heterogeneous category may include patients with AMA-negative PBC or small duct PSC.[13,22,23]

The goals of this review are to indicate the features in patients with otherwise classical AIH that suggest an overlap syndrome, describe the clinical and histologic findings that support the designation of an overlap syndrome, and indicate how the cholestatic features can affect outcome and management strategies.

CLINICAL INDICATIONS OF AN OVERLAP SYNDROME

The main clinical findings that raise suspicion of an overlap syndrome in a patient with AIH are marked elevation of the serum alkaline phosphatase or γ-glutamyl transferase (GGT) level, the presence of AMA, histologic findings of bile duct injury or loss, concurrent inflammatory bowel disease, and recalcitrance to conventional corticosteroid therapy (**Table 2**).[13,14]

- The serum alkaline phosphatase level is increased more than 2-fold the upper limit of the normal (ULN) range in only 21% of patients with classical AIH, and no patients with AIH have serum alkaline phosphatase levels more than 4-fold ULN.[24] A serum alkaline phosphatase level increased 2-fold ULN or greater in an adult with AIH should raise the suspicion of an overlap syndrome.[24]
- The serum GGT level can also reflect an atypical cholestatic component. The serum GGT level is commonly increased in classical AIH, but its failure to improve during conventional corticosteroid treatment suggests a strong cholestatic element.[25] A sustained or increasing serum GGT level above the ULN during immunosuppressive therapy should generate suspicion of an overlap syndrome.[26]
- AMA occurs in 6% to 18% of patients with AIH.[27–29] These AMA-positive patients with otherwise classical features of AIH should be evaluated as a possible overlap syndrome with PBC by expert histologic assessment.[1,19] These patients warrant the designation of an overlap syndrome with PBC only if they have histologic findings of bile duct destruction or loss (**Fig. 3**).[1,30]
- Histologic findings of destructive cholangitis (florid duct lesion; see **Fig. 3**), bile duct loss (**Fig. 4**), or fibrous obliterative cholangitis (**Fig. 5**) in a patient with AIH compels further assessment regardless of the clinical phenotype.[1,4,16,19,31] The assessment should include serum GGT level, AMA determination, and endoscopic cholangiopathy (ERC) or MR cholangiopathy (MRC). These patients may have an overlap syndrome with PBC, PSC, AMA-negative PBC, or small duct PSC.[13,14]
- Forty-one percent of patients with AIH and concurrent inflammatory bowel disease have focal biliary strictures and dilations by cholangiography.[32] Cholestatic laboratory changes or histologic findings of bile duct injury or loss may be absent, especially in children,[33] and the presence of inflammatory bowel disease alone is sufficient indication for performing ERC or MRC.[13,14,32] Patients with an abnormal cholangiogram have an overlap syndrome between AIH and PSC, and they frequently have a poor response to conventional corticosteroid therapy.[11,34,35] Liver biopsy assessment may not be necessary to diagnose this overlap syndrome if the ERC or MRC findings are typical of PSC.[12,36,37]
- The laboratory indices of liver inflammation typically improve within 2 weeks of corticosteroid therapy,[38] and they normalize in 39% to 90% of patients within 3 to 6 months.[39–41] Laboratory tests worsen in 7% of patients during therapy (treatment failure)[42] or improve but not to normal levels in 14% (incomplete

Table 2
Clues to an overlap syndrome

Clinical Clue	Features	Implication
Serum AP >2-fold ULN at presentation	Present in only 21% with AIH[24] Rarely ≥4-fold ULN in AIH[24]	Unusual cholestatic component in AIH[17,24] Justifies histologic examination and AMA[24] Consider ERC or MRC[13,14,17,24]
Serum GGT > ULN unimproved or worse during therapy	Common in AIH at entry[25] Usually improves during therapy[26]	Consider cholestatic component if unchanged or worse during therapy[25,26] Justifies histologic examination and AMA[13] ERC or MRC if unchanged or worse[13,26]
AMA at presentation or later	Occurs in 6%–18% of AIH[11,24,27,46]	Requires histologic examination[1,11] Bile duct injury suggests PBC overlap[1,11] Could be serologic finding only[28,46]
Histologic findings of bile duct injury or loss	Liver tissue examination shows[1,19,31,53] Destructive cholangitis Ductopenia Periductal fibrosis Fibrous obliterative cholangitis	Justifies serologic test for AMA[1,13,24] ERC or MRC if AMA negative[13,14,21]
Concurrent inflammatory bowel disease	Abnormal ERC in 41%[32] May have no cholestatic findings[33]	Perform ERC or MRC in all patients[13,14,32] Focal strictures and dilations confirm PSC[20] Liver biopsy if normal cholangiography[36,37]
Recalcitrance to corticosteroid therapy (treatment failure or incomplete response)	Treatment failure in 7% of AIH[42] Incomplete response in 14%[40]	Reevaluate original diagnosis[42] Perform liver biopsy, AMA, and MRC[42]

Abbreviations: AIH, autoimmune hepatitis; AMA, antimitochondrial antibodies; AP, alkaline phosphatase; ERC, endoscopic retrograde cholangiography; GGT, gamma glutamyl transferase; MRC, MR cholangiography; PBC, primary biliary cholangitis; PSC, primary sclerosing cholangitis; ULN, upper limit of the normal range.

response).[40] Patients with a suboptimal response to standard therapy for AIH (treatment failure or incomplete response) should have their original diagnosis reevaluated for possible alternative diagnoses or concurrent factors (drug-induced liver disease, fatty liver disease, viral infection, or overlap syndrome).[42]

CAVEATS REGARDING THE DIAGNOSIS OF OVERLAP SYNDROMES

The diagnosis of an overlap syndrome can be confounded by an abnormal cholangiogram reflective of advanced hepatic fibrosis, the presence of AMA without other cholestatic features, histologic findings of nondestructive cholangitis, and the application of scoring systems inappropriate for the diagnosis (**Table 3**).

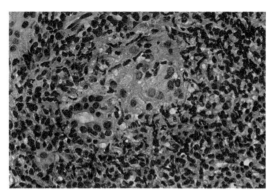

Fig. 3. Destructive cholangitis. Lymphocytes and histiocytes surround, infiltrate, and damage an interlobular bile duct. The presence of destructive cholangitis in a patient with otherwise classical features of autoimmune hepatitis suggests an overlap syndrome between autoimmune hepatitis and primary biliary cholangitis. Original magnification ×400; hematoxylin and eosin stain.

- Cholangiographic changes of PSC occur in less than 2% of adults with classical AIH, and ERC or MRC is not warranted in these patients unless they have concurrent inflammatory bowel disease or recalcitrance to conventional corticosteroid therapy.[43] Hepatic fibrosis may distort the intrahepatic biliary tree and suggest an overlap syndrome with PSC, and it may account for an erroneous perception of bile duct injury.[43] An abnormal MRC has been reported in 10% of adults with AIH,[44] but the frequency of bile duct changes in AIH by MRC has been similar to that in nonautoimmune liver diseases and associated mainly with advanced hepatic fibrosis.[43] The role of cholangiography may be greater in

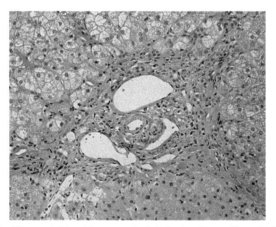

Fig. 4. Ductopenia. The portal tract has an arteriole but not an adjacent bile duct. The presence of ductopenia in a patient with otherwise classical features of autoimmune hepatitis suggests an overlap syndrome between autoimmune hepatitis and primary biliary cholangitis or primary sclerosing cholangitis. Original magnification ×400; hematoxylin and eosin stain. (*From* Czaja AJ, Carpenter HA. Optimizing diagnosis from the medical liver biopsy. Clin Gastroenterol Hepatol 2007;5(8):904; with permission.)

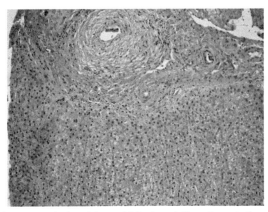

Fig. 5. Fibrous obliterative cholangitis. A thick rim of fibrosis encircles an obliterated bile duct. Periductal fibrosis of any extent in a patient with otherwise classical features of autoimmune hepatitis suggests an overlap syndrome between autoimmune hepatitis and primary sclerosing cholangitis. Original magnification ×200; hematoxylin and eosin stain. (*From* Czaja AJ, Carpenter HA. Optimizing diagnosis from the medical liver biopsy. Clin Gastroenterol Hepatol 2007;5(8):904; with permission.)

children with AIH because 50% of these patients have an autoimmune sclerosing cholangitis that can result in progressive bile duct injury and shortened transplant-free survival.[33,45]

- The presence of AMA in patients with AIH is insufficient for diagnosing an overlap syndrome with PBC. AMA may appear during the course of AIH or disappear during therapy without manifesting other features of PBC.[27] These patients lack a cholestatic clinical phenotype. Their histologic findings may be typical of AIH without features of PBC[28] or disclose focal cholangitis as frequently as AMA-negative patients (100% vs 85%).[46] The AMA in these patients may persist for 12 to 27 years without progression to classical PBC,[27,28] and these patients commonly respond to conventional corticosteroid therapy.[11,27,28]

- Histologic findings of nondestructive lymphocytic cholangitis are present in 9% of patients with classical AIH,[19] and the presence of this histologic finding does not constitute an overlap syndrome. Lymphocytes may aggregate around and infiltrate interlobular or septal bile ducts without destroying them **(Fig. 6)**.[19] Lymphocytic cholangitis occurs with similar frequencies in PBC (9%), PSC (6%), and AIH (9%), and this nondestructive inflammatory response does not designate an overlap syndrome.[19]

- Diagnostic scoring systems have not been developed for the overlap syndromes, and the revised comprehensive and simplified scoring systems promulgated by the International Autoimmune Hepatitis Group are not discriminative diagnostic indices that can be used for this purpose.[12] These scoring systems have not been validated prospectively for the diagnosis of AIH,[47] and they lack diagnostic sensitivity for designating an overlap syndrome.[48] The revised comprehensive scoring system supports the presence of AIH in only 54% of patients diagnosed with an overlap syndrome by clinical judgment, and the simplified scoring system accords with clinical judgment in only 62%.[48] Liver tissue examination has performed better than the scoring systems in supporting the designation of an overlap syndrome, and clinical judgment remains the gold standard for the diagnosis.[13,14,48,49]

Table 3
Caveats regarding diagnosis of overlap syndromes

Caveat	Features	Implications
ERC or MRC findings falsely suggest PSC	Hepatic fibrosis distorts biliary tree[43] No focal biliary strictures and dilations[43]	PSC wrongly diagnosed[43,44] MRC abnormal in 10% AIH[44] PSC in only 1.7% AIH[43]

AMA without cholestatic phenotype or progressive bile duct injury or loss	AMA in 6%–18% with AIH[24,27,28,46]
	AMA can persist, appear, or disappear[27]
	Persistent AMA for 12–27 y[28,46]
	Histologic findings
	  Typical AIH not PBC[28]
	  Focal cholangitis as frequently in AMA[+] and AMA[-] AIH[27,46]
	  Does not progress to typical PBC[28,46]
		AMA without cholestatic phenotype or bile duct injury insufficient for overlap[27,28]
		AMA alone does not alter diagnosis or treatment of AIH[27]
		Responds to steroid therapy[11,27]

Lymphocytic nondestructive cholangitis insufficient for overlap diagnosis	Dense lymphocytic aggregation around interlobular and septal bile ducts[19] Unassociated with decreased or damaged bile ducts[19]	Insufficient for overlap[19] Similar frequencies in classical PBC, PSC, and AIH[19]
Misuse of diagnostic scoring systems of IAIHG	Diagnostic scoring systems of IAIHG not discriminative indices[12] Lack prospective validation for AIH[47] Not designed for overlap detection[6,7,12] Low sensitivity for AIH in overlaps[48]	Diagnostic scoring systems of IAIHG should not be used for overlap diagnosis[12,48] Histologic examination is a major independent diagnostic factor[48,49] Clinical judgment is diagnostic gold standard[13,14,48,49]

Abbreviations: AIH, autoimmune hepatitis; AMA, antimitochondrial antibodies; ERC, endoscopic retrograde cholangiography; IAIHG, International Autoimmune Hepatitis Group; MRC, MR cholangiography; PBC, primary biliary cholangitis; PSC, primary sclerosing cholangitis.

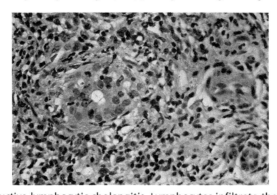

Fig. 6. Nondestructive lymphocytic cholangitis. Lymphocytes infiltrate the bile duct epithelium without destroying it. The finding lacks diagnostic specificity, and the finding by itself does not constitute an overlap syndrome. Original magnification ×400; hematoxylin and eosin stain.

DIAGNOSIS OF THE AUTOIMMUNE HEPATITIS–PRIMARY BILIARY CHOLANGITIS OVERLAP SYNDROME

The Paris criteria for the diagnosis of the AIH-PBC overlap syndrome[15] has been endorsed by the European Association for the Study of the Liver (EASL) with the stipulation that all patients must have interface hepatitis (see **Table 1**).[12,36] They must also have a serum alanine aminotransferase level of 5-fold the ULN or greater, serum immunoglobulin G level of 2-fold the ULN or greater, or the presence of smooth muscle antibodies. The features of AIH must be accompanied by 2 of 3 features of PBC, including a serum alkaline phosphatase level of 2-fold the ULN or greater, or a GGT level of 5-fold the ULN or greater, AMA, or florid duct lesions on histologic examination (see **Fig. 3**).[12,36]

The performance parameters of the Paris criteria have been excellent when compared with clinical judgment (sensitivity, 92%; specificity, 97%),[50] but all patients with the overlap syndrome may not be detected by the Paris criteria.[51] Patients may have serum alkaline phosphatase levels of less than 2-fold the ULN and isolated or transient features of mild bile duct injury.[11] Patients outside the Paris criteria may respond better to conventional corticosteroid therapy than those satisfying the Paris criteria,[11,15] and this outcome justifies efforts to expand the diagnostic criteria to include these corticosteroid-responsive individuals.[51] The frequency of the overlap syndrome between AIH and PBC has been 1% among patients with PBC who have been diagnosed by the Paris criteria,[51] 7% among patients with AIH who have been diagnosed mainly by clinical judgment,[11] and 14% in a retrospective experience involving 5 centers spanning 21 years.[18] Ethnicity may influence the frequency of occurrence as Hispanic patients more commonly have an overlap syndrome of AIH and PBC than non-Hispanics (31% vs 13%).[52]

DIAGNOSIS OF THE AUTOIMMUNE HEPATITIS–PRIMARY SCLEROSING CHOLANGITIS OVERLAP SYNDROME

Patients with AIH who have focal strictures and dilations of the biliary tree by ERC or MRC have an overlap syndrome with PSC (see **Table 1**). The frequency of occurrence varies with the indications for performing cholangiography. Forty-one percent of patients with AIH and concurrent inflammatory bowel disease have cholangiographic changes of PSC,[32] 50% of children with AIH have findings by ERC that indicate autoimmune sclerosing cholangitis,[33] and 1.7% to 10.0% of adults with classical AIH have biliary changes by MRC (albeit associated mainly with advanced hepatic fibrosis).[43,44] The histologic findings may disclose portal edema or fibrosis, ductopenia (see **Fig. 4**), ductal tortuosity, ductular proliferation, cholate stasis, increased stainable hepatic copper, periductal fibrosis, or rarely, fibrous obliterative cholangitis (see **Fig. 5**).[1,16,19,31,53]

DIAGNOSIS OF THE AUTOIMMUNE HEPATITIS–CHOLESTATIC OVERLAP SYNDROME

Patients with AIH who have cholestatic features that cannot be categorized as PBC or PSC have an overlapping cholestatic syndrome that may represent AMA-negative PBC[23,54] or small duct PSC (see **Table 1**).[22] These patients may have been previously classified as having autoimmune cholangitis.[21,55–57] Serum alkaline phosphatase levels are typically less than 2-fold the ULN, AMA are absent, ERC or MRC is normal, and destructive cholangitis reminiscent of PBC (see **Fig. 3**) or portal fibrosis, portal edema, or ductopenia reminiscent of PSC may be present (see **Fig. 4**).[1,11,14,21] The frequency of this overlap syndrome in a large cohort of patients with AIH is 11%.[11]

Enzyme immunoassays that are specific for PBC, including antibodies to gp210, sp100, or individual mitochondrial antigens, have been demonstrated in 35% of AMA-negative patients with cholestatic phenotypes, and they can support the diagnosis of AMA-negative PBC in some patients within this heterogeneous subgroup.[58,59]

MANAGEMENT OF THE OVERLAP SYNDROMES

The management of the overlap syndromes has not been established by controlled clinical trial.[12] Management has been empiric, and recommendations have included treatment with corticosteroids,[11,13,14] ursodeoxycholic acid (UDCA; 13–15 mg/kg per day),[60] and corticosteroids in combination with UDCA (**Table 4**).[12,36,37] Therapies should be individualized and guided by the severity of the cholestatic findings at presentation (serum alkaline phosphatase and GGT levels, histologic findings of bile duct injury or loss, and cholangiographic findings) and by the response to treatment.[13,14]

- Patients with AIH and overlapping features of PBC who satisfy the Paris criteria have equivalent manifestations of AIH and PBC, and treatment with prednisone or prednisolone (30 mg/d tapered over 4 weeks to 10 mg/d), azathioprine (50 mg/d), and UDCA (13–15 mg/kg per day) has been superior to corticosteroids alone or UDCA alone in a limited clinical experience.[15] Other clinical experiences have supported the responsiveness of this overlap syndrome to combination therapy,[18,61] and this regimen has been endorsed by EASL.[12,36] A metaanalysis of 8 clinical trials found that combination therapy was superior to UDCA alone in improving liver tests.[62] Frequencies of death, need for liver transplantation, and other adverse events were similar in patients receiving combination therapy or UDCA alone by this same metaanalysis.[62] The combination regimen of UDCA with budesonide has not been compared with the regimen using UDCA in combination with prednisone or prednisolone.
- Patients with AIH and overlapping features of PBC who are outside the Paris criteria have predominately AIH with background features of PBC.[11] These patients can respond as well to conventional therapy with prednisone or prednisolone (30 mg/d tapered over 4 weeks to 10 mg/d) in combination with azathioprine (50 mg/d) as patients with classical AIH, and this regimen can be instituted and later modified according to response.[11,13,14,51]
- Patients with predominately PBC and features of AIH that approximate the Paris criteria may improve laboratory tests (median percentages) and histologic findings of lobular inflammation (3 of 9 patients) on UDCA alone (13–15 mg/kg per day), but the experience has been small (12 patients).[60] The combination of corticosteroids, azathioprine, and UDCA (13–15 mg/kg per day) has been preferred, especially in patients with moderate to severe interface hepatitis.[61]
- Therapy with cyclosporine (5–6 mg/kg per day), tacrolimus (4–8 mg/d), or mycophenolate mofetil (2 g/d) has been used empirically as a salvage or second-line therapy for 13 patients with the overlap syndrome of AIH and PBC who were nonresponders to the standard regimens.[18,61] Three of 5 patients receiving cyclosporine improved, 3 of 4 patients receiving tacrolimus responded in variable degrees, and 3 of 3 patients receiving mycophenolate mofetil had complete or partial responses.[61] In another retrospective study, 2 patients receiving cyclosporine and UDCA improved.[18]
- Patients with AIH and overlapping features of PSC have a variable response to corticosteroids[11,35,63,64] and little or no response to UDCA.[64] Treatment with

Table 4
Treatment regimens and outcomes for overlap syndromes

Overlap Syndrome	Treatment Regimens	Outcomes
AIH-PBC overlap (satisfying Paris criteria)	Combination therapy[12,15,18,36,61,66]: Prednisone or prednisolone (30 mg/d tapered to 10 mg/d) Azathioprine (50 mg/d) UDCA (13–15 mg/kg per day) Alternative empiric therapies[76]: Budesonide (9 mg/d), azathioprine (50 mg/d), UDCA (13–15 mg/kg per day)[76] Cyclosporine (3 mg/kg per day)[75] Mycophenolate mofetil (1–3 g/d)[74] UDCA only (13–15 mg/kg per day)[60]	Combination therapy: Improves laboratory tests and prevents fibrosis[15,66] 5-y transplant-free survival, 100%[50] 10-y survival, 92%[13,50] Budesonide and UDCA combination: 3 of 4 patients failed[76] Cyclosporine: 3 patients improved[18,75] Mycophenolate mofetil improvement[74]: 57% of azathioprine nonresponsive 63% of azathioprine intolerant UDCA only: 12 patients[60] Laboratory better (median percent) Histologic improvement, 3 of 9 patients
AIH-PBC overlap (AP<2-fold ULN and outside Paris criteria)	Conventional therapy for AIH[11,13,14,51]: Prednisone or prednisolone (30 mg/d tapered to 10 mg/d) Azathioprine (50 mg/d)	Similar to classical AIH[11,13,51,67,68]: Improvement, 81% (vs 86%) Treatment failure, 14% (vs 9%)
AIH-PSC overlap	Combination triple therapy[12,36,37,65]: Prednisone or prednisolone (0.5 mg/kg per day tapered to 10–15 mg) Azathioprine (50–75 mg/d) UDCA (13–15 mg/d) AVOID high dose UDCA[70] Individualized standard therapy for AIH[63]: Prednisolone, 20–80 mg/d, reduced to 7.5–10 mg/d maintenance Azathioprine, 75–150 mg/d	Combination triple therapy[65]: Less transplantation, malignancy, and mortality vs classical PSC Individualized standard therapy for AIH[63]: Laboratory improvement, 5 of 5 patients Alternative therapies Cyclosporine: salvaged 1 patient[90] Mycophenolate mofetil: ineffective in 6 of 8 children with ASC[73]
AIH-undefined cholestatic overlap (possible AMA-negative PBC or small duct PSC)	Individualized by cholestatic features and response to chosen regimen[13,14] Corticosteroids, UDCA, and combination triple therapy are considerations[13,14]	Corticosteroids[11,21] Rare complete response UDCA alone[21] Improvement, 12% Corticosteroids, azathioprine, UDCA[13,14] Poorly documented

Abbreviations: AIH, autoimmune hepatitis; AMA, antimitochondrial antibodies; AP, alkaline phosphatase; ASC, autoimmune sclerosing cholangitis; PBC, primary biliary cholangitis; PSC, primary sclerosing cholangitis; UDCA, ursodeoxycholic acid; ULN, upper limit of normal range.

prednisone or prednisolone (0.5 mg/kg per day tapered to 10–15 mg/d), azathioprine (50–75 mg/d), and UDCA (13–15 mg/d) has improved the outcomes in these patients (frequency of transplantation, malignancy, and death) compared with adults with classical PSC,[65] and immunosuppressive therapy in combination with UDCA has been recommended by EASL[36] and the American Association for the Study of the Liver, despite the absence of strong clinical evidence.[12,37]

- Highly individualized therapy with corticosteroids (prednisolone, 20–80 mg/d, tapered to 7.5–10 mg/d maintenance) and azathioprine (75–150 mg/d) in combination or as a single maintenance regimen have improved laboratory tests and maintained survival in 5 patients with AIH and PSC during a follow-up interval ranging from 2 to 21 years (mean, 9.8).[63] This empiric management regimen has been superseded by the recommendations of EASL and the American Association for the Study of the Liver.[12,36,37]

- Patients with AIH and a cholestatic phenotype that may reflect AMA-negative PBC or small duct PSC respond poorly to the administration of corticosteroids or UDCA alone. Corticosteroid therapy rarely induces laboratory and histologic resolution,[11] and UDCA alone improves manifestations in only 12%.[21] The liver societies have not promulgated management recommendations for this population, and therapy typically is based on strategies dictated by the predominant manifestations at presentation (inflammatory vs cholestatic) and the response to the initial schedule. Combination therapy with prednisone or prednisolone (30 mg/d tapered over 4 weeks to 10 mg/d), azathioprine (50 mg/d), and UDCA (13–15 mg/kg per day) should be considered in patients recalcitrant to single drug therapy (corticosteroids or UDCA) or with prominent inflammatory and cholestatic findings at presentation.

TREATMENT OUTCOMES

Combination therapy with prednisone or prednisolone, azathioprine and UDCA has significantly improved serum alkaline phosphatase ($P<.05$), GGT ($P = .02$), and alanine aminotransferase ($P = .02$) levels in patients satisfying Paris criteria for the overlap syndrome of AIH and PBC (see **Table 4**).[15,66] Hepatic fibrosis has not progressed during 3 years of combination therapy,[66] the 5-year transplant-free survival has been 100%,[50] and the 10-year survival has been 92%.[13,50] Laboratory resolution (67 vs 27%) has also occurred more commonly than in patients treated with corticosteroids or UDCA alone, albeit the experience has been small.[15] Patients with AIH and overlapping background features of PBC who are outside the Paris criteria commonly respond to conventional corticosteroid therapy for classical AIH. These patients experience clinical, laboratory, and histologic improvement as commonly as patients with classical AIH (81 vs 86%) and fail treatment as infrequently (14 vs 9%).[11,13,51,67,68]

Treatment outcomes in patients with the overlap syndrome of AIH and PSC have been variable, possibly because of the severity or advanced nature of the PSC at the time of discovery (see **Table 4**). Whereas conventional corticosteroid therapy for AIH has been uniformly effective in some patients with this diagnosis,[63] most experiences indicate a poor response to this management strategy.[11,35] Laboratory and histologic improvement to normal or near-normal occurs less frequently than in classical AIH (22 vs 64%), disease progression (treatment failure) is more common (33 vs 10%), and death from liver failure or requirement for liver transplantation is more often (33 vs 8%).[11,13,14] Survival has been poorer in these patients than in those with the overlap syndrome of AIH and PBC,[35] and they have justified the alternative treatment strategy of immunosuppressive therapy in combination with UDCA.[12,36,37] Laboratory features can improve on combination therapy, and survival has been maintained during a mean observation period of 93 months.[13,65,69] Hepatic fibrosis, however, has progressed and cirrhosis has developed in 75% within 12 years.[13,69]

Treatment outcomes of patients with AIH and an undefined cholestatic syndrome have also been variable and unsatisfactory (see **Table 4**).[11,14] Conventional corticosteroid therapy has failed to normalize laboratory tests in 88% to 100% of patients, disease progression has occurred in 17%, and liver transplantation has been required in 33%.[11,14] UDCA administered alone or in combination with corticosteroids has had similarly poor results. The administration of UDCA alone has induced laboratory and histologic improvement in only 12%.[14,21] The heterogeneity of the cholestatic syndromes that comprise this overlap population may contribute to these outcomes, and future improvements in diagnosis may reclassify these patients into more treatable subpopulations.

CAVEATS REGARDING TREATMENT

Poor treatment results are the principal motivations for modifying treatment regimens, but unestablished salvage therapies introduce another level of empiricism to the original empiric strategy. High doses of UDCA (28–30 mg/kg per day) may have untoward consequences.[70–72] Mycophenolate mofetil has been ineffective in children with AIH and autoimmune sclerosing cholangitis,[73] and the drug has been beneficial in some adults with AIH and PBC.[74] Calcineurin inhibitors have been useful in isolated individuals with AIH and PBC,[75] whereas budesonide in combination with UDCA has been ineffective or toxic in patients with hepatic fibrosis, especially in individuals with AIH and PBC.[76] Importantly, the salvage therapies require experience in their safe administration, and they each may introduce their own drug-related complications.

- The administration of high doses of UDCA (28–30 mg/kg per day) to patients with PSC has increased the frequency of adverse clinical events, including mortality and the need for liver transplantation.[70] High levels of lithocholic acid, the hepatotoxic metabolite of UDCA, may have contributed to these consequences, and such treatment should be avoided in all management strategies.[13,71]
- Mycophenolate mofetil (1–3 g/d) is the next-generation purine antagonist that has been used as frontline[26,77] and salvage therapy for AIH.[78–81] Remission occurred in 57% of patients with AIH and PBC who did not respond to regimens with azathioprine, and it was achieved in 63% of patients who were intolerant of azathioprine.[74] In contrast, 6 of 8 children with AIH and autoimmune sclerosing cholangitis did not respond to therapy with mycophenolate mofetil.[73] Treatment with mycophenolate mofetil is contraindicated in patients who are pregnant or contemplating pregnancy because of it teratogenic effects on the migration of the fetal cranial neural crest.[82,83] Other side effects are similar to those of azathioprine, including cytopenia.[83]
- Budesonide (3 mg 3 times per daily) is a next-generation glucocorticoid, and its use in combination with azathioprine (50 mg/d) and UDCA (13–15 mg/kg per day) in 4 patients with features of AIH and PBC failed to improve laboratory indices in 3 patients, one of whom also had a severe allergic reaction.[76] Patients with advanced hepatic fibrosis or cirrhosis are at risk for budesonide-related complications,[84] and they may not respond to treatment with budesonide.[76,85,86]
- The calcineurin inhibitors have been used as frontline and salvage therapies for patients with classical AIH.[83,87–89] Three reports have indicated that patients with an overlap syndrome may also respond.[18,75,90] One patient

with AIH and PSC responded to therapy with cyclosporine,[12,90] 1 patient with AIH and PBC who was refractory to corticosteroid therapy improved with cyclosporine,[75] and 2 patients with AIH and PBC responded to cyclosporine in combination with UDCA.[18] These limited anecdotal experiences are insufficient to endorse the routine administration of calcineurin inhibitors as a salvage therapy, but they do support further evaluation of this possibility.

OVERVIEW

Patients with AIH may have cholestatic features that are outside the boundaries of the classical disease (AMA, increased serum alkaline phosphatase level ≥2-fold ULN, histologic changes of bile duct injury or loss, and focal biliary strictures and dilations by ERC or MRC).[11,14,91,92] These features may be reminiscent of patients with PBC, PSC, AMA-negative PBC, or small duct PSC, and they have been designated as overlap syndromes.[13,30] The true nature of these syndromes is unclear. They may represent inflammatory forms of classical PBC or PSC,[67] cholestatic forms of classical AIH,[13] or 2 concurrent diseases.[93]

AIH does not have disease-specific clinical, laboratory, and histologic features,[2] and the occurrence of these nonspecific inflammatory and immune-mediated features in patients with PBC or PSC is insufficient to declare the concurrence of 2 separate diseases or a new pathologic entity.[13] The rarity that 2 diseases such as PBC and PSC occur together[94–98] supports the concept that the overlap syndromes reflect the concurrence of nonspecific inflammatory and immune-mediated findings in a disease otherwise characterized by highly specific diagnostic features (AMA, florid duct lesions, ductopenia, or focal biliary strictures and dilations by ERC or MRC). In this context, the overlap syndromes may all be forms of PBC or PSC with varying degrees of inflammatory and immune-mediated manifestations that have clinical penetrance as AIH. Alternatively, the overlap syndromes could reflect 2 concurrent diseases, transitional stages in the emergence of a single classical disease, or a distinct phenotype with its own pathogenic mechanisms.[13,93]

The diagnosis is based mainly on the detection of clinical, laboratory, or histologic features that are discordant with classical AIH. The presence of the serum alkaline phosphatase level greater than 2-fold ULN, AMA, histologic changes of bile duct injury or loss, concurrent inflammatory bowel disease, and recalcitrance to corticosteroid therapy are key clues to the diagnosis.[13,14] Treatment is empiric and directed by the predominant manifestations of the disease (inflammatory vs cholestatic; AIH vs PBC or PSC).[12] Immunosuppressive therapy in combination with UDCA (13–15 mg/kg per day) has been recommended by the liver societies for most patients, but management strategies can be individualized.[12,13,36,37,99,100]

REFERENCES

1. Carpenter HA, Czaja AJ. The role of histologic evaluation in the diagnosis and management of autoimmune hepatitis and its variants. Clin Liver Dis 2002;6: 685–705.
2. Manns MP, Czaja AJ, Gorham JD, et al. Diagnosis and management of autoimmune hepatitis. Hepatology 2010;51:2193–213.
3. Czaja AJ. Diagnosis and management of autoimmune hepatitis. Clin Liver Dis 2015;19:57–79.
4. Czaja AJ, Carpenter HA. Sensitivity, specificity, and predictability of biopsy interpretations in chronic hepatitis. Gastroenterology 1993;105:1824–32.

5. Czaja AJ. Diagnosis and management of autoimmune hepatitis: current status and future directions. Gut Liver 2016;10:177–203.
6. Alvarez F, Berg PA, Bianchi FB, et al. International Autoimmune Hepatitis Group Report: review of criteria for diagnosis of autoimmune hepatitis. J Hepatol 1999; 31:929–38.
7. Hennes EM, Zeniya M, Czaja AJ, et al. Simplified criteria for the diagnosis of autoimmune hepatitis. Hepatology 2008;48:169–76.
8. Czaja AJ. Performance parameters of the diagnostic scoring systems for autoimmune hepatitis. Hepatology 2008;48:1540–8.
9. Czaja AJ, Carpenter HA. Validation of scoring system for diagnosis of autoimmune hepatitis. Dig Dis Sci 1996;41:305–14.
10. Boberg KM, Fausa O, Haaland T, et al. Features of autoimmune hepatitis in primary sclerosing cholangitis: an evaluation of 114 primary sclerosing cholangitis patients according to a scoring system for the diagnosis of autoimmune hepatitis. Hepatology 1996;23:1369–76.
11. Czaja AJ. Frequency and nature of the variant syndromes of autoimmune liver disease. Hepatology 1998;28:360–5.
12. Boberg KM, Chapman RW, Hirschfield GM, et al. Overlap syndromes: the International Autoimmune Hepatitis Group (IAIHG) position statement on a controversial issue. J Hepatol 2011;54:374–85.
13. Czaja AJ. The overlap syndromes of autoimmune hepatitis. Dig Dis Sci 2013;58: 326–43.
14. Czaja AJ. Cholestatic phenotypes of autoimmune hepatitis. Clin Gastroenterol Hepatol 2014;12:1430–8.
15. Chazouilleres O, Wendum D, Serfaty L, et al. Primary biliary cirrhosis-autoimmune hepatitis overlap syndrome: clinical features and response to therapy. Hepatology 1998;28:296–301.
16. Dienes HP, Erberich H, Dries V, et al. Autoimmune hepatitis and overlap syndromes. Clin Liver Dis 2002;6:349–62, vi.
17. Czaja AJ. Variant forms of autoimmune hepatitis. Curr Gastroenterol Rep 1999; 1:63–70.
18. Heurgue A, Vitry F, Diebold MD, et al. Overlap syndrome of primary biliary cirrhosis and autoimmune hepatitis: a retrospective study of 115 cases of autoimmune liver disease. Gastroenterol Clin Biol 2007;31:17–25.
19. Ludwig J, Czaja AJ, Dickson ER, et al. Manifestations of nonsuppurative cholangitis in chronic hepatobiliary diseases: morphologic spectrum, clinical correlations and terminology. Liver 1984;4:105–16.
20. Wiesner RH, LaRusso NF. Clinicopathologic features of the syndrome of primary sclerosing cholangitis. Gastroenterology 1980;79:200–6.
21. Czaja AJ, Carpenter HA, Santrach PJ, et al. Autoimmune cholangitis within the spectrum of autoimmune liver disease. Hepatology 2000;31:1231–8.
22. Angulo P, Maor-Kendler Y, Lindor KD. Small-duct primary sclerosing cholangitis: a long-term follow-up study. Hepatology 2002;35:1494–500.
23. Invernizzi P, Crosignani A, Battezzati PM, et al. Comparison of the clinical features and clinical course of antimitochondrial antibody-positive and -negative primary biliary cirrhosis. Hepatology 1997;25:1090–5.
24. Kenny RP, Czaja AJ, Ludwig J, et al. Frequency and significance of antimitochondrial antibodies in severe chronic active hepatitis. Dig Dis Sci 1986;31: 705–11.
25. Muratori P, Granito A, Quarneti C, et al. Autoimmune hepatitis in Italy: the Bologna experience. J Hepatol 2009;50:1210–8.

26. Zachou K, Gatselis N, Papadamou G, et al. Mycophenolate for the treatment of autoimmune hepatitis: prospective assessment of its efficacy and safety for induction and maintenance of remission in a large cohort of treatment-naive patients. J Hepatol 2011;55:636–46.

27. Montano-Loza AJ, Carpenter HA, Czaja AJ. Frequency, behavior, and prognostic implications of antimitochondrial antibodies in type 1 autoimmune hepatitis. J Clin Gastroenterol 2008;42:1047–53.

28. O'Brien C, Joshi S, Feld JJ, et al. Long-term follow-up of antimitochondrial antibody-positive autoimmune hepatitis. Hepatology 2008;48:550–6.

29. Czaja AJ. Performance parameters of the conventional serological markers for autoimmune hepatitis. Dig Dis Sci 2011;56:545–54.

30. Czaja AJ. Diagnosis and management of the overlap syndromes of autoimmune hepatitis. Can J Gastroenterol 2013;27:417–23.

31. Ludwig J, MacCarty RL, LaRusso NF, et al. Intrahepatic cholangiectases and large-duct obliteration in primary sclerosing cholangitis. Hepatology 1986;6: 560–8.

32. Perdigoto R, Carpenter HA, Czaja AJ. Frequency and significance of chronic ulcerative colitis in severe corticosteroid-treated autoimmune hepatitis. J Hepatol 1992;14:325–31.

33. Gregorio GV, Portmann B, Karani J, et al. Autoimmune hepatitis/sclerosing cholangitis overlap syndrome in childhood: a 16-year prospective study. Hepatology 2001;33:544–53.

34. Ben-Ari Z, Czaja AJ. Autoimmune hepatitis and its variant syndromes. Gut 2001; 49:589–94.

35. Al-Chalabi T, Portmann BC, Bernal W, et al. Autoimmune hepatitis overlap syndromes: an evaluation of treatment response, long-term outcome and survival. Aliment Pharmacol Ther 2008;28:209–20.

36. Beuers U, Boberg KM, Chapman RW, et al. EASL Clinical Practice Guidelines: management of cholestatic liver diseases. J Hepatol 2009;51:237–67.

37. Chapman R, Fevery J, Kalloo A, et al. Diagnosis and management of primary sclerosing cholangitis. Hepatology 2010;51:660–78.

38. Czaja AJ, Rakela J, Ludwig J. Features reflective of early prognosis in corticosteroid-treated severe autoimmune chronic active hepatitis. Gastroenterology 1988;95:448–53.

39. Kanzler S, Lohr H, Gerken G, et al. Long-term management and prognosis of autoimmune hepatitis (AIH): a single center experience. Z Gastroenterol 2001; 39:339–41, 344–8.

40. Czaja AJ. Rapidity of treatment response and outcome in type 1 autoimmune hepatitis. J Hepatol 2009;51:161–7.

41. Manns MP, Woynarowski M, Kreisel W, et al. Budesonide induces remission more effectively than prednisone in a controlled trial of patients with autoimmune hepatitis. Gastroenterology 2010;139:1198–206.

42. Montano-Loza AJ, Carpenter HA, Czaja AJ. Features associated with treatment failure in type 1 autoimmune hepatitis and predictive value of the model of end-stage liver disease. Hepatology 2007;46:1138–45.

43. Lewin M, Vilgrain V, Ozenne V, et al. Prevalence of sclerosing cholangitis in adults with autoimmune hepatitis: a prospective magnetic resonance imaging and histological study. Hepatology 2009;50:528–37.

44. Abdalian R, Dhar P, Jhaveri K, et al. Prevalence of sclerosing cholangitis in adults with autoimmune hepatitis: evaluating the role of routine magnetic resonance imaging. Hepatology 2008;47:949–57.

45. Mieli-Vergani G, Vergani D. Autoimmune liver diseases in children - What is different from adulthood? Best Pract Res Clin Gastroenterol 2011;25:783–95.
46. Nezu S, Tanaka A, Yasui H, et al. Presence of antimitochondrial autoantibodies in patients with autoimmune hepatitis. J Gastroenterol Hepatol 2006;21: 1448–54.
47. Yeoman AD, Westbrook RH, Al-Chalabi T, et al. Diagnostic value and utility of the simplified International Autoimmune Hepatitis Group (IAIHG) criteria in acute and chronic liver disease. Hepatology 2009;50:538–45.
48. Gatselis NK, Zachou K, Papamichalis P, et al. Comparison of simplified score with the revised original score for the diagnosis of autoimmune hepatitis: a new or a complementary diagnostic score? Dig Liver Dis 2010;42:807–12.
49. Papamichalis PA, Zachou K, Koukoulis GK, et al. The revised international auto-immune hepatitis score in chronic liver diseases including autoimmune hepatitis/overlap syndromes and autoimmune hepatitis with concurrent other liver disorders. J Autoimmune Dis 2007;4:3.
50. Kuiper EM, Zondervan PE, van Buuren HR. Paris criteria are effective in diagnosis of primary biliary cirrhosis and autoimmune hepatitis overlap syndrome. Clin Gastroenterol Hepatol 2010;8:530–4.
51. Bonder A, Retana A, Winston DM, et al. Prevalence of primary biliary cirrhosis-autoimmune hepatitis overlap syndrome. Clin Gastroenterol Hepatol 2011;9: 609–12.
52. Levy C, Naik J, Giordano C, et al. Hispanics with primary biliary cirrhosis are more likely to have features of autoimmune hepatitis and reduced response to ursodeoxycholic Acid than non-Hispanics. Clin Gastroenterol Hepatol 2014; 12:1398–405.
53. Ludwig J, Barham SS, LaRusso NF, et al. Morphologic features of chronic hepatitis associated with primary sclerosing cholangitis and chronic ulcerative colitis. Hepatology 1981;1:632–40.
54. Michieletti P, Wanless IR, Katz A, et al. Antimitochondrial antibody negative primary biliary cirrhosis: a distinct syndrome of autoimmune cholangitis. Gut 1994; 35:260–5.
55. Taylor SL, Dean PJ, Riely CA. Primary autoimmune cholangitis. An alternative to antimitochondrial antibody-negative primary biliary cirrhosis. Am J Surg Pathol 1994;18:91–9.
56. Goodman ZD, McNally PR, Davis DR, et al. Autoimmune cholangitis: a variant of primary biliary cirrhosis. Clinicopathologic and serologic correlations in 200 cases. Dig Dis Sci 1995;40:1232–42.
57. Sherlock S. Ludwig Symposium on biliary disorders. Autoimmune cholangitis: a unique entity? Mayo Clin Proc 1998;73:184–90.
58. Muratori P, Muratori L, Gershwin ME, et al. 'True' antimitochondrial antibody-negative primary biliary cirrhosis, low sensitivity of the routine assays, or both? Clin Exp Immunol 2004;135:154–8.
59. Milkiewicz P, Buwaneswaran H, Coltescu C, et al. Value of autoantibody analysis in the differential diagnosis of chronic cholestatic liver disease. Clin Gastroenterol Hepatol 2009;7:1355–60.
60. Joshi S, Cauch-Dudek K, Wanless IR, et al. Primary biliary cirrhosis with additional features of autoimmune hepatitis: response to therapy with ursodeoxycholic acid. Hepatology 2002;35:409–13.
61. Ozaslan E, Efe C, Heurgue-Berlot A, et al. Factors associated with response to therapy and outcome of patients with primary biliary cirrhosis with features of autoimmune hepatitis. Clin Gastroenterol Hepatol 2014;12:863–9.

62. Zhang H, Yang J, Zhu R, et al. Combination therapy of ursodeoxycholic acid and budesonide for PBC-AIH overlap syndrome: a meta-analysis. Drug Des Devel Ther 2015;9:567–74.

63. McNair AN, Moloney M, Portmann BC, et al. Autoimmune hepatitis overlapping with primary sclerosing cholangitis in five cases. Am J Gastroenterol 1998;93: 777–84.

64. Olsson R, Glaumann H, Almer S, et al. High prevalence of small duct primary sclerosing cholangitis among patients with overlapping autoimmune hepatitis and primary sclerosing cholangitis. Eur J Intern Med 2009;20:190–6.

65. Floreani A, Rizzotto ER, Ferrara F, et al. Clinical course and outcome of autoimmune hepatitis/primary sclerosing cholangitis overlap syndrome. Am J Gastroenterol 2005;100:1516–22.

66. Chazouilleres O, Wendum D, Serfaty L, et al. Long term outcome and response to therapy of primary biliary cirrhosis-autoimmune hepatitis overlap syndrome. J Hepatol 2006;44:400–6.

67. Lohse AW, zum Buschenfelde KH, Franz B, et al. Characterization of the overlap syndrome of primary biliary cirrhosis (PBC) and autoimmune hepatitis: evidence for it being a hepatitic form of PBC in genetically susceptible individuals. Hepatology 1999;29:1078–84.

68. Tanaka A, Harada K, Ebinuma H, et al. Primary biliary cirrhosis - autoimmune hepatitis overlap syndrome: a rationale for corticosteroids use based on a nation-wide retrospective study in Japan. Hepatol Res 2011;41:877–86.

69. Luth S, Kanzler S, Frenzel C, et al. Characteristics and long-term prognosis of the autoimmune hepatitis/primary sclerosing cholangitis overlap syndrome. J Clin Gastroenterol 2009;43:75–80.

70. Lindor KD, Kowdley KV, Luketic VA, et al. High-dose ursodeoxycholic acid for the treatment of primary sclerosing cholangitis. Hepatology 2009;50:808–14.

71. Sinakos E, Marschall HU, Kowdley KV, et al. Bile acid changes after high-dose ursodeoxycholic acid treatment in primary sclerosing cholangitis: relation to disease progression. Hepatology 2010;52:197–203.

72. Imam MH, Sinakos E, Gossard AA, et al. High-dose ursodeoxycholic acid increases risk of adverse outcomes in patients with early stage primary sclerosing cholangitis. Aliment Pharmacol Ther 2011;34:1185–92.

73. Aw MM, Dhawan A, Samyn M, et al. Mycophenolate mofetil as rescue treatment for autoimmune liver disease in children: a 5-year follow-up. J Hepatol 2009;51: 156–60.

74. Baven-Pronk AM, Coenraad MJ, van Buuren HR, et al. The role of mycophenolate mofetil in the management of autoimmune hepatitis and overlap syndromes. Aliment Pharmacol Ther 2011;34:335–43.

75. Duclos-Vallee JC, Hadengue A, Ganne-Carrie N, et al. Primary biliary cirrhosis-autoimmune hepatitis overlap syndrome. Corticoresistance and effective treatment by cyclosporine A. Dig Dis Sci 1995;40:1069–73.

76. Efe C, Ozaslan E, Kav T, et al. Liver fibrosis may reduce the efficacy of budesonide in the treatment of autoimmune hepatitis and overlap syndrome. Autoimmun Rev 2012;11:330–4.

77. Zachou K, Gatselis NK, Arvaniti P, et al. A real-world study focused on the long-term efficacy of mycophenolate mofetil as first-line treatment of autoimmune hepatitis. Aliment Pharmacol Ther 2016;43(10):1035–47.

78. Czaja AJ. Mycophenolate mofetil to the rescue in autoimmune hepatitis: a fresh sprout on the decision tree. J Hepatol 2009;51:8–10.

79. Czaja AJ, Carpenter HA. Empiric therapy of autoimmune hepatitis with myco-phenolate mofetil: comparison with conventional treatment for refractory dis-ease. J Clin Gastroenterol 2005;39:819–25.
80. Devlin SM, Swain MG, Urbanski SJ, et al. Mycophenolate mofetil for the treat-ment of autoimmune hepatitis in patients refractory to standard therapy. Can J Gastroenterol 2004;18:321–6.
81. Fallatah HI, Akbar HO. Mycophenolate mofetil as a rescue therapy for autoim-mune hepatitis patients who are not responsive to standard therapy. Expert Rev Gastroenterol Hepatol 2011;5:517–22.
82. Lin AE, Singh KE, Strauss A, et al. An additional patient with mycophenolate mo-fetil embryopathy: cardiac and facial analyses. Am J Med Genet A 2011;155A: 748–56.
83. Czaja AJ. Drug choices in autoimmune hepatitis: part B - nonsteroids. Expert Rev Gastroenterol Hepatol 2012;6:617–35.
84. Geier A, Gartung C, Dietrich CG, et al. Side effects of budesonide in liver cirrhosis due to chronic autoimmune hepatitis: influence of hepatic metabolism versus portosystemic shunts on a patient complicated with HCC. World J Gas-troenterol 2003;9:2681–5.
85. Czaja AJ, Lindor KD. Failure of budesonide in a pilot study of treatment-dependent autoimmune hepatitis. Gastroenterology 2000;119:1312–6.
86. Czaja AJ. Drug choices in autoimmune hepatitis: part A - steroids. Expert Rev Gastroenterol Hepatol 2012;6:603–15.
87. Malekzadeh R, Nasseri-Moghaddam S, Kaviani MJ, et al. Cyclosporin A is a promising alternative to corticosteroids in autoimmune hepatitis. Dig Dis Sci 2001;46:1321–7.
88. Van Thiel DH, Wright H, Carroll P, et al. Tacrolimus: a potential new treatment for autoimmune chronic active hepatitis: results of an open-label preliminary trial. Am J Gastroenterol 1995;90:771–6.
89. Czaja AJ. Autoimmune hepatitis: focusing on treatments other than steroids. Can J Gastroenterol 2012;26:615–20.
90. Lawrence SP, Sherman KE, Lawson JM, et al. A 39 year old man with chronic hepatitis. Semin Liver Dis 1994;14:97–105.
91. Czaja AJ. Overlap syndrome of primary biliary cirrhosis and autoimmune hepa-titis: a foray across diagnostic boundaries. J Hepatol 2006;44:251–2.
92. Czaja AJ. The variant forms of autoimmune hepatitis. Ann Intern Med 1996;125: 588–98.
93. Poupon R. Autoimmune overlapping syndromes. Clin Liver Dis 2003;7:865–78.
94. Burak KW, Urbanski SJ, Swain MG. A case of coexisting primary biliary cirrhosis and primary sclerosing cholangitis: a new overlap of autoimmune liver diseases. Dig Dis Sci 2001;46:2043–7.
95. Kingham JG, Abbasi A. Co-existence of primary biliary cirrhosis and primary sclerosing cholangitis: a rare overlap syndrome put in perspective. Eur J Gas-troenterol Hepatol 2005;17:1077–80.
96. Jeevagan A. Overlap of primary biliary cirrhosis and primary sclerosing cholan-gitis - a rare coincidence or a new syndrome. Int J Gen Med 2010;3:143–6.
97. Oliveira EM, Oliveira PM, Becker V, et al. Overlapping of primary biliary cirrhosis and small duct primary sclerosing cholangitis: first case report. J Clin Med Res 2012;4:429–33.
98. Floreani A, Motta R, Cazzagon N, et al. The overlap syndrome between primary biliary cirrhosis and primary sclerosing cholangitis. Dig Liver Dis 2015;47:432–5.

99. Lindor KD, Gershwin ME, Poupon R, et al. AASLD Practice Guidelines. Primary biliary cirrhosis. Hepatology 2009;50:291–308.
100. Gleeson D, Heneghan MA. British Society of Gastroenterology (BSG) guidelines for management of autoimmune hepatitis. Gut 2011;60:1611–29.

Morphologic Subtypes of Hepatocellular Carcinoma

Michael S. Torbenson, MD

KEYWORDS

- Hepatocellular carcinoma subtypes • Carcinosarcoma
- Clear cell hepatocellular carcinoma • Cirrhotomimetic hepatocellular carcinoma
- Diffuse hepatocellular carcinoma • Fibrolamellar carcinoma
- Sarcomatoid hepatocellular carcinoma • Scirrhous hepatocellular carcinoma

KEY POINTS

- Hepatocellular carcinomas show substantial morphologic variability.
- This morphologic variability segregates into distinct entities.
- These entities are called subtypes and have unique clinical, biological, and molecular findings.

INTRODUCTION

Hepatocellular carcinomas are malignant epithelial neoplasms that originate in the liver and show exclusively or primarily hepatic differentiation. However, hepatocellular carcinomas are not homogenous and within this broad definition there are many distinctive subtypes. These subtypes are important for several reasons. First, they are important to recognize in surgical pathology as part of the acceptable spectrum of changes for a diagnosis of hepatocellular carcinoma. As part of this, some of the variants present specific diagnostic pitfalls. For example, the scirrhous variant can resemble a cholangiocarcinoma. Second, the variants provide prognostic information beyond that contained in tumor grade. Third, morphologic findings predict genetic findings, not exclusively, but with sufficient strength that including morphology improves the quality of molecular studies. As 1 example, a specific microdeletion is found in fibrolamellar carcinoma. Finally, it seems reasonable to believe that hepatocellular carcinoma subtypes, define by both morphology and genetics, will be increasingly relevant to prognosis and to therapy in the future.

GROWTH PATTERN VERSUS SUBTYPE

There are 4 major growth patterns in hepatocellular carcinomas: trabecular (70%), solid (20%), pseudoglandular/acinar (10%), and macrotrabecular (1%).[1] Of note,

Department of Laboratory Medicine and Pathology, Mayo Clinic Rochester, Rochester, MN, USA
E-mail address: Torbenson.Michael@mayo.edu

Gastroenterol Clin N Am 46 (2017) 365–391
http://dx.doi.org/10.1016/j.gtc.2017.01.009
0889-8553/17/© 2017 Elsevier Inc. All rights reserved.

gastro.theclinics.com

these growth patterns should not be equated with subtypes. In addition to these 4 main growth patterns, some hepatocellular carcinomas have nodules that show distinctly different tumor morphology within the same tumor mass, a finding often called "nodule within a nodule." In these cases, one of the nodules often shows higher grade cytology, suggesting tumor evolution that led to the emergence of a more aggressive clone. In other cases, multiple morphologies of similar grades can be present, perhaps representing genetic instability without significant selection pressure.

DEFINITION OF A HEPATOCELLULAR CARCINOMA SUBTYPE

Hepatocellular carcinoma subtypes, when fully developed, have 4 primary elements.[2] Of course, each of the 4 elements will not be fully or equally developed when a subtype is first defined, but each of these 4 elements will develop over time.

1. Reproducible histologic findings on hematoxylin and eosin (H&E) staining. The subtype should have a histologic pattern that is strong enough to strongly suggest the diagnosis on H&E examination. The core set of histologic findings in most subtypes will not be absolutely specific, but should have high sensitivity to be useful.
2. Additional testing that helps to confirm the diagnosis of a specific subtype in cases with compatible H&E findings. These confirmatory testing can be immunohistochemistry, fluorescence in situ hybridization, or other molecular studies.
3. Clinical correlates. The type and strength of the clinical correlates varies considerably among subtypes. In some cases, clinical findings may be similar to conventional hepatocellular carcinomas.
4. Unique molecular findings. These findings are often incorporated into step 2, being used as the foundation for confirmatory testing.

Using this approach, 12 reasonably well-established subtypes and 6 proposed subtypes have been defined, together constituting approximately 35% of all hepatocellular carcinomas (**Table 1**). These subtypes and their definitions are discussed further herein. It is anticipated that better definitions will develop over time for some or all of these subtypes, and that is a good thing. What has not been a good thing is that many authors have written many papers on hepatocellular carcinoma subtypes using idiosyncratic definitions, which makes the literature challenging to interpret and can seriously muddle the field. Studies should as much as possible use a common reference definition as part of the study design. If the authors have a refinement on the definition, that is excellent and will hopefully advance the field, but it is best practice to include both the reference definition and the refined definition in the study design and data analysis, so that the published data can be reasonably synthesized.

MOLECULAR SUBTYPES

An alternative approach is to rely solely on molecular findings to define hepatocellular carcinoma subtypes, an approach fully embraced by most of the molecular papers on hepatocellular carcinoma. However, this approach has been disappointing to date. It is not the case that molecular subtypes do not contain, for example, prognostic information, but instead that they contain less information than the current approach of stage, grade, and morphologic subtype. In part this reflects the widespread genetic variability that can be seen within a single hepatocellular carcinoma, leading to many subclones, and, perhaps surprisingly, evidence that these clones are often not under strong Darwinian type selection pressure.[3]

Table 1
Hepatocellular carcinoma subtypes

Subtype	Frequency in Surgical Pathology Specimens (%)	Prognosis[a]
Steatohepatitic	20	Similar
Clear cell	7	Better
Scirrhous	4	Similar to better
Cirrhotomimetic	1	Worse
Combined hepatocellular-cholangiocarcinoma	1	Worse
Fibrolamellar carcinoma	1	Similar to better
Combined hepatocellular and neuroendocrine	<1	Worse
Granulocyte colony-stimulating factor producing	<1	Worse
Sarcomatoid	<1	Worse
Carcinosarcoma	<1	Worse
Carcinosarcoma with osteoclast-like giant cells	<1	Worse
Lymphocyte rich	<1	Better
Provisional subtypes		
Chromophobe	1–2	Unclear
Combined hepatocellular-cholangiocarcinoma with stem cell features	<1	Unclear
Lipid rich	<1	Unclear
Myxoid	<1	Unclear
Syncytial giant cell	<1	Unclear
Transitional cell	<1	Unclear

[a] Compared with conventional hepatocellular carcinoma.

MAJOR HEPATOCELLULAR CARCINOMA SUBTYPES

Occasionally a case can have features that could lead to classification in either of 2 different categories. For example, some cirrhotomimetic hepatocellular carcinomas also show clear cell morphology. In this setting, the subtype with the worse prognosis is used for primary classification and in this example the primary classification would be cirrhotomimetic. The frequency of each subtype (see **Table 1**) is shown for surgical pathology specimens. The frequency can be quite different in autopsy studies, which tend to be enriched for poorly differentiated subtypes, such as carcinosarcomas and sarcomatoid hepatocellular carcinomas.

All of the subtypes can be found in cirrhotic and noncirrhotic livers, with the exception of fibrolamellar carcinoma, which is found only in noncirrhotic livers. With the exception of the steatohepatitic variant of hepatocellular carcinoma, which is associated with the metabolic syndrome and alcohol-induced liver disease, none of the subtypes have well-defined, specific etiologic associations.

Carcinosarcoma

Definition and hematoxylin and eosin findings

Carcinosarcomas have both a malignant epithelial component and a malignant mesenchymal component (**Fig. 1**). The epithelial component is hepatocellular

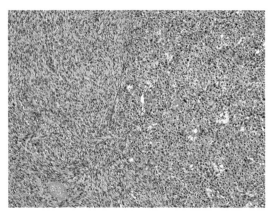

Fig. 1. Carcinosarcoma A component of fibrosarcoma is seen on the left, hepatocellular carcinoma on the right (hematoxylin-eosin).

carcinoma, usually moderately to poorly differentiated. The sarcomatous component shows morphologic or immunohistochemical evidence of mesenchymal differentiation, such as leiomyosarcoma, rhabdomyosarcoma, chondrosarcoma, fibrosarcoma, or osteosarcoma.

Confirmatory tests
Immunostains can document lineage differentiation in the sarcomatous component. The sarcomatous component is typically keratin negative. Vimentin positivity is seen in both carcinosarcomas and sarcomatoid hepatocellular carcinomas and does not distinguish these 2 subtypes.

Clinical findings
Older age at presentation.

Molecular findings
Molecular data are limited. One study found that both components shared a *TP53* mutation, but also had additional specific mutations in the different morphologies, including *PIK3CA* mutations in the hepatocellular carcinoma component and *FGFR3* mutations in the sarcoma component.[4]

Other findings
A subset of carcinosarcomas secrete granulocyte colony-stimulating factor and have numerous intratumoral neutrophils.[5]

Differential
Sarcomatoid hepatocellular carcinoma is often confused with carcinosarcoma because both tumors have a spindle cell component. The findings in the spindle cell component separate these 2 entities (**Table 2**). Adult hepatoblastomas are theoretically in the differential (see **Table 2**), but it remains controversial if this entity truly exists.

Carcinosarcoma with Osteoclast-like Giant Cells

Definition and hematoxylin and eosin findings
These tumors have a hepatocellular component, which can vary from well-differentiated to poorly differentiated, plus a sarcomatous component. Thus, it would

Table 2
Differential for carcinosarcoma

Feature	Carcinosarcoma	Sarcomatoid Hepatocellular Carcinoma	Hepatoblastoma
Age	Often elderly	Often elderly	Almost all <5
Epithelial component	Hepatocellular carcinoma, usually moderately to poorly differentiated	Hepatocellular carcinoma, usually moderately to poorly differentiated	Various morphologies, most with fetal or embryonal patterns
Spindle cell nuclear cytology	Often different between the 2 components	Often similar between the 2 components	Different between the 2 components
Spindle cell component morphology	Specific mesenchymal lineage	Nondescript spindle cells without specific mesenchymal lineage	Nondescript spindle cells, often with osteoid formation
Spindle cell component immunostains	Vimentin positive Keratin negative	Vimentin positive Keratin positive	Vimentin positive Keratin negative

not be unreasonable to classify these cases as a variant of carcinosarcoma, but given their unique findings they are usually classified separately. The sarcomatous component shows the following triad of findings.[1,6–10] (1) The sarcoma component is composed of mononuclear spindled cells (**Fig. 2**) that are negative for markers of specific mesenchymal linage differentiation, keratins, and markers of hepatic differentiation.[2] (2) Benign giant cells are scattered throughout the tumor. These giant cells are large and look like osteoclasts, having up to 30 nuclei. They stain strongly for CD68 and other markers of osteoclast like differentiation.[3,6,7] (3) Resection specimens commonly show extensive hemorrhage, cystic change, necrosis, and numerous pigment-laden macrophages, although these changes can be less evident on biopsy specimens.

Confirmatory tests
Immunostains on the sarcomatous component (see above) should confirm the H&E findings.

Clinical findings
Limited data.

Molecular findings
Limited data.

Differential
Rare cholangiocarcinomas and metastatic carcinomas can also have a similar sarcomatous component with osteoclast-like giant cells.

Cirrhotomimetic Hepatocellular Carcinoma

Definition and hematoxylin and eosin findings
This subtype is defined by the gross findings, where the liver is involved extensively by tumor that grows as numerous small nodules, which blend in almost imperceptibly with the background liver, being about the same size and the same color (**Fig. 3**). Because of this distinctive growth pattern, the tumor burden is invariably underestimated on both imaging and gross examination, often substantially. Essentially all cirrhotomimetic hepatocellular carcinomas arise in cirrhotic livers, befitting their name, but very rare cases with an identical growth pattern can occur in noncirrhotic livers,

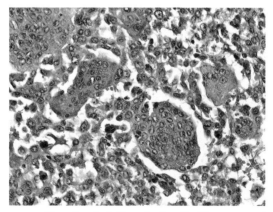

Fig. 2. Carcinosarcoma with osteoclast like giant cells. The sarcomatous component is composed of small mononuclear tumor cells, but they are admixed with benign osteoclast like giant cells. Hemosiderin deposits are also evident (hematoxylin-eosin).

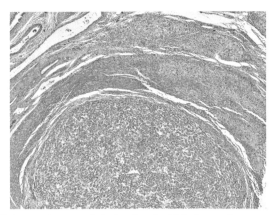

Fig. 3. Hepatocellular carcinoma, cirrhotomimetic. This tumor is composed of numerous small nodules that are similar in size to cirrhotic nodules (hematoxylin-eosin).

with numerous small tumor nodules spread throughout the liver, often seeming to originate as deposits in the portal veins.

The tumor nodules will often coalesce focally into a larger ill-defined mass, which is still consistent with a diagnosis of cirrhotomimetic hepatocellular carcinoma as long as the core pattern is seen, with extensive involvement of the liver by numerous small nodules of hepatocellular carcinoma. Most of the nodules will be less than 2 cm. There is no minimum number of nodules required, but in almost all cases there are more than 20 small nodules of tumor. Of note, the term cirrhotomimetic hepatocellular carcinoma should not be used for a case solely because there was tumor evident by histologic examination that was not evident by imaging studies or gross examination.

Histologically, these tumors look much like a conventional hepatocellular carcinoma and stain in a conventional fashion with markers of hepatic differentiation. They are typically moderately to poorly differentiated and can show clear cell change, fatty change, and have bile production. Clear cell change may be associated with a better prognosis,[11] but these cases should still be classified as cirrhotomimetic.

Confirmatory tests
None.

Clinical findings
Autopsy studies suggest the distinctive growth pattern results from early tumor colonization of the large hilar portal vein branches, leading to subsequent seeding of the rest of the liver.[12,13] However, the full explanation is likely more complicated and presumably reflects tumor-specific genetic changes, because many cases of hepatocellular carcinoma involve the hilar branches of the portal veins but do not have a cirrhotomimetic growth pattern.

Molecular findings
None.

Other findings
In a subset of cases, the background livers can show moderate to marked iron accumulation, but it is unclear if this reflects an association with genetic iron overload versus a secondary finding. Anecdotal experience suggests there is no strong association with *HFE* mutations.

Differential
Cirrhotomimetic hepatocellular carcinomas should be distinguished from conventional hepatocellular carcinomas that have satellite nodules (seen in about 40% of conventional hepatocellular carcinoma surgical pathology specimens), including when satellite nodules were not evident on imaging studies. The satellite nodules in conventional hepatocellular carcinomas tend to be located close to the dominant nodule, usually within a few centimeters, and lack the widely dispersed pattern seen with cirrhotomimetic hepatocellular carcinomas. In addition, the numbers of satellite nodules in conventional hepatocellular carcinomas are fewer than 5 in 90% of cases and fewer than 10 in essentially all cases.[14]

Clear Cell Hepatocellular Carcinoma

Definition and hematoxylin and eosin findings
The tumor cells have abundant clear cytoplasm that is filled with glycogen (**Fig. 4**). In many cases, not all of the tumor cells will have clear cytoplasm, leading to the need for a threshold minimum to define this subtype. There is a lot of variation in the definitions used in the literature, but a minimum requirement of at least 50% clear cells is suggested, with a more pure group of tumors achieved using a requirement of at least 80% of clear cells. Of note, a primary classification of clear cell carcinoma is not used in tumors composed of multiple adjacent nodules with distinctly different morphologies, even when one of the nodule shows clear cell change.

Most clear cell hepatocellular carcinomas are well-differentiated or moderately differentiated. Tumor cells can also have fat in addition to the glycogen, with steatosis found in one-third of cases.[15] Clear cell hepatocellular carcinomas are positive for the usual markers of hepatic differentiation, including HepPar1, Arginase1, and albumin in situ hybridization.

Confirmatory tests
None.

Clinical findings
The prognosis is better than conventional hepatocellular carcinoma.

Molecular findings
Limited data.

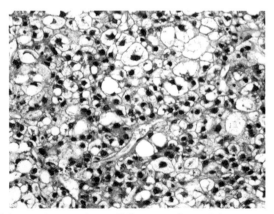

Fig. 4. Hepatocellular carcinoma, clear cell (hematoxylin-eosin).

Other findings
Compared with conventional hepatocellular carcinomas, clear cell hepatocellular carcinomas tend to be smaller,[16,17] better differentiated,[16] and have lower rates of vascular invasion.[16–18]

Differential
Clear cell carcinomas from other organs, such as the kidney or ovary, can metastasize to the liver and immunostains are useful in these cases. Immunostains for PAX8 are negative and markers of hepatic differentiation are positive. Clear cell carcinomas of the kidney are HepPar1 negative,[19] but 35% of clear cell carcinomas of the ovary can be focally HepPar1 positive,[20] so other stains such as arginase can be helpful.

The differential also includes lipid-rich hepatocellular carcinomas, a very rare subtype where the tumor cells also seem to be clear on low-power examination. However, on high-power examination, the tumor cells are filled with tiny lipid droplets and not glycogen. Other tumors that can enter the differential include benign adrenal rests and epithelioid angiomyolipomas, which can sometimes show a clear cell type change. Immunostains will sort out these differentials as needed.

Combined Hepatocellular Carcinoma–Cholangiocarcinoma

Definition and hematoxylin and eosin findings
Combined hepatocellular carcinoma–cholangiocarcinomas have 2 distinct epithelial components (**Fig. 5**), which should be located together in 1 nodule or in immediately adjacent nodules. The term double primary is used when the hepatocellular carcinoma component is clearly separated from the cholangiocarcinoma component by intervening nonneoplastic liver.

The hepatocellular carcinoma is typically moderately to poorly differentiated and otherwise largely unremarkable. The cholangiocarcinoma likewise shows the usual morphologic findings of a conventional cholangiocarcinoma. Transition zones can be seen between the 2 components but are usually narrow. The hepatocellular carcinoma is positive for the typical markers of hepatocellular differentiation such as HepPar1 and arginase 1, whereas the cholangiocarcinoma component is positive for typical biliary type keratins, such as CK19 and CK7, but negative for markers of hepatocellular differentiation. In resection specimens, the approximate percent of each

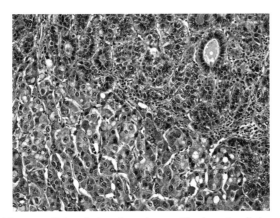

Fig. 5. Combined hepatocellular–cholangiocarcinoma. The hepatocellular carcinoma component is on the bottom left, and the cholangiocarcinoma is in the upper right (hematoxylin-eosin).

component should be conveyed, because some cases are predominately 1 component with only a small amount of the other.

Confirmatory tests

Immunostains are needed to confirm the H&E impression, because the H&E findings in some cases can suggest areas of biphenotypic differentiation that are not confirmed by immunostains.

Clinical findings

Serum CA19-9 levels and serum alpha-fetoprotein (AFP) levels are increased in about 50% of individuals with this tumor type.[21] The elevated CA19-9 levels reflect the cholangiocarcinoma component and AFP the hepatocellular carcinoma component.

The frequency of lymph node disease at presentation is higher than with conventional hepatocellular carcinomas. For example, 1 study found regional lymph node metastases in 2% of hepatocellular carcinoma, 13% of combined hepatocellular carcinoma–cholangiocarcinomas, and 21% of cholangiocarcinomas.[22] For this reason, hilar lymph node dissection is performed when the diagnosis of a combined tumor is known before surgery.

The overall prognosis falls in between that of cholangiocarcinoma and hepatocellular carcinoma.[23,24] Combined tumors are staged in the American Joint Committee on Cancer's system using the cholangiocarcinoma protocol because the cholangiocarcinoma component tends to drive prognosis. Nonetheless, these combined tumors are sufficiently distinct from cholangiocarcinomas that a unique staging system should be developed in the future.

Molecular findings

No consistent findings to date.

Differential

The most common mistake is basing a diagnosis of a combined tumor on immunostain findings only, without the morphologic correlates. This can happen in both directions, because conventional hepatocellular carcinomas can express CK7 (30%) or CK19 (15%) or CK20 (10%), whereas cholangiocarcinoma can express HepPar1 (5%–10%) or glypican 3 (5%–10%) or arginase (1%–5%). The staining in these cases is often focal or patchy, but can lead the unwary into a misdiagnosis of mixed tumor. A clearly distinct morphologic component is mandatary for the diagnosis of this subtype.

The differential includes double primary carcinomas, which have 2 distinctly different nodules of hepatocellular and cholangiocarcinoma, with intervening nonneoplastic hepatic parenchyma. The frequency of double primary carcinomas is 0.2%.[25] Overall, the cholangiocarcinoma component tends to drive the prognosis,[25] but each component should be graded and staged separately.

Combined Hepatocellular and Neuroendocrine Carcinoma

Definition and hematoxylin and eosin findings

This tumor has a component of hepatocellular carcinoma and a component of neuroendocrine carcinoma (**Fig. 6**). Just like with combined hepatocellular carcinoma and cholangiocarcinoma, the 2 components should be evident on the H&E and confirmed by immunostains. The 2 components should be located together. If the 2 components instead are separate nodules with intervening normal hepatic parenchyma, then they are classified as separate primaries.

The hepatocellular component is usually well-differentiated to moderately differentiated with no unusual findings and a typical staining pattern with markers of hepatic

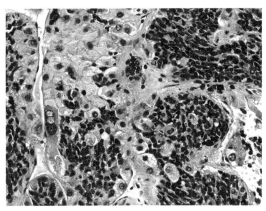

Fig. 6. Combined hepatocellular–neuroendocrine carcinoma. The hepatocellular carcinoma tumor sinusoids are spread wide by small cell neuroendocrine carcinoma (hematoxylin-eosin).

differentiation. The neuroendocrine component shows a small cell morphology in most cases, although a large cell morphology can also be seen. Neuroendocrine markers like synaptophysin and chromogranin are positive. The neuroendocrine component is usually found admixed with the hepatocellular component, often growing in the sinusoids. The relative proportion of each component varies, but most cases are primarily hepatocellular with a smaller component of neuroendocrine tumor. Despite this, metastatic disease is often purely neuroendocrine.

Confirmatory tests
Both components should be evident on H&E and confirmed by immunostains. The morphologic findings of 2 distinct components are necessary and a diagnosis of a combined tumor should not be based solely on immunostain results in a monomorphic tumor. As an example, focal synaptophysin or CD56 staining can be found in some conventional hepatocellular carcinomas.

Clinical findings
No distinct findings to date.

Molecular findings
Limited to no data.

Fibrolamellar Carcinoma

Definition and hematoxylin and eosin findings
Fibrolamellar carcinoma are composed of large eosinophilic cells with prominent nucleoli and abundant intratumoral fibrosis (**Fig. 7**). The collagen is often deposited in parallel bands, providing the genesis for the "lamellar" part of the tumor's name "fibrolamellar" (**Fig. 8**), but in other cases the collagen has a more haphazard deposition pattern. The distinctive fibrosis is also commonly present in metastatic disease. The fibrosis in fibrolamellar carcinomas often shows heterogeneity. In fact, about 10% of cases have areas that show a solid growth pattern with little or no fibrosis. These solid areas of growth are part of the spectrum of findings in fibrolamellar carcinoma and do not indicate a mixed conventional hepatocellular carcinoma and fibrolamellar carcinoma.[26]

Fibrolamellar carcinomas also commonly have pale bodies and hyaline bodies, but neither are specific for fibrolamellar carcinoma. Other findings include intratumoral

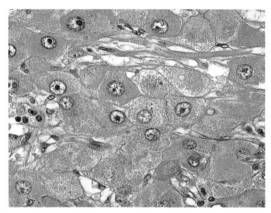

Fig. 7. Fibrolamellar carcinoma. The tumor cells have abundant pink cytoplasm with prominent nucleoli (hematoxylin-eosin).

cholestasis and variably dilated psuedoglands, which result from dilated bile canaliculi. In some cases, the psuedoglands are much larger and produce mucinous material that is Alcian blue positive and often weakly to moderately mucicarmine positive.[27] Nonetheless, these cases are not called combined cholangiocarcinoma–fibrolamellar carcinoma. The background livers are essentially normal by light microscopy.[28]

Fibrolamellar carcinomas are positive for the major markers of hepatic differentiation, such as HepPar1, arginase, and albumin in situ hybridization. Glypican 3 is positive in about 50% of cases and AFP stains are negative. Immunostains are negative for chromogranin and synaptophysin.[29,30]

Confirmatory tests
The H&E diagnosis in some cases can be straightforward, but many cases have overlapping features with conventional hepatocellular carcinomas and the diagnosis strongly benefits from combining morphology with confirmatory tests. Sometimes, there is hesitancy to use confirmatory tests. However, using tests to confirm the diagnosis does not indicate diagnostic weakness, but instead shows an awareness of the challenges in this area and a commitment to getting the diagnosis right. Molecular

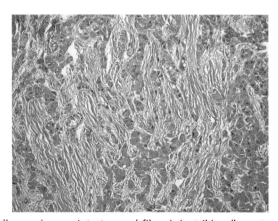

Fig. 8. Fibrolamellar carcinoma. Intratumoral fibrosis is striking (hematoxylin-eosin).

testing focuses on detecting a characteristic deletion leading to *DNAJB1-PRKACA* gene fusion and can include DNA based testing for the deletion itself or RNA testing for the resulting fusion transcript. In paraffin-embedded tissues, RNA degradation can lead to false-negative testing, giving advantages to fluorescence in situ hybridization as a diagnostic test. The *DNAJB1-PRKACA* microdeletion is a defining feature of this tumor, found in more than 99% of all cases tested to date.

If molecular testing is not available, then immunostains can confirm the diagnosis. Coexpression of CD68 (KP-1 clone) and CK7 is highly specific for the diagnosis when combined with morphology. Staining can be patchy, but the stains still perform very well on biopsy material. When using these stains to confirm the diagnosis, the internal controls should be brightly positive to ensure robust stain performance. The benign bile ducts in the background liver are CK7 positive and the Kupffer cells within the tumor and non tumor tissue are CD68 positive.

Clinical findings
Serum AFP levels can be mildly elevated,[31,32] but are essentially never greater than 200 ng/mL. In contrast with hepatocellular carcinomas in cirrhotic livers, the gender distribution in fibrolamellar carcinoma is about equal.[32–34] Tumors occur in younger individuals, with 80% presenting between the ages of 10 and 35 years.[35] The overall prognosis is similar to that seen in conventional hepatocellular carcinomas without underlying liver disease,[30,36] although a very modest survival benefit was still observed in some studies.[37,38]

Molecular findings
Fibrolamellar carcinomas are characterized by the activation of protein kinase A, which results in almost all cases from microdeletions on chromosome 19,[39] leading to a fusion between the *DNAJB1* gene and the *PRKACA* gene. *PRKACA* encodes one of the catalytic units of the enzyme protein kinase A and the fusion leads to overexpression of this enzyme.

Other findings
Fibrolamellar carcinomas can rarely cooccur in the same liver with benign hepatic adenomas, most commonly type 1 hepatic adenomas with liver fatty acid binding protein loss.[35,40–42] The data are unclear as to whether this finding implies a shared risk factor or is coincidental. A minority of fibrolamellar carcinomas also induce a secondary, reactive nodular hyperplasia at their periphery. Most fibrolamellar carcinomas are cytologically homogenous, but rare tumors acquire additional mutations leading to tumor progression, with a distinct nodule of conventional-appearing hepatocellular carcinoma growing within the fibrolamellar carcinoma.[43] These cases are not mixed tumors, but instead represent tumor progression.

Differential
The differential includes conventional hepatocellular carcinoma, scirrhous hepatocellular carcinoma, neuroendocrine carcinoma metastatic to the liver (some cases can have very similar tumor cytology), and cholangiocarcinoma in cases where the psuedoglands are prominent. In most cases, the correct diagnosis is achieved readily when it is based on the combination of morphologic findings plus molecular testing.

Granulocyte Colony-Stimulating Factor Producing Hepatocellular Carcinoma

Definition and hematoxylin and eosin findings
This subtype is characterized by production of granulocyte colony-stimulating factor, leading to marked infiltrates by neutrophils (**Fig. 9**). The hepatocellular carcinoma is

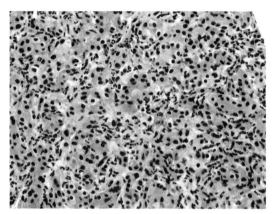

Fig. 9. Hepatocellular carcinoma, granulocyte colony-stimulating factor producing. Numerous neutrophils infiltrate the tumor (hematoxylin-eosin).

poorly differentiated in most cases and focal areas of sarcomatoid dedifferentiation are common.[44,45]

Confirmatory tests
Immunostains for granulocyte colony-stimulating factor are useful to confirm the diagnosis, but are not available widely.

Clinical findings
Most cases occur in older individuals and the prognosis is poor.[5,44–46] As a result of the granulocyte colony-stimulating factor production by the tumor, most individuals present with markedly elevated peripheral white blood cell counts. Other common findings include elevated serum interleukin-6 levels[5,44–46] and elevated serum C-reactive protein levels.[5,44–47]

Molecular findings
Limited data.

Differential
Granulocyte colony-stimulating factor can also be produced by cholangiocarcinomas[48] and metastatic carcinomas,[49] so the hepatocellular carcinoma component should be proven by morphology and immunostains.

Lymphocyte-Rich Hepatocellular Carcinoma and Lymphoepithelioma-like Hepatocellular Carcinoma

Definition and hematoxylin and eosin findings
Both lymphocyte-rich hepatocellular carcinomas and lymphoepithelioma-like hepatocellular carcinomas have striking lymphocytic infiltrates as their defining feature, but they differ in the grade of the hepatocellular carcinoma: well-differentiated to moderately differentiated in lymphocyte-rich hepatocellular carcinomas (**Fig. 10**) and poorly differentiated in lymphoepithelioma-like hepatocellular carcinomas (**Fig. 11**). In both entities, the lymphocytic infiltrates are striking on the H&E stains, with more lymphocytes than tumor cells. In lymphocyte-rich hepatocellular carcinomas, routine markers of hepatic differentiation such as arginase and HepPar1 are positive. In lymphoepithelioma-like hepatocellular carcinomas, markers of hepatic differential can be focal and a broad panel is often needed to prove hepatic differentiation. It is unclear if lymphoepithelioma-like hepatocellular carcinoma is simply a high-grade

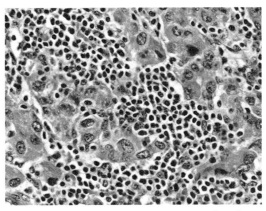

Fig. 10. Hepatocellular carcinoma, lymphocyte rich. Numerous lymphocytes infiltrate the tumor (hematoxylin-eosin).

version of lymphocyte-rich hepatocellular carcinoma, but it is reasonable to keep these entities separate until this point is clarified.

Confirmatory tests
None.

Clinical findings
Limited data.

Molecular findings
The distinctive morphology does not result from microsatellite instability.[50] Lymphoepithelioma-like carcinomas in other organs are often positive for Epstein–Barr virus, but this is not the case in lymphocyte-rich and lymphoepithelioma-like hepatocellular carcinomas. All cases to date are negative for Epstein–Barr virus by in situ hybridization.[50–54] It is true that low levels of Epstein–Barr virus DNA can be detected by polymerase chain reaction,[55] but the same holds true for conventional

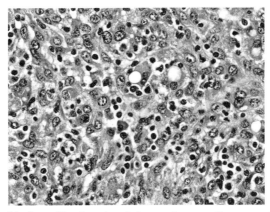

Fig. 11. Lymphoepithelioma-like hepatocellular carcinomas. Numerous lymphocytes infiltrate the tumor and the poorly differentiated carcinoma is hard to see on the hematoxylin and eosin staining (hematoxylin-eosin).

hepatocellular carcinomas[56] and this finding by itself does not indicate a role for Epstein–Barr virus.

Other findings
The inflammatory cells have been examined in a number of studies and all have reached the same basic conclusion: the infiltrates are composed predominately of CD4- and CD8-positive T cells, along with scattered germinal centers that contain B cells.[50,53]

Differential
Some conventional hepatocellular carcinomas are misclassified as lymphocyte-rich tumors when they have dense but focal areas of inflammation or when they have a more generalized but still mild lymphocytosis. Cholangiocarcinomas and metastatic disease can have also have lymphocyte rich morphologies, so immunostains are used to prove hepatic differentiation.

Sarcomatoid Hepatocellular Carcinoma

Definition and hematoxylin and eosin findings
Sarcomatoid hepatocellular carcinomas are conventional hepatocellular carcinomas with a component showing a spindle cell morphology (**Fig. 12**). The amount of spindle cell change ranges from 1% to 80%, but is usually a minor component.[57] The spindle cell component should not have evidence for specific mesenchymal differentiation by morphology or by immunostains; if it does, then the tumor is classified as a carcinosarcoma. A definite hepatocellular carcinoma component is required for this diagnosis and can be poorly differentiated, requiring immunostains to identify hepatic differentiation.

Confirmatory tests
The spindle cell component is usually negative for hepatic markers, but should be vimentin positive and keratin positive.

Clinical findings
Similar risk factors to conventional hepatocellular carcinoma.

Molecular findings
Limited data.

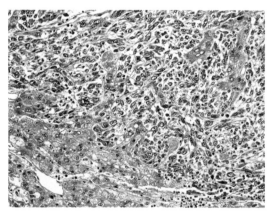

Fig. 12. Hepatocellular carcinoma, sarcomatoid. The spindled cells were vimentin and keratin positive (hematoxylin-eosin).

Other findings
The frequency of sarcomatoid change is much higher in autopsy studies and can approach 10%,[58] because autopsy studies are often enriched for advanced stage tumors, Chemoembolization therapy can also induce or select for sarcomatoid changes.[58]

Differential
This tumor is differentiated from carcinosarcomas by the spindle cell component, as discussed previously (see **Table 2**).

Scirrhous Hepatocellular Carcinoma

Definition and hematoxylin and eosin findings
This subtype is defined by abundant and diffuse intratumoral fibrosis (**Fig. 13**). The fibrosis should involve at least 50% of the tumor and in most cases involves essentially the entire tumor. The fibrosis is dense, making up at least 25% of the surface area in most low-power fields, with bands or broad sheets of fibrosis. The fibrosis sometimes divides the tumor into clusters of adjacent smaller subnodules. Within this fibrosis, the tumor grows as thin trabeculae in most cases, although the trabeculae can also be thicker and more bulbous. Most scirrhous cases are well-differentiated to moderately differentiated. Scirrhous hepatocellular carcinomas are often located beneath the liver capsule and are most common in noncirrhotic livers.[59–61] Cytoplasmic inclusions are common and can include hyaline bodies and pale bodies.[62] Fatty change or clear cell change can also be seen.[62]

Confirmatory tests
None.

Clinical findings
Similar to conventional hepatocellular carcinoma.

Molecular findings
Limited data.

Other findings
The scirrhous subtype of hepatocellular carcinoma differs from conventional hepatocellular carcinoma with regard to immunohistochemical findings. First, reticulin stains

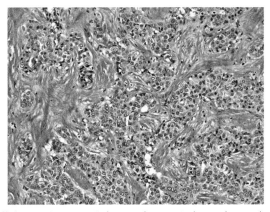

Fig. 13. Hepatocellular carcinoma, scirrhous subtype. A dense desmoplastic background is seen (hematoxylin-eosin).

rarely will not show convincing loss of reticulin. Second, HepPar staining is often focal or absent, with only about 40% to 60% of cases staining positive.[63,64] Arginase is positive in 85% of cases and glypican 3 in 80% of cases.[64]

Differential

The differential includes fibrolamellar carcinoma, cholangiocarcinoma, and metastatic disease. Fibrolamellar carcinoma and scirrhous hepatocellular carcinoma are both CK7 positive,[65] but only fibrolamellar carcinomas consistently express CD68.[66,67] Molecular testing is also very helpful in this situation.[26] Positive staining with markers of hepatic differentiation will exclude cholangiocarcinoma and metastatic disease, although a panel of stains is often needed for this purpose.

Steatohepatitic Hepatocellular Carcinoma

Definition and hematoxylin and eosin findings

The tumor cells in this variant show steatohepatitis (**Fig. 14**), with macrovesicular steatosis, lymphocytic inflammation, balloon cells, Mallory-Denk bodies, and pericellular fibrosis.[68,69] To qualify for this diagnosis, fat alone is not enough, because there also has to be evidence of injury (inflammation or ballooned tumor cells) as well as pericellular fibrosis. The fibrosis is often best seen on trichrome stains. The steatohepatitis should be a dominant part of the histology, present in at least 50% of the tumor. Most cases are well-differentiated to moderately differentiated and will stain like a conventional hepatocellular carcinoma.

Confirmatory tests

None.

Clinical findings

This subtype is strongly associated with the metabolic syndrome or with chronic alcohol use. The background, nonneoplastic liver typically shows fatty liver disease.[68,70,71]

Molecular findings

These tumors are less likely than conventional hepatocellular carcinomas to have activation of the beta-catenin pathway, with fewer beta-catenin mutations and fewer cases showing strong and diffuse glutamine synthesis staining.[72]

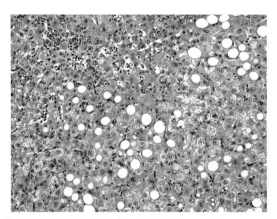

Fig. 14. Hepatocellular carcinoma, steatohepatitic subtype. This tumor shows macrovesicular steatosis, ballooned hepatocytes, and lymphocytic inflammation (hematoxylin-eosin).

Other findings

The steatohepatitic variant of hepatocellular carcinoma in rare cases is found in livers that have no fatty change in the nonneoplastic parenchyma.[73] In these cases, the steatohepatitic morphology likely represents tumor-specific genetic or epigenetic changes and not a response to the metabolic syndrome or alcohol use, as is true for most cases of steatohepatitic hepatocellular carcinoma.

Differential

In some cases, the tumor can be mistaken for steatohepatitis alone. The correct diagnosis results from recognizing the architectural and cytologic atypia of the cancer. Focal nodular hyperplasia can occasionally can show steatohepatitic changes and should also be excluded by the usual methods.

PROVISIONAL SUBTYPES OF HEPATOCELLULAR CARCINOMA

These subtypes are provisional because published data are limited to a few papers.

Combined Hepatocellular Carcinoma–Cholangiocarcinoma with Stem Cell Features

The 2010 World Health Organization classification of liver tumors[74] introduced a separate classification for tumors called combined hepatocellular carcinoma–cholangiocarcinomas with stem cell features (**Table 3**). The stem cell–like features could be found in either or both of the epithelial components. Subsequent studies have attempted to use this classification system, but have encountered significant difficulties and the classification will need to be refined. In many cases, these terms have been applied to either hepatocellular carcinomas or cholangiocarcinomas that are not combined tumors. The literature is still interesting and valuable, but has to be read very carefully because the authors in many cases use the same terminology for what are clearly different tumors. As a brief summary, there are 3 stem cell–like variants: typical (**Fig. 15**), intermediate cell (**Fig. 16**), and cholangiocellular (**Fig. 17**). The first 2 variants

Table 3
Combined hepatocellular–cholangiocarcinoma with stem cell features, based on 2010 WHO-based definitions

Subtype	H&E and Immunohistochemical Features
Typical	Core histology: HCC component has a peripheral rim of smaller cells with a high nuclear to cytoplasmic ratio and hyperchromatic nuclei. Stains: The usual markers of hepatocellular differentiation are positive in the HCC. The peripheral cells can be positive for CK7, CK19, and often CD56, c-Kit, and EpCAM.
Intermediate cell	Core histology: Small oval cells with mild to focally moderate cytologic atypia, often hard to classify as hepatic or biliary on morphology, but are positive for hepatic markers. Stains: Coexpression of markers of hepatocellular and biliary differentiation, for example, HepPar1, CK19, and CEA. CKit expression is common.
Cholangiolocellular	Core histology: Cholangiocarcinoma morphology with small cells and mild cytologic atypia, growing in a branching, anastomosing cord like pattern. Small tubular structures can be seen. Stains: Positive for CK19, CK7, CD56, c-Kit, and EpCAM but negative for makers of hepatic differentiation.

Abbreviations: HCC, hepatocellular carcinoma; H&E, hematoxylin and eosin; WHO, World Health Organization.

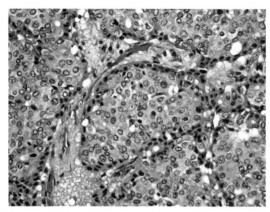

Fig. 15. Combined hepatocellular–cholangiocarcinoma, with stem cell features. The typical subtype (type 1) shows a thin rim of small basophilic cells surrounding more conventional nests of hepatocellular carcinoma cells (hematoxylin-eosin).

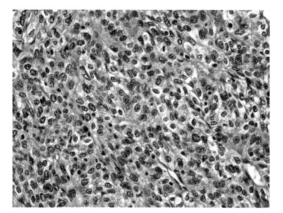

Fig. 16. Combined hepatocellular–cholangiocarcinoma, with stem cell features. The intermediate cell subtype (type 2) shows basophilic cells that are oval to slightly spindled and are difficult to classify based on morphology alone (hematoxylin-eosin).

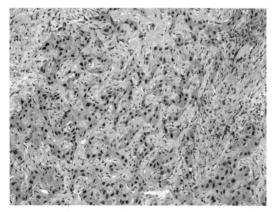

Fig. 17. Combined hepatocellular–cholangiocarcinoma, with stem cell features. The cholangiolocellular subtype (type 3) shows interanastomosing cords of biliary type cells (hematoxylin-eosin).

have primarily hepatic differentiation, and the third subtype has primarily cholangio-carcinoma differentiation.

Chromophobe Hepatocellular Carcinoma

Chromophobe hepatocellular carcinomas are characterized by tumor cells with amphophilic to eosinophilic cytoplasm and generally bland nuclear changes, but with scattered tumor cells showing striking nuclear pleomorphism (**Fig. 18**). This sub-type of hepatocellular carcinoma is strongly associated with alternative lengthening of telomeres,[2] where tumor cells maintain their telomeres by a telomere-independent mechanism that involves homologous recombination of the telomeres.[75]

Hepatocellular Carcinoma with Syncytial Giant Cells

In this subtype, the tumors cells have numerous syncytial multinucleated giant cells, similar to those seen in infantile giant cell hepatitis (**Fig. 19**). Despite the multinuclea-tion, the tumor is well-differentiated and lacks the bizarre, atypical multinucleated giant cells of some poorly differentiated hepatocellular carcinomas.[76]

Lipid-Rich Hepatocellular Carcinoma

Lipid-rich hepatocellular carcinomas have clear cytoplasm that results from lipid accu-mulation, with numerous tiny droplets of fat (**Fig. 20**).[77] These changes should be diffuse, although occasional larger droplets of fat are acceptable. The differential in-cludes adrenal rests as well as metastatic carcinomas, such as neuroendocrine car-cinoma, which have lipid-rich variants.

Myxoid Hepatocellular Carcinoma

This subtype is well-differentiated to moderately differentiated and purely hepatitic with a trabecular growth pattern, but the trabeculae are spread apart by myxoid ma-terial within the sinusoids (**Fig. 21**). There is no evidence for cholangiocarcinoma by either morphology or immunostains.[78] The tumor cells stain strongly with HepPar1 and Arginase and typically show loss of liver fatty acid binding protein staining with strong and diffuse positivity for glutamine synthetase.

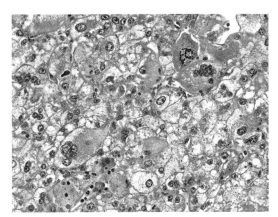

Fig. 18. Hepatocellular carcinoma, chromophobe subtype. Scattered very atypical cells are present in the background of tumor cells with bland nuclear cytology and abundant clear to eosinophilic cytoplasm (hematoxylin-eosin).

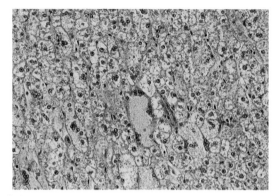

Fig. 19. Hepatocellular carcinoma with syncytial giant cells. These tumors tend to be very well-differentiated despite the giant cell change (hematoxylin-eosin).

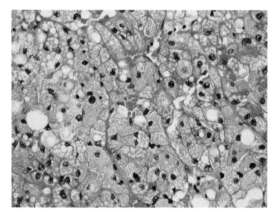

Fig. 20. Hepatocellular carcinoma, lipid-rich subtype. The tumor cytoplasm is filled with numerous small droplets of fat (hematoxylin-eosin).

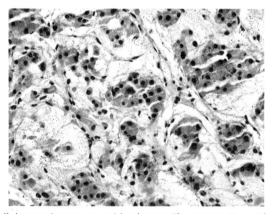

Fig. 21. Hepatocellular carcinoma, myxoid subtype. The tumor sinusoids are distended by abundant myxoid material that was Alcian blue positive and weakly mucicarmine positive (hematoxylin-eosin).

Transitional Liver Cell Tumor

Conventional hepatocellular carcinomas in older children and adolescents sometimes have focal areas that resemble the fetal or embryonal growth patterns of hepatoblastoma.[79] These foci can be subjective, making it challenging to confidently separate them from conventional hepatocellular carcinomas.

REFERENCES

1. Nzeako UC, Goodman ZD, Ishak KG. Comparison of tumor pathology with duration of survival of North American patients with hepatocellular carcinoma. Cancer 1995;76:579–88.
2. Wood LD, Heaphy CM, Daniel HD, et al. Chromophobe hepatocellular carcinoma with abrupt anaplasia: a proposal for a new subtype of hepatocellular carcinoma with unique morphological and molecular features. Mod Pathol 2013;26:1586–93.
3. Ling S, Hu Z, Yang Z, et al. Extremely high genetic diversity in a single tumor points to prevalence of non-Darwinian cell evolution. Proc Natl Acad Sci U S A 2015;112:E6496–505.
4. Luchini C, Capelli P, Fassan M, et al. Next-generation histopathologic diagnosis: a lesson from a hepatic carcinosarcoma. J Clin Oncol 2014;32:e63–6.
5. Aita K, Seki K. Carcinosarcoma of the liver producing granulocyte-colony stimulating factor. Pathol Int 2006;56:413–9.
6. Lee KB. Sarcomatoid hepatocellular carcinoma with mixed osteoclast-like giant cells and chondroid differentiation. Clin Mol Hepatol 2014;20:313–6.
7. Kuwano H, Sonoda T, Hashimoto H, et al. Hepatocellular carcinoma with osteoclast-like giant cells. Cancer 1984;54:837–42.
8. Hood DL, Bauer TW, Leibel SA, et al. Hepatic giant cell carcinoma. An ultrastructural and immunohistochemical study. Am J Clin Pathol 1990;93:111–6.
9. Sasaki A, Yokoyama S, Nakayama I, et al. Sarcomatoid hepatocellular carcinoma with osteoclast-like giant cells: case report and immunohistochemical observations. Pathol Int 1997;47:318–24.
10. Tanahashi C, Nagae H, Nukaya T, et al. Combined hepatocellular carcinoma and osteoclast-like giant cell tumor of the liver: possible clue to histogenesis. Pathol Int 2009;59:813–6.
11. Clayton EF, Malik S, Bonnel A, et al. Liver transplantation and cirrhotomimetic hepatocellular carcinoma: classification and outcomes. Liver Transpl 2014;20:765–74.
12. Okuda K, Noguchi T, Kubo Y, et al. A clinical and pathological study of diffuse type hepatocellular carcinoma. Liver 1981;1:280–9.
13. Kanematsu M, Semelka RC, Leonardou P, et al. Hepatocellular carcinoma of diffuse type: MR imaging findings and clinical manifestations. J Magn Reson Imaging 2003;18:189–95.
14. Plessier A, Codes L, Consigny Y, et al. Underestimation of the influence of satellite nodules as a risk factor for post-transplantation recurrence in patients with small hepatocellular carcinoma. Liver Transpl 2004;10:S86–90.
15. Yang SH, Watanabe J, Nakashima O, et al. Clinicopathologic study on clear cell hepatocellular carcinoma. Pathol Int 1996;46:503–9.
16. Li T, Fan J, Qin LX, et al. Risk factors, prognosis, and management of early and late intrahepatic recurrence after resection of primary clear cell carcinoma of the liver. Ann Surg Oncol 2011;18:1955–63.

17. Xu W, Ge P, Liao W, et al. Edmondson grade predicts survival of patients with primary clear cell carcinoma of liver after curative resection: a retrospective study with long-term follow-up. Asia Pac J Clin Oncol 2016. [Epub ahead of print].

18. Liu Z, Ma W, Li H, et al. Clinicopathological and prognostic features of primary clear cell carcinoma of the liver. Hepatol Res 2008;38:291–9.

19. Murakata LA, Ishak KG, Nzeako UC. Clear cell carcinoma of the liver: a comparative immunohistochemical study with renal clear cell carcinoma. Mod Pathol 2000;13:874–81.

20. Fan Z, van de Rijn M, Montgomery K, et al. Hep par 1 antibody stain for the differential diagnosis of hepatocellular carcinoma: 676 tumors tested using tissue microarrays and conventional tissue sections. Mod Pathol 2003;16:137–44.

21. Li R, Yang D, Tang CL, et al. Combined hepatocellular carcinoma and cholangiocarcinoma (biphenotypic) tumors: clinical characteristics, imaging features of contrast-enhanced ultrasound and computed tomography. BMC Cancer 2016; 16:158.

22. Yin X, Zhang BH, Qiu SJ, et al. Combined hepatocellular carcinoma and cholangiocarcinoma: clinical features, treatment modalities, and prognosis. Ann Surg Oncol 2012;19:2869–76.

23. Yeh MM. Pathology of combined hepatocellular-cholangiocarcinoma. J Gastroenterol Hepatol 2010;25:1485–92.

24. Lee JH, Chung GE, Yu SJ, et al. Long-term prognosis of combined hepatocellular and cholangiocarcinoma after curative resection comparison with hepatocellular carcinoma and cholangiocarcinoma. J Clin Gastroenterol 2011;45:69–75.

25. Cao J, Huang L, Liu C, et al. Double primary hepatic cancer (hepatocellular carcinoma and intrahepatic cholangiocarcinoma) in a single patient: a clinicopathologic study of 35 resected cases. J Gastroenterol Hepatol 2013;28:1025–31.

26. Graham RP, Jin L, Knutson DL, et al. DNAJB1-PRKACA is specific for fibrolamellar carcinoma. Mod Pathol 2015;28(6):822–9.

27. Goodman ZD, Ishak KG, Langloss JM, et al. Combined hepatocellular-cholangiocarcinoma. A histologic and immunohistochemical study. Cancer 1985;55:124–35.

28. Klein WM, Molmenti EP, Colombani PM, et al. Primary liver carcinoma arising in people younger than 30 years. Am J Clin Pathol 2005;124:512–8.

29. Ward SC, Huang J, Tickoo SK, et al. Fibrolamellar carcinoma of the liver exhibits immunohistochemical evidence of both hepatocyte and bile duct differentiation. Mod Pathol 2010;23:1180–90.

30. Kakar S, Burgart LJ, Batts KP, et al. Clinicopathologic features and survival in fibrolamellar carcinoma: comparison with conventional hepatocellular carcinoma with and without cirrhosis. Mod Pathol 2005;18:1417–23.

31. Darcy DG, Malek MM, Kobos R, et al. Prognostic factors in fibrolamellar hepatocellular carcinoma in young people. J Pediatr Surg 2015;50:153–6.

32. Ang CS, Kelley RK, Choti MA, et al. Clinicopathologic characteristics and survival outcomes of patients with fibrolamellar carcinoma: data from the fibrolamellar carcinoma consortium. Gastrointest Cancer Res 2013;6:3–9.

33. Eggert T, McGlynn KA, Duffy A, et al. Fibrolamellar hepatocellular carcinoma in the USA, 2000-2010: a detailed report on frequency, treatment and outcome based on the Surveillance, Epidemiology, and End Results database. United European Gastroenterol J 2013;1:351–7.

34. El-Serag HB, Davila JA. Is fibrolamellar carcinoma different from hepatocellular carcinoma? A US population-based study. Hepatology 2004;39:798–803.

35. Torbenson M. Fibrolamellar carcinoma: 2012 update. Scientifica (Cairo) 2012; 2012:15.
36. Njei B, Konjeti VR, Ditah I. Prognosis of patients with fibrolamellar hepatocellular carcinoma versus conventional hepatocellular carcinoma: a systematic review and meta-analysis. Gastrointest Cancer Res 2014;7:49–54.
37. Pinna AD, Iwatsuki S, Lee RG, et al. Treatment of fibrolamellar hepatoma with subtotal hepatectomy or transplantation. Hepatology 1997;26:877–83.
38. Mayo SC, Mavros MN, Nathan H, et al. Treatment and prognosis of patients with fibrolamellar hepatocellular carcinoma: a national perspective. J Am Coll Surg 2014;218:196–205.
39. Honeyman JN, Simon EP, Robine N, et al. Detection of a recurrent DNAJB1-PRKACA chimeric transcript in fibrolamellar hepatocellular carcinoma. Science 2014;343:1010–4.
40. LeBrun DP, Silver MM, Freedman MH, et al. Fibrolamellar carcinoma of the liver in a patient with Fanconi anemia. Hum Pathol 1991;22:396–8.
41. Terracciano LM, Tornillo L, Avoledo P, et al. Fibrolamellar hepatocellular carcinoma occurring 5 years after hepatocellular adenoma in a 14-year-old girl: a case report with comparative genomic hybridization analysis. Arch Pathol Lab Med 2004;128:222–6.
42. Graham RP, Terracciano LM, Meves A, et al. Hepatic adenomas with synchronous or metachronous fibrolamellar carcinomas: both are characterized by LFABP loss. Mod Pathol 2016;29(6):607–15.
43. Seitz G, Zimmermann A, Friess H, et al. Adult-type hepatocellular carcinoma in the center of a fibrolamellar hepatocellular carcinoma. Hum Pathol 2002;33: 765–9.
44. Kohno M, Shirabe K, Mano Y, et al. Granulocyte colony-stimulating-factor-producing hepatocellular carcinoma with extensive sarcomatous changes: report of a case. Surg Today 2012;43(4):439–45.
45. Araki K, Kishihara F, Takahashi K, et al. Hepatocellular carcinoma producing a granulocyte colony-stimulating factor: report of a resected case with a literature review. Liver Int 2007;27:716–21.
46. Amano H, Itamoto T, Emoto K, et al. Granulocyte colony-stimulating factor-producing combined hepatocellular/cholangiocellular carcinoma with sarcomatous change. J Gastroenterol 2005;40:1158–9.
47. Joshita S, Nakazawa K, Koike S, et al. A case of granulocyte-colony stimulating factor-producing hepatocellular carcinoma confirmed by immunohistochemistry. J Korean Med Sci 2010;25:476–80.
48. Takenaka M, Akiba J, Kawaguchi T, et al. Intrahepatic cholangiocarcinoma with sarcomatous change producing granulocyte-colony stimulating factor. Pathol Int 2013;63:233–5.
49. Shimakawa T, Asaka S, Usuda A, et al. Granulocyte-colony stimulating factor (G-CSF)-producing esophageal squamous cell carcinoma: a case report. Int Surg 2014;99:280–5.
50. Chan AW, Tong JH, Pan Y, et al. Lymphoepithelioma-like hepatocellular carcinoma: an uncommon variant of hepatocellular carcinoma with favorable outcome. Am J Surg Pathol 2015;39:304–12.
51. Emile JF, Adam R, Sebagh M, et al. Hepatocellular carcinoma with lymphoid stroma: a tumour with good prognosis after liver transplantation. Histopathology 2000;37:523–9.
52. Chen CJ, Jeng LB, Huang SF. Lymphoepithelioma-like hepatocellular carcinoma. Chang Gung Med J 2007;30:172–7.

53. Patel KR, Liu TC, Vaccharajani N, et al. Characterization of Inflammatory (Lymphoepithelioma-like) hepatocellular carcinoma: a study of 8 cases. Arch Pathol Lab Med 2014;138:1193–202.

54. Nemolato S, Fanni D, Naccarato AG, et al. Lymphoepitelioma-like hepatocellular carcinoma: a case report and a review of the literature. World J Gastroenterol 2008;14:4694–6.

55. Si MW, Thorson JA, Lauwers GY, et al. Hepatocellular lymphoepithelioma-like carcinoma associated with Epstein Barr virus: a hitherto unrecognized entity. Diagn Mol Pathol 2004;13:183–9.

56. Li W, Wu BA, Zeng YM, et al. Epstein-Barr virus in hepatocellular carcinogenesis. World J Gastroenterol 2004;10:3409–13.

57. Nishi H, Taguchi K, Asayama Y, et al. Sarcomatous hepatocellular carcinoma: a special reference to ordinary hepatocellular carcinoma. J Gastroenterol Hepatol 2003;18:415–23.

58. Kojiro M, Sugihara S, Kakizoe S, et al. Hepatocellular carcinoma with sarcomatous change: a special reference to the relationship with anticancer therapy. Cancer Chemother Pharmacol 1989;23(Suppl):S4–8.

59. Fujii T, Zen Y, Harada K, et al. Participation of liver cancer stem/progenitor cells in tumorigenesis of scirrhous hepatocellular carcinoma–human and cell culture study. Hum Pathol 2008;39:1185–96.

60. Lee JH, Choi MS, Gwak GY, et al. Clinicopathologic characteristics and long-term prognosis of scirrhous hepatocellular carcinoma. Dig Dis Sci 2012;57:1698–707.

61. Kim GJ, Rhee H, Yoo JE, et al. Increased expression of CCN2, epithelial membrane antigen, and fibroblast activation protein in hepatocellular carcinoma with fibrous stroma showing aggressive behavior. PLoS One 2014;9:e105094.

62. Kurogi M, Nakashima O, Miyaaki H, et al. Clinicopathological study of scirrhous hepatocellular carcinoma. J Gastroenterol Hepatol 2006;21:1470–7.

63. Sugiki T, Yamamoto M, Aruga A, et al. Immunohistological evaluation of single small hepatocellular carcinoma with negative staining of monoclonal antibody Hepatocyte Paraffin 1. J Surg Oncol 2004;88:104–7.

64. Krings G, Ramachandran R, Jain D, et al. Immunohistochemical pitfalls and the importance of glypican 3 and arginase in the diagnosis of scirrhous hepatocellular carcinoma. Mod Pathol 2013;26:782–91.

65. Matsuura S, Aishima S, Taguchi K, et al. 'Scirrhous' type hepatocellular carcinomas: a special reference to expression of cytokeratin 7 and hepatocyte paraffin 1. Histopathology 2005;47:382–90.

66. Limaiem F, Bouraoui S, Sboui M, et al. Fibrolamellar carcinoma versus scirrhous hepatocellular carcinoma: diagnostic usefulness of CD68. Acta Gastroenterol Belg 2015;78:393–8.

67. Ross HM, Daniel HD, Vivekanandan P, et al. Fibrolamellar carcinomas are positive for CD68. Mod Pathol 2011;24:390–5.

68. Salomao M, Remotti H, Vaughan R, et al. The steatohepatitic variant of hepatocellular carcinoma and its association with underlying steatohepatitis. Hum Pathol 2012;43:737–46.

69. Salomao M, Yu WM, Brown RS Jr, et al. Steatohepatitic hepatocellular carcinoma (SH-HCC): a distinctive histological variant of HCC in hepatitis C virus-related cirrhosis with associated NAFLD/NASH. Am J Surg Pathol 2010;34:1630–6.

70. Shibahara J, Ando S, Sakamoto Y, et al. Hepatocellular carcinoma with steatohepatitic features: a clinicopathological study of Japanese patients. Histopathology 2014;64:951–62.

71. Jain D, Nayak NC, Kumaran V, et al. Steatohepatitic hepatocellular carcinoma, a morphologic indicator of associated metabolic risk factors: a study from India. Arch Pathol Lab Med 2013;137:961–6.
72. Ando S, Shibahara J, Hayashi A, et al. beta-catenin alteration is rare in hepatocellular carcinoma with steatohepatitic features: immunohistochemical and mutational study. Virchows Arch 2015;467:535–42.
73. Yeh MM, Liu Y, Torbenson M. Steatohepatitic variant of hepatocellular carcinoma in the absence of metabolic syndrome or background steatosis: a clinical, pathological, and genetic study. Hum Pathol 2015;46:1769–75.
74. Bosman F, Carneiro F, Hruban RH, et al. WHO classification of tumors of the digestive system. Lyon (France): IARC; 2010.
75. Heaphy CM, Subhawong AP, Hong SM, et al. Prevalence of the alternative lengthening of telomeres telomere maintenance mechanism in human cancer subtypes. Am J Pathol 2011;179:1608–15.
76. Atra A, Al-Asiri R, Wali S, et al. Hepatocellular carcinoma, syncytial giant cell: a novel variant in children: a case report. Ann Diagn Pathol 2007;11:61–3.
77. Orikasa H, Ohyama R, Tsuka N, et al. Lipid-rich clear-cell hepatocellular carcinoma arising in non-alcoholic steatohepatitis in a patient with diabetes mellitus. J Submicrosc Cytol Pathol 2001;33:195–200.
78. Salaria SN, Graham RP, Aishima S, et al. Primary hepatic tumors with myxoid change: morphologically unique hepatic adenomas and hepatocellular carcinomas. Am J Surg Pathol 2015;39:318–24.
79. Prokurat A, Kluge P, Kosciesza A, et al. Transitional liver cell tumors (TLCT) in older children and adolescents: a novel group of aggressive hepatic tumors expressing beta-catenin. Med Pediatr Oncol 2002;39:510–8.

Hepatitis E Virus and the Liver

Clinical Settings and Liver Pathology

Daniela Lenggenhager, MD, Achim Weber, MD*

KEYWORDS

- Liver • Hepatitis • Hepatitis E virus (HEV) • Histology

KEY POINTS

- Hepatitis E virus (HEV), a fecally-orally transmitted RNA virus, occurring endemically as well as sporadically, is a leading cause of acute hepatitis worldwide.
- Of the 4 major genotypes infecting humans, genotypes 1 and 2 are restricted to humans, whereas genotypes 3 and 4 also are zoonosis.
- Hepatitis E is generally self-limited, presenting similar to other forms of acute hepatitis, but rarely leads to fulminant liver failure, or takes a chronic course in immunocompromised individuals.
- Hepatitis E displays a spectrum of histological changes which, besides the typical acute (cholestatic) hepatitis pattern, also comprises fulminant cases with (sub)-total necrosis and chronic hepatitis prone to fibrosis development.
- Awareness of HEV, familiarity with its clinical and histopathologic spectrum, and knowledge of diagnostic tools will enable clinicians and pathologists to reliably and promptly diagnose HEV.

INTRODUCTION

Hepatitis E virus (HEV) infection, although already described in a large outbreak that took place in Delhi, India, more than 60 years ago,[1] and long known as a leading cause of acute hepatitis worldwide, only in recent years has experienced increased awareness, and is now globally recognized as a significant health problem.[2,3] If nothing else, the increased interest in HEV is due to the fact that HEV is also known to be highly prevalent in industrialized countries[4,5] with seroprevalence rates of up to more than 30% in France.[6] In developed countries, the virus is generally transmitted zoonotically, and may take a chronic course in immunocompromised patients.[7,8] Accordingly,

Disclosure: The authors have no conflict of interest. This work was supported by an intramural grant from the Center Of Clinical Research (ZKF) Innovation Pool to A. Weber.

Department of Pathology and Molecular Pathology, University and University Hospital Zurich, Schmelzbergstrasse 12, Zurich 8091, Switzerland

* Corresponding author.

E-mail address: achim.weber@usz.ch

Gastroenterol Clin N Am 46 (2017) 393–407
http://dx.doi.org/10.1016/j.gtc.2017.01.010
0889-8553/17/© 2017 Elsevier Inc. All rights reserved.

clinicians as well as pathologists are increasingly challenged with the differential diagnosis of HEV infection in their daily practice, requiring knowledge of clinical presentation and histopathologic changes to reliably come to this diagnosis in due time. Herein, we aim to provide an overview on the basic, clinical, and pathologic aspects of HEV with a focus on histopathology, by reviewing the current literature, illustrated with cases observed in our own practice.

HEPATITIS E VIRUS
Virology and Genotypes

The HEV is a small, nonenveloped, positive-strand RNA virus of the family *Hepeviridae*, genus *Orthohepevirus*.[9] Its 7.2-kb genome comprises 3 open reading frames (ORF): ORF1 coding for a nonstructural protein responsible for viral replication, ORF2 coding for a capsid protein, and ORF3 coding for a small phosphoprotein required for viral particle secretion. ORF2 and ORF3 are extensively overlapping, and this overlapping sequence is highly conserved intragenotypically and intergenotypically. Besides the 7.2-kb full-length RNA from which the ORF1 protein (~190 kDa) is transcribed, a 2.2-kb subgenomic RNA is generated during HEV genome replication, allowing the expression of ORF3 protein (13 kDa) and ORF2 protein (72 kDa).[10]

HEV strains infecting humans belong to a single serotype, and have been classified into 4 major genotypes (**Table 1**).[10,11] Whereas HEV genotypes (GT) 1 and 2 (GT1 and GT2) are restricted to humans, genotypes 3 and 4 (GT3 and GT4) are also zoonosis, which have been detected in a wide range of species including their main reservoir in domestic pigs, deer, wild boars, and other game animals, but also oysters and bivalves. In line, HEV genotypes circulating in humans and animals of the same geographic areas have been demonstrated to be closely related phylogenetically[12] (**Box 1**).

Global Distribution

The global distribution of HEV varies considerably.[13,14] Whereas HEV GT1 and GT2 are mainly restricted to endemic regions such as Asia, Africa, and Central

Table 1
Hepatitis E virus genotypes

	Genotype 1 (GT1)	Genotype 2 (GT2)	Genotype 3 (GT3)	Genotype 4 (GT4)
Geographic distribution	Endemic regions, for example, Asia, Africa, Central America	Endemic regions, mainly Africa and Central America	Worldwide	Southeast Asia, China
Spread	Contaminated drinking water	Contaminated food or drinking water	Consumption of uncooked or undercooked contaminated meat	Consumption of uncooked or undercooked contaminated meat
Transmission	Fecally-orally	Fecally-orally	(Fecally)-orally, blood products	(Fecally)-orally
Host	Restricted to humans	Restricted to humans	Humans and zoonotical transmission	Humans and zoonotical transmission
Reservoir	Humans	Humans	Animals	Animals

Box 1
Hepatitis E Virus (HEV)

- Small, nonenveloped, positive-strand RNA virus of the family *Hepeviridae*, genus *Orthohepevirus*
- Single serotype, but 4 major genotypes (GT) infecting humans: GT1 and GT2 (restricted to humans), GT3 and GT4 (also zoonosis)
- 7.2-kb genome with 3 ORFs: ORF1, coding for a nonstructural protein responsible for viral replication; ORF2, coding for a capsid protein; and ORF3 (extensively overlapping with ORF2), coding for a small phosphoprotein required for viral particle secretion

---

America, GT3 is distributed worldwide, and GT4 is mainly present in Southeast Asia and China. Remarkably, Southwestern France has been identified as a hyperendemic region with an HEV GT3 seroprevalence rate of greater than 50%.[5,15] While GT1 and GT2 are typical waterborne infections mainly acquired by contaminated drinking water, autochthonous infections with GT3 and GT4 mostly result from the consumption of uncooked or undercooked contaminated meat (**Fig. 1**).

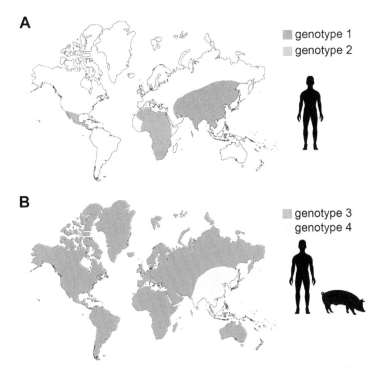

Fig. 1. Global distribution of hepatitis E virus (HEV). Main geographic distribution of the HEV genotypes infecting humans. (*A*) Endemic, waterborne infections caused by genotypes 1 and 2 (restricted to humans). (*B*) Sporadic infections caused by genotypes 3 and 4 (also constituting zoonosis). Genotype 3 occurs worldwide and is hyperendemic in a region in Southwest France.

HEPATITIS E VIRUS INFECTION: CLINICAL SETTINGS
Clinical Manifestations of Hepatitis E

Clinical manifestations of hepatitis E are highly variable, displaying a broad spectrum ranging from asymptomatic or subclinical presentations to acute liver failure with a potentially fatal outcome. Irrespective of the genotype, the majority of HEV infections remain asymptomatic. If clinically apparent, hepatitis E infection mostly presents as an acute, self-limiting disease, but also may take a chronic course.[7,8,13,16] Among other factors, the course of hepatitis E is considerably determined by the patients' immune status and preexisting liver diseases (**Table 2**).[17]

Acute Hepatitis E

Acute hepatitis E typically manifests 2 to 6 weeks after infection with symptoms including nausea and vomiting, malaise/lethargy, abdominal pain, loss of appetite, fever, and jaundice.[13,16,18] Clinical presentation of typical acute HEV infection is similar to those observed with other forms of acute (viral) hepatitis, although hepatitis E seems to be more severe compared with hepatitis A, and prolonged cholestasis has been described in a significant proportion of patients.[19] Although epidemic outbreaks of hepatitis E are characteristic for resources-limited countries, frequently caused by fecally contaminated drinking water, naturally sporadic cases also occur throughout endemic regions. As a result of traveling, HEV infections acquired in HEV-endemic areas are occasionally imported into non–HEV-endemic countries (**Fig. 2**), a scenario that, parallel to a prospectively increasing travel activity, might be observed more frequently in the future. However, locally acquired cases of autochthonous HEV GT3 (or GT4) are typical for developed countries, the majority of which are asymptomatic, and when clinically apparent usually last for 4 to 6 weeks before resolving.[13]

Because the clinical features of acute HEV infection are similar to those observed in other forms of acute hepatitis, the differential diagnosis is broad and comprises in particular acute viral hepatitis caused by virus other than HEV, and especially drug-induced liver injury.[20] Remarkably, middle-aged to elderly men seem to represent a risk group; they have been reported to be particularly prone to developing symptomatic autochthonous acute hepatitis E.[13] Although a fatal course of hepatitis E is rarely observed in the general population, HEV GT1 infection during pregnancy may take a severe course with significant maternal, fetal, and neonatal morbidity and high mortality rates of up to 25%.[21,22] Moreover, patients with preexisting liver diseases are prone to develop acute or subacute liver failure, and thus are at higher risk to take a fatal course.[23,24]

Chronic Hepatitis E

Because hepatitis E is mostly a self-limited disease, the majority of patients eliminate the virus spontaneously and recover clinically and biochemically within a few weeks. However, immunocompromised patients are at risk to develop persistent HEV infection and chronic hepatitis. After 2 seminal papers from France reporting chronic HEV infection in transplant recipients,[7,25] chronic HEV infections have also been documented in further collectives of (solid organ) transplant recipients, patients with HIV infection or hematologic malignancies undergoing chemotherapy.[26–29] Chronic hepatitis in immunocompromised patients is mainly caused by GT3 (less frequently GT4) infection, and confers a significant risk for the development of fibrosis, cirrhosis, and loss the liver graft.[7,29,30] However, the clinical

Table 2
Clinical settings of HEV infection

	Epidemic HEV Infection	Subgroup: Pregnant women	Nonepidemic HEV Infection	Subgroup: Patients with preexisting liver disease	Subgroup: Immunocompromised individuals
GT	GT1, GT2	GT1, GT2	GT3 and GT4	GT3	Mainly GT3 (few GT4 cases documented)
Patients group	Younger patients	Women, reproductive age	Older patients	Older patients, frequently alcohol disease	Any age
Clinical presentation	Ranging from asymptomatic/subclinical to fulminant	Risk for fulminant hepatitis	Ranging from asymptomatic/subclinical to symptomatic	Acute deterioration of a preexisting chronic liver disease	Rarely symptomatic
Course	Usually self-limited disease with viral clearance, no chronic course, no development of cirrhosis	Higher risk for fatal outcome (in particular in 3rd trimester)	Usually self-limited disease with viral clearance, no chronic course, no development of cirrhosis	Higher risk for fatal outcome	Viral clearance might fail, and disease might take a chronic course, risk for developing fibrosis and cirrhosis
Liver test abnormalities	Remarkable, ALT typically > 1000 IU/L at time of diagnosis				Less remarkable, ALT typically << 1000 IU/L

Abbreviations: ALT, alanine aminotransferase; GT, genotype; HEV, hepatitis E virus.

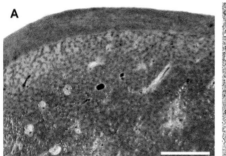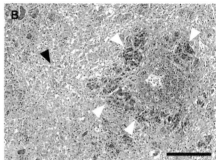

Fig. 2. Liver explant from a 26-year-old patient with fulminant epidemic hepatitis E virus genotype 1 infection after a trip to India. (*A*) Macroscopy of the liver explant with subtotal parenchymal necrosis and tissue collapse resulting in a low liver weight of 660 g (scale bar, 1 cm). (*B*) Microscopic findings of the liver explant with only few viable cells (*white arrowheads*) in the periportal area and panlobular necrosis with collapse around the central vein (*black arrowhead*; hematoxylin and eosin stain, scale bar 200 μm).

course of chronic hepatitis E in immunocompromised patients is often asymptomatic or unremarkable, going along with only mildly to modestly abnormal liver function tests.[13]

Extrahepatic Manifestation of Hepatitis E

Despite its primarily hepatotropic nature, HEV most likely also infects cells other than hepatocytes, and extrahepatic manifestations of HEV are increasingly recognized.[10] These might be caused directly or indirectly, that is, immune mediated, and are best documented for neurologic symptoms including neuritis, Guillain-Barré syndrome and neuropathy, but also include hematologic abnormalities such as thrombocytopenia, lymphocytosis, or lymphopenia.[18,31]

Laboratory Diagnosis of Hepatitis E

Clinical suspicion of hepatitis E can be verified by laboratory tests either indirectly by screening sera for the patient's immune response, or directly by molecular detection of HEV RNA, for example, in blood or stool samples. If HEV-specific immunoglobulin M antibodies are detected, thereby raising suspicion of acute hepatitis E, then this can be further confirmed by demonstrating rising immunoglobulin G antibody levels, or molecular testing. In general, antibody-based serologic testing for HEV remains challenging and is less robust compared with molecular testing.[32–34] Detection of HEV RNA is important for establishing, confirming, and monitoring (in particular in cases of chronic hepatitis) the diagnosis of hepatitis E. Because the extensively overlapping ORF2/ORF3 sequence is highly conserved intergenotypically and intragenotypically, it constitutes an ideal target region for molecular testing.[10,35] A variety of polymerase chain reaction-based assays have been established targeting this region for the detection of HEV RNA, not only in blood and stool, but also other materials.[29,35–38] Owing to a comparatively short viremic period of about 3 weeks, and an additional 2 weeks period in which the virus is detectable in stool samples, a negative test for HEV RNA does not exclude recent infection[39] (**Box 2**).

Box 2
Diagnostic tools for HEV infection

Serum-based diagnostics
- HEV-specific IgM antibodies: postulated for the diagnosis of acute HEV infection
- HEV-specific IgG antibodies: >3-fold increase considered to confirm the diagnosis of acute HEV infection
- Antibody-based serologic testing for HEV remains challenging
- PCR-based molecular detection of HEV RNA: most assays target the intergenotypically and intragenotypically highly conserved, extensively overlapping ORF2/ORF3 sequence
- PCR-based molecular detection of HEV RNA: more robust compared with antibody-based serologic testing; also applicable to test stool samples

Tissue-based diagnostics
- Histology (H&E staining)
- PCR-based molecular detection of HEV RNA in tissue samples: robust, useful and reliable ancillary tool, applied to cases in which serum-based testing was not performed
- In situ hybridization of HEV RNA in tissue samples: still experimental, not routinely performed
- Immunohistochemistry: performed by some laboratories, awaiting systematic evaluation

Abbreviations: H&E, hematoxylin and eosin; HEV, hepatitis E virus; IgM, immunoglobulin M; ORF, open reading frame; PCR, polymerase chain reaction.

HEPATITIS E VIRUS INFECTION: LIVER PATHOLOGY
Histology of Acute Epidemic Hepatitis E Virus Infection (Genotypes 1 and 2)

Because acute hepatitis E in developing countries is mostly a clinical diagnosis, liver biopsies are rarely performed in relation to the number of actual cases. In contrast, histology is proportionally more often taken for the diagnostic workup of travel-related cases of hepatitis E, for example, after visiting India,[40] Asia, Africa, or Central America. However, liver histology has also been well-documented in several large epidemic outbreaks, including one that took place in 1955/1956 in Delhi, India,[41] and another that took place in the late 1970 in Kashmir,[42] as well as in a series of 11 postmortal biopsies taken from patients who had developed fatal acute fulminant hepatitis E.[43] Collectively, the histologic changes described in these reports are similar to those found in hepatitis A with either a more inflammatory (also designated "classical" or "standard") pattern of hepatitis, or a more cholestatic (also designated "obstructive") variant. In detail, the following histopathologic features were found: a variable amount of mixed portal and lobular inflammation, prominent Kupffer cells, ballooning degeneration, and liver cell necrosis, varying from single cell apoptosis to more severe forms with bridging and submassive hepatic necrosis. Pseudorosette formation as well as hepatocytic and intracanalicular bile stasis were frequently observed in the more cholestatic variants. Bridging necrosis or (sub)total necrosis and cholangiolar proliferation with bile plugs within dilated cholangioles has been reported in severe cases. Besides diagnostic biopsies performed on travel-related cases of hepatitis E, pathologists in industrialized countries are confronted with liver explants in rare cases of imported fulminant HEV infection with liver failure requiring liver transplantation.

This is illustrated by a case we recently observed of a 26-year-old woman who had developed fulminant travel-related hepatitis owing to infection with HEV GT1 after a trip to India.[37] Macroscopy of the liver explant displayed extensive parenchymal collapse and necrosis (liver weight of 660 g; see **Fig. 2**A). Histology revealed panlobular necrosis, with parenchymal collapse and a few remaining viable parenchymal cells mostly around portal tracts (see **Fig. 2**B).

Histology of Acute Autochthonous Hepatitis E Virus Infection (Genotype 3)

Reports on histologic changes owing to documented acute autochthonous HEV infection are rather rare; in the past, HEV infection has been underrecognized[31] and recently the majority of cases are diagnosed serologically without liver biopsy. However, owing to an increased awareness of autochthonous HEV infection in the recent past, the number of reports including histopathology of hepatitis E has increased in recent years, frequently based on biopsies which had been taken early in the diagnostic workup before the results of blood testing when differential diagnosis was still open.[37,44–46] Collectively, histopathologic features of acute autochthonous HEV infection with GT3 are similar to those described in HEV infection with GT1 with the classical picture of acute hepatitis with lobular and portal inflammation and interface hepatitis. However, some differences depending on the clinical context have been noticed.

Immunocompetent patients typically reveal a significant lobular disarray with ballooning degeneration of hepatocytes and occasional rosette formation as well as spotty necrosis, sometimes with central and even portal–central necrosis. The portal tracts are markedly expanded by bile ductular proliferation and a mixed inflammatory cell infiltrate composed of lymphocytes, plasma cells, and histiocytes, but also a considerable number of polymorphs with neutrophils and eosinophils, also involving the bile ducts.[44,46] Drebber and colleagues[45] mention the absence of fibrosis (feature of chronic hepatitis), whereas Malcolm and colleagues[44] describe a zonal distribution pattern of inflammatory cells in the portal tracts with polymorphs being more pronounced at the periphery/interface and the lymphohistiocytic component (including plasma cells) dominating centrally. They also observed a variable degree of hepatocytic and canalicular bilirubinostasis.

Immunosuppressed organ transplant recipients are reported to generally show milder lobular as well as portal inflammation. Kamar and colleagues[7] describe lobular inflammation with spotty necrosis that include acidophil bodies but without ballooning and only mildly to moderately expanded portal tracts with an inflammatory infiltrate composed mainly of lymphocytes, hypothesizing that these findings could be related to the immunosuppressive therapy in those transplant recipients. In our own study, we noticed a lack of cholestasis and lobular disarray, again indicative of less extensive damage.[29]

In patients with underlying/preexisting cirrhosis, the histopathologic findings of acute hepatitis E are nonspecific and consistent with an acute insult to an underlying cirrhotic process, and easily can be mistaken for alcoholic hepatitis in the context of established ethanolic cirrhosis.[3,46,47]

A typical histology of acute autochthonous HEV GT3 infection is illustrated in **Fig. 3** showing the case of a 52-year-old previously healthy patient who got sick after ingestion of presumably undercooked pork. Histologically, the portal tracts are extended with bile ductular proliferations, mixed inflammatory infiltrates and marked interface activity as well as lobular inflammation with prominent lobular disarray (**Fig. 3**A). In line with the patient's lack of preexisting liver disease, the Sirius red staining reveals no significant fibrosis or cirrhosis indicative of any preexisting chronic liver disease (see **Fig. 3**B). The portal inflammatory infiltrate is mixed and consists of lots of lymphocytes, some histiocytes and plasma cells, as well as some eosinophils and neutrophils. Furthermore, the bile duct branches

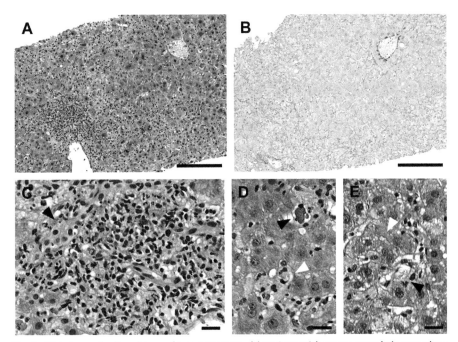

Fig. 3. Histology of a liver biopsy from a 52-year-old patient with acute autochthonous hepatitis E virus genotype 3 infection, presumably after ingestion of undercooked pork meat. (*A*) Overview revealing severe portal inflammation with pronounced interface hepatitis as well as lobular inflammation with significant lobular disarray (hematoxylin and eosin [H&E] stain, scale bar 200 μm). (*B*) Overview revealing no significant fibrosis (Sirius red stain, scale bar 200 μm). (*C*) High-power view displaying mixed inflammatory infiltrates in the portal tract with bile duct damage (*black arrowhead*; H&E stain, scale bar 20 μm). (*D*) High power view displaying spotty apoptotic hepatocytes (*black arrowhead*) and confluent hepatocyte necrosis cleared by macrophages (*white arrowhead*) (H&E stain, scale bar 20 μm). (*E*) Bilirubinostasis (*black arrowhead*) and pseudorosettes formation (*white arrowhead*) (H&E stain, scale bar 20 μm).

are affected by the inflammation and display degenerative/reactive changes of the bile duct epithelium (see **Fig. 3**C). There is significant lobular inflammation with signs of recent as well as older hepatocyte damage that range from spotty hepatocyte apoptosis to areas of piecemeal necrosis already cleared by macrophages (see **Fig. 3**D), as well as pseudorosette formation and bilirubinostasis (see **Fig. 3**E).

Histology of Chronic Hepatitis E Virus (Genotype 3) Infection in Immunocompromised Patients

As outlined, in the last years chronic HEV infection has been recognized as a relevant differential diagnosis of abnormal liver function tests developing in immunocompromised patients, especially solid organ transplant recipients. The threshold to perform a liver biopsy on these patients is rather low, especially on liver transplant recipients because the differential diagnosis is broad and in particular transplant rejection has to be ruled out histologically.

Histologic patterns of chronic hepatitis E overlap with those observed in other chronic viral hepatitis B or C infection. They include portal hepatitis with mild to dense lymphocytic infiltrates, mostly no relevant interface hepatitis and lobular activity with variable degree of piecemeal necrosis, mainly consisting of single-cell apoptosis without significant inflammation, and eventually development of fibrosis.[7,27,29,48] The capacity for fibrosis was well-shown in a patient we recently described who had experienced a de novo HEV infection after liver transplantation for cirrhosis owing to α1-antitypsin deficiency, and subsequently developed liver fibrosis, which was reflected in a series of 5 liver biopsies taken over a period of 38 months. The same case also remarkably illustrates the wide spectrum of inflammatory activity observable during HEV infection in the patient ranging from nearly nonreactive to significant inflammatory activity.[29]

Histologic changes representative of chronic HEV (GT3) infection in immunocompromised patients are illustrated in **Fig. 4** showing the case of a 66-year-old patient with liver transplantation 2 years and 9 months before the diagnosis of chronic hepatitis E. Histology reveals a preserved architecture and a mostly portal mononuclear inflammation (see **Fig. 4**A), predominantly composed of lymphocytes (see **Fig. 4**B). Whereas overt lobular inflammatory infiltrates are lacking, scattered apoptotic hepatocytes are found indicating ongoing activity (see **Fig. 4**C), next to small aggregates of ceroid laden macrophages in the lobular compartment indicative of prior hepatocyte damage (see **Fig. 4**D). Furthermore, portal and periportal fibrosis with few portoportal septa has developed in this case (**Box 3**; see **Fig. 4**E).

Histologic Differential Diagnoses of Hepatitis E

The various histopathologic patterns in the context of HEV infection described show that histopathologic changes are far from being pathognomonic for hepatitis E, but similar as the clinical presentation, are highly overlapping with other causes of hepatitis. The most important histopathologic differential diagnosis that, depending on the particular histopathologic pattern, to be considered are listed in **Table 3**.

Ancillary Tools for Histology in Hepatitis E

Because histopathologic changes related to HEV infection are highly overlapping with other causes of hepatitis, ancillary tools are needed to come to an accurate diagnosis. Polymerase chain reaction-based molecular tests targeting the ORF2/ORF3 gene region have been adopted for the detection of HEV RNA in formalin-fixed, paraffin-embedded tissues and successfully applied to routinely processed liver specimens by several pathology laboratories, including ours.[29,37,45] Molecular testing for HEV RNA on a liver biopsy thus remains an option for retrospective analyses or cases in which blood samples are no longer available for serologic testing. Although localization studies suggest themselves to be applied to liver tissues, so far only a few studies on HEV proteins and HEV RNA in the liver are reported. These include the detection of swine HEV RNA by in situ hybridization[49] and protein by immunohistochemistry,[50] the detection of HEV ORF2 and ORF3 proteins in human liver tissues by immunohistochemistry,[51] or the detection of HEV ORF3 protein in humanized mice.[52] However, not all of the images displayed in these reports withstand a critical examination with respect to specificity of signals shown. There is clearly a need for a systematic and comprehensive evaluation of immunohistochemistry (**Fig. 5**) and in situ hybridization for visualizing HEV proteins and RNA in human liver tissues, and determining the value of these tools in a diagnostic setting.

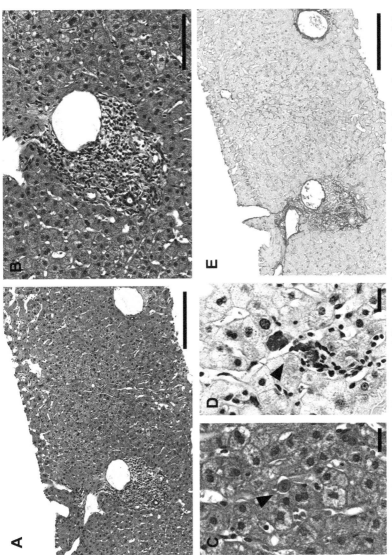

Fig. 4. Histology of a liver biopsy from a 66-year-old patient with liver transplantation 2 years and 9 months before a diagnosis of chronic hepatitis E virus genotype 3 infection presumably acquired by autochthonous infection. (A) Overview revealing predominantly portal inflammation and preserved lobular architecture (hematoxylin and eosin [H&E] stain, scale bar 200 μm). (B) Detailed view with a mononuclear inflammatory infiltrate in the portal tract without interface hepatitis (H&E, scale bar 100 μm). (C) High-power view displaying few scattered apoptotic hepatocytes (arrowhead) reflecting minimal activity (H&E stain, scale bar 20 μm) and (D) small lobular aggregates of ceroid-laden macrophages, indicative of preceded hepatocyte damage (Diastase-periodic acid Schiff stain, scale bar 20 μm). (E) Overview showing portal and periportal fibrosis with short septae (Sirius red stain, scale bar 200 μm).

> **Box 3**
> **Histologic features of hepatitis E**
>
> Fulminant liver failure
> - Panlobular necrosis
> - Parenchymal collapse
> - Bilirubinostasis
> - Clearing by ceroid-laden macrophages
>
> Acute hepatitis E
> - Mixed lobular and portal inflammation and interface activity (lymphocytes, plasma cells, histiocytes, neutrophil and eosinophil granulocytes)
> - Lobular disarray and increased number of Kupffer cells
> - Ballooned hepatocytes and pseudorosettes formation
> - Variable degree of hepatocyte necrosis (single apoptotic bodies/spotty necrosis/bridging necrosis)
> - Cholangitis and ductular proliferation
> - Hepatocytic and intracanalicular bilirubinostasis
>
> Chronic hepatitis E
> - Mononuclear portal based inflammation (predominantly lymphocytes), lacking or low interface activity
> - Single scattered apoptotic hepatocytes
> - Fibrosis development

SUMMARY

Our perception of hepatitis E has dramatically changed during the last years from a disease traditionally regarded to be only relevant in developing countries, over the "new kid on the block" status in industrialized countries starting about 2 decades ago, to a disease now clearly recognized as a leading cause of acute hepatitis worldwide, thus constituting a globally significant health problem. In the past, hepatitis E has been unrecognized or misdiagnosed in industrialized countries, and it presumably still is even today. This is due to the fact that the clinical and histologic presentations of hepatitis E are highly overlapping with hepatitis of other etiology, in particular non-E viral hepatitis and drug-induced liver injury, and far from specific or even characteristic. Clinical manifestations of hepatitis E are highly variable, including mainly

Table 3
Most relevant differential diagnosis of hepatitis E virus infection based on histologic patterns

Fulminant Liver Failure	Acute Hepatitis	Chronic Hepatitis
DILI, toxins	Viral non-E hepatotropic viruses (eg, HAV), and nonhepatotropic viruses (eg, EBV)	Viral non-E hepatotropic viruses (HBV, HCV)
Viral non-E hepatotropic viruses (eg, HBV), and nonhepatotropic viruses (eg, adenovirus)	Autoimmune hepatitis	Liver transplanted patients: rejection, recurrence of primary viral hepatitis (HCV)
Autoimmune hepatitis	DILI, toxins	
Metabolic disorders (eg, Wilsons' disease)		

Abbreviations: DILI, drug-induced liver injury; EBV, Epstein–Barr virus; HAV, hepatitis A virus; HBV, hepatitis B virus; HCV, hepatitis C virus.

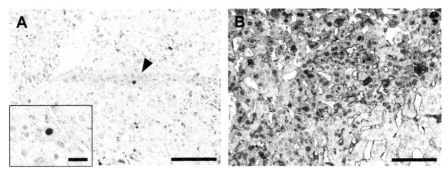

Fig. 5. Ancillary diagnostic tools for histology. (*A*) and (*B*) immunohistochemistry with hepatitis E virus open reading frame 2 antibody, ranging from (*A*) only single scattered positive nuclear (*arrowhead and insert*) or cytoplasmic (not shown) signals to (*B*) larger geographic areas with numerous hepatocytes with nuclear and/or cytoplasmic signals (scale bars 100 μm; insert scale bar 20 μm).

asymptomatic/subclinical presentations or acute, self-limiting hepatitis. Rarely, HEV presents as acute liver failure with a potentially fatal outcome. In immunocompromised individuals, chronic hepatitis is also found. Accordingly, a broad spectrum of histopathologic patterns of hepatitis E is observed comprising acute hepatitis potentially associated with cholestasis and/or variable degree of necrosis, and chronic hepatitis in immunocompromised individuals with potential fibrosis development. Thus, diagnosis of hepatitis E is expected to remain challenging in the near future. Increased awareness of hepatitis E and familiarity with diagnostics tools, in particular molecular testing for HEV RNA, and a low threshold for testing, will enable clinicians and pathologists to come to the diagnosis reliably and timely.

REFERENCES

1. Viswanathan R. Epidemiology. Indian J Med Res 1957;45(Suppl.):1–29.
2. Purcell RH, Emerson SU. Hepatitis E: an emerging awareness of an old disease. J Hepatol 2008;48(3):494–503.
3. Dalton HR, Bendall R, Ijaz S, et al. An emerging infection in developed countries. Lancet Infect Dis 2008;8(11):698–709.
4. Kuniholm MH, Purcell RH, McQuillan GM, et al. Epidemiology of hepatitis E virus in the United States: results from the Third National Health and Nutrition Examination Survey, 1988-1994. J Infect Dis 2009;200(1):48–56.
5. Mansuy JM, Gallian P, Dimeglio C, et al. A nationwide survey of hepatitis E viral infection in French blood donors. Hepatology 2016;63(4):1145–54.
6. Hartl J, Otto B, Madden RG, et al. Hepatitis E Seroprevalence in Europe: a meta-analysis. Viruses 2016;8(8).
7. Kamar N, Selves J, Mansuy JM, et al. Hepatitis E virus and chronic hepatitis in organ-transplant recipients. N Engl J Med 2008;358(8):811–7.
8. Kamar N, Garrouste C, Haagsma EB, et al. Factors associated with chronic hepatitis in patients with hepatitis E virus infection who have received solid organ transplants. Gastroenterology 2011;140(5):1481–9.
9. Smith DB, Simmonds P, International Committee on Taxonomy of Viruses Hepeviridae Study Group, et al. Consensus proposals for classification of the family Hepeviridae. J Gen Virol 2014;95(Pt 10):2223–32.

10. Debing Y, Moradpour D, Neyts J, et al. Update on hepatitis E virology: implications for clinical practice. J Hepatol 2016;65(1):200–12.
11. Lu L, Li C, Hagedorn CH. Phylogenetic analysis of global hepatitis E virus sequences: genetic diversity, subtypes and zoonosis. Rev Med Virol 2006;16(1):5–36.
12. Legrand-Abravanel F, Mansuy JM, Dubois M, et al. Hepatitis E virus genotype 3 diversity, France. Emerg Infect Dis 2009;15(1):110–4.
13. Kamar N, Bendall R, Legrand-Abravanel F, et al. Hepatitis E. Lancet 2012; 379(9835):2477–88.
14. Aggarwal R, Jameel S. Hepatitis E. Hepatology 2011;54(6):2218–26.
15. Mansuy JM, Bendall R, Legrand-Abravanel F, et al. Hepatitis E virus antibodies in blood donors, France. Emerg Infect Dis 2011;17(12):2309–12.
16. Hoofnagle JH, Nelson KE, Purcell RH. Hepatitis E. N Engl J Med 2012;367(13): 1237–44.
17. Hamid SS, Atiq M, Shehzad F, et al. Hepatitis E virus superinfection in patients with chronic liver disease. Hepatology 2002;36(2):474–8.
18. Woolson KL, Forbes A, Vine L, et al. Extra-hepatic manifestations of autochthonous hepatitis E infection. Aliment Pharmacol Ther 2014;40(11–12):1282–91.
19. Chau TN, Lai ST, Tse C, et al. Epidemiology and clinical features of sporadic hepatitis E as compared with hepatitis A. Am J Gastroenterol 2006;101(2):292–6.
20. Davern TJ, Chalasani N, Fontana RJ, et al. Acute hepatitis E infection accounts for some cases of suspected drug-induced liver injury. Gastroenterology 2011; 141(5):1665–72.e1-9.
21. Khuroo MS, Teli MR, Skidmore S, et al. Incidence and severity of viral hepatitis in pregnancy. Am J Med 1981;70(2):252–5.
22. Krain LJ, Atwell JE, Nelson KE, et al. Fetal and neonatal health consequences of vertically transmitted hepatitis E virus infection. Am J Trop Med Hyg 2014;90(2): 365–70.
23. Peron JM, Bureau C, Poirson H, et al. Fulminant liver failure from acute autochthonous hepatitis E in France: description of seven patients with acute hepatitis E and encephalopathy. J Viral Hepat 2007;14(5):298–303.
24. Kumar Acharya S, Kumar Sharma P, Singh R, et al. Hepatitis E virus (HEV) infection in patients with cirrhosis is associated with rapid decompensation and death. J Hepatol 2007;46(3):387–94.
25. Gerolami R, Moal V, Colson P. Chronic hepatitis E with cirrhosis in a kidney-transplant recipient. N Engl J Med 2008;358(8):859–60.
26. Dalton HR, Bendall RP, Keane FE, et al. Persistent carriage of hepatitis E virus in patients with HIV infection. N Engl J Med 2009;361(10):1025–7.
27. Haagsma EB, Niesters HG, van den Berg AP, et al. Prevalence of hepatitis E virus infection in liver transplant recipients. Liver Transpl 2009;15(10):1225–8.
28. Gerolami R, Moal V, Picard C, et al. Hepatitis E virus as an emerging cause of chronic liver disease in organ transplant recipients. J Hepatol 2009;50(3):622–4.
29. Protzer U, Bohm F, Longerich T, et al. Molecular detection of hepatitis E virus (HEV) in liver biopsies after liver transplantation. Mod Pathol 2015;28(4):523–32.
30. Behrendt P, Steinmann E, Manns MP, et al. The impact of hepatitis E in the liver transplant setting. J Hepatol 2014;61(6):1418–29.
31. Dalton HR, Kamar N, van Eijk JJ, et al. Hepatitis E virus and neurological injury. Nat Rev Neurol 2016;12(2):77–85.
32. Khudyakov Y, Kamili S. Serological diagnostics of hepatitis E virus infection. Virus Res 2011;161(1):84–92.

33. El-Sayed Zaki M, El-Deen Zaghloul MH, El Sayed O. Acute sporadic hepatitis E in children: diagnostic relevance of specific immunoglobulin M and immunoglobulin G compared with nested reverse transcriptase PCR. FEMS Immunol Med Microbiol 2006;48(1):16–20.
34. Huang S, Zhang X, Jiang H, et al. Profile of acute infectious markers in sporadic hepatitis E. PLoS One 2010;5(10):e13560.
35. Aggarwal R. Diagnosis of hepatitis E. Nat Rev Gastroenterol Hepatol 2013;10(1): 24–33.
36. Jothikumar N, Cromeans TL, Robertson BH, et al. A broadly reactive one-step real-time RT-PCR assay for rapid and sensitive detection of hepatitis E virus. J Virol Methods 2006;131(1):65–71.
37. Chijioke O, Bawohl M, Springer E, et al. Hepatitis e virus detection in liver tissue from patients with suspected drug-induced liver injury. Front Med (Lausanne) 2015;2:20.
38. Gyarmati P, Mohammed N, Norder H, et al. Universal detection of hepatitis E virus by two real-time PCR assays: TaqMan and Primer-Probe Energy Transfer. J Virol Methods 2007;146(1–2):226–35.
39. Chauhan A, Jameel S, Dilawari JB, et al. Hepatitis E virus transmission to a volunteer. Lancet 1993;341(8838):149–50.
40. Friedman LS, Lee SR, Nelson SB, et al. Case 36-2016. N Engl J Med 2016; 375(21):2082–92.
41. Gupta DN, Smetana HF. The histopathology of viral hepatitis as seen in the Delhi epidemic (1955-56). Indian J Med Res 1957;45(Suppl.):101–13.
42. Khuroo MS. Study of an epidemic of non-A, non-B hepatitis. Possibility of another human hepatitis virus distinct from post-transfusion non-A, non-B type. Am J Med 1980;68(6):818–24.
43. Agrawal V, Goel A, Rawat A, et al. Histological and immunohistochemical features in fatal acute fulminant hepatitis E. Indian J Pathol Microbiol 2012;55(1):22–7.
44. Malcolm P, Dalton H, Hussaini HS, et al. The histology of acute autochthonous hepatitis E virus infection. Histopathology 2007;51(2):190–4.
45. Drebber U, Odenthal M, Aberle SW, et al. Hepatitis E in liver biopsies from patients with acute hepatitis of clinically unexplained origin. Front Physiol 2013;4: 351.
46. Peron JM, Danjoux M, Kamar N, et al. Liver histology in patients with sporadic acute hepatitis E: a study of 11 patients from South-West France. Virchows Arch 2007;450(4):405–10.
47. Lockwood GL, Fernandez-Barredo S, Bendall R, et al. Hepatitis E autochthonous infection in chronic liver disease. Eur J Gastroenterol Hepatol 2008;20(8):800–3.
48. Kamar N, Abravanel F, Selves J, et al. Influence of immunosuppressive therapy on the natural history of genotype 3 hepatitis-E virus infection after organ transplantation. Transplantation 2010;89(3):353–60.
49. Choi C, Chae C. Localization of swine hepatitis E virus in liver and extrahepatic tissues from naturally infected pigs by in situ hybridization. J Hepatol 2003; 38(6):827–32.
50. Ha SK, Chae C. Immunohistochemistry for the detection of swine hepatitis E virus in the liver. J Viral Hepat 2004;11(3):263–7.
51. Gupta P, Jagya N, Pabhu SB, et al. Immunohistochemistry for the diagnosis of hepatitis E virus infection. J Viral Hepat 2012;19(2):e177–83.
52. Sayed IM, Verhoye L, Cocquerel L, et al. Study of hepatitis E virus infection of genotype 1 and 3 in mice with humanised liver. Gut 2016:1–10.

Hepatic Progenitor Cells
An Update

Matthias Van Haele, MD, Tania Roskams, MD, PhD*

KEYWORDS

- Hepatic progenitor cell • Liver stem cell • Liver progenitor cell • Liver regeneration
- Liver niche

KEY POINTS

- During normal liver homeostasis, the HPC and its niche are in a quiescent state. A significant activation and contribution to liver regeneration are seen after severe liver damage.
- The interaction among HPCs, the HPC niche, cytokines, chemokines, and growth factors is critical for the activation of the HPC compartment.
- Senescence of the parenchymal compartment after chronic liver injury is clearly an essential requirement for the proliferation of the HPCs.
- Recent evidence suggests the existence of other niches with potent stemness. However, further research of these subjects is required for better insights.

INTRODUCTION

The liver is an intriguing organ because of its impressive regenerative capacity after considerable damage. This damage can be toxic, genetic, metabolic, viral, or immunologic. When this occurs in an unchallenged healthy liver, the loss of hepatocytes is replenished by the remaining mature and functional hepatocytes.[1] One of the exemplary illustrations, and also a classic animal model, is the recovery after a partial hepatectomy (HPx) in rats and mice. Over the years, many research groups have created various animal models to induce liver damage and regeneration. They studied both the self-renewal capacity of hepatocytes and cholangiocytes after liver injury, and possible differentation towards stem/progenitor cells in the liver. These stem/progenitor cells, called oval cells in rodent models, has the ability to differentiate into cholangiocytes or hepatocytes when regular liver homeostasis becomes compromised, such as by toxic inhibition of the proliferative capacity of hepatocytes or senescence in the setting of chronic liver diseases. The complicated process of regeneration is driven by many different cytokines and growth factors. In clinical practice, the regenerative

Disclosure Statement: The authors have nothing to disclose.
Liver Research Unit, Department of Imaging and Pathology, KU Leuven and University Hospitals Leuven, Minderbroederstraat 12, 3000 Leuven, Belgium
* Corresponding author.
E-mail address: tania.roskams@uzleuven.be

Gastroenterol Clin N Am 46 (2017) 409–420
http://dx.doi.org/10.1016/j.gtc.2017.01.011
0889-8553/17/© 2017 Elsevier Inc. All rights reserved.

capacity of the liver is well known in living donor liver transplantation, which was first performed from adult to child and nowadays also from adult to adult.[2,3] Despite this success, there is still a significant shortage of liver transplants. A study in the United Kingdom showed that 19% of adult nonurgent registrants died within 1 year awaiting a graft.[4] For this reason, researchers are investigating the possibility of cell-based therapy. Next to isolated hepatocytes, stem/progenitor cells are potential candidates. Thanks to the increasing knowledge of stem cells, various potential targets are suggested.[5,6] Stem cells that have been investigated in the light of liver regeneration are hepatic progenitor cells (HPC), mesenchymal stem cells, and bone marrow cells. This article focuses on the HPC and its niche.

HEPATIC PROGENITOR CELLS

The hepatocyte is a parenchymal cell with a long life cycle, which is responsible for liver regeneration under normal conditions.[7] When the regenerative capacity of the hepatocyte is compromised, because of senescence, which is indicated by p16 and p21 immunohistochemical positivity, it is accepted that a population of HPCs is activated.[8–10] This activation aids in the regeneration process.[11,12] The extent and the specific contribution of these cells in liver regeneration are not entirely clear. HPCs are located in the smallest part of the biliary tree, the canals of Hering, which are also known as the transition zone between the terminal segment of the bile duct epithelium and the hepatocytes.[13,14] This is a strategic location because of its regenerative possibilities toward hepatocytes or cholangiocytes. A difficulty for existing research in this domain is the widespread use of a diffuse nomenclature for these HPCs and its related reaction. Intermediate hepatobiliary cell, liver progenitor cell, liver stem cell, or atypical ductular cell are some examples of regularly used terms.[15–17] The term "oval cells" is used in many articles, and is the equivalent of HPCs in rodents.[18,19] Another phenomenon is the so-called ductular reaction. This ductular reaction is histologically recognized as the proliferation of ductular structures in the portal triad.[20] It is seen in a variety of liver diseases, ranging from acute to chronic injuries (**Fig. 1**). The ductular reaction is thought to harbor the HPC compartment.[20–23] The study by Yoon

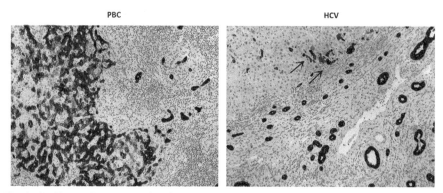

Fig. 1. (*Left*) Histologic example of an extensive ductular reaction, lymphocytic infiltration, and cholestasis in primary biliary cholangitis (PBC). In this chronic and progressive cholestatic disease, we stained the diffuse bile ductular reaction and cholate stasis with cytokeratin 7 (original magnification ×100). (*Right*) A case of hepatitis C virus (HCV) at a later stage with accompanying ductular proliferation. Note the differentiation process from strong- to weak-stained cytokeratin-7-positive cells toward the damaged hepatic compartment (*arrows*) (original magnification ×200).

and colleagues[24] concluded that the progeny of the HPC in chronic viral hepatitis is derived from the ductular reaction. When one combines these histologic findings with the measurements of telomere lengths in epithelial cell adhesion molecule (EpCAM)(+) hepatocytes versus EpCAM(−) hepatocytes and the gene-expression profiles of the HPCs found by our group (Spee and colleagues), these data support the connection of the HPCs and the ductular reaction in virtually all human liver diseases.[24–28] In addition, we found in these cryopreserved liver tissue of human patients a strong activation of the Wnt pathway in specimens with known acute necrotizing hepatitis after hepatitis C infection (hepatocyte loss).[25] This was in contrast to the high activation of the Notch signaling in primary biliary cholangitis (cholangiocyte loss).

IDENTIFICATION OF THE HEPATIC PROGENITOR CELL

When using the standard hematoxylin and eosin staining, HPCs are not distinguishable in their surrounding environment because of their inconspicuous morphology. These small epithelial cells have a remarkable oval-shaped nucleus with a limited amount of cytoplasm. Several stainings, such as EpCAM, macrophage inhibitory cytokine-1-1C3, prominin-1, neuronal cell adhesion molecule/CD56, sex-determining region Y-box 9, cytokeratin-7, and cytokeratine-19 (CK19), have shown positivity in these cells.[25,29–31] Despite the existence of an extensive staining panel, no exclusive staining for the sole use of targeting the HPC has been found. This is acceptable when understanding the continuous pathophysiologic changes of the HPC after activation and its presumed bilineage potential of differentiation toward hepatocytes and biliary epithelial cells (BECs). The pathway of differentiation depends on the cell type that endured the most damage during the injury, as is seen in hepatitis, where the regeneration is stimulated toward the hepatocellular compartment. If the disease is particularly focused on cholangiocytes, as observed in primary biliary cholangitis or primary sclerosing cholangitis, the regeneration is mainly stimulated toward BECs.[32–34]

However, the level of contribution of the HPC to liver homeostasis is still in debate. It has been established that the turnover rate of cells that are responsible for the natural homeostasis of an organ is much slower in the liver compared with the epidermis or the gastrointestinal tract.[35,36] It has been shown that the turnover of noninjured hepatocytes occurs after several months at least.[37] Because of this slow turnover rate, many studies have used the Cre/loxP recombination technique allowing one to target specific DNA alterations that can be triggered by an external stimulus. Furuyama and colleagues[38] used this tamoxifen-inducible genetic lineage tracing system on a mouse model. The initially labeled cholangiocytes were tagged by the inducible recombinase CreERT2, which was inserted in the region of the Sox9 locus. They found an expansion of the Sox9-positive cells in the whole liver parenchyma during liver regeneration, demonstrating the role of Sox9-positive stem/progenitor cells to be a source of newly generated hepatocytes. The study of Furuyama and colleagues[38] also supported the "streaming liver hypothesis," which was first proposed by Zajicek and colleagues[39] in 1985. They suggested the existence of stem/progenitor cell compartment near the periportal area with a regenerative capacity of distributing cells toward the pericentral region. In contrast, two other lineage-tracing studies that were using osteopontin and Sox9, could not support the same results to confirm the streaming liver hypothesis.[40,41] Comparable results were observed after fate-tracing of hepatocytes based on a Cre recombination and activation by an adenoassociated viral vector.[42,43] Subsequently, a study from Español-Suñer and colleagues[40] in mice followed the fate of stem/progenitor cells and biliary cells after several types of induced liver injuries. No contribution of stem/progenitor cells to the liver regeneration was seen after partial

HPx, acute and chronic exposure to carbon tetrachloride, or after a 3,5-diethoxycarbonyl-1,4-dihydrocollidine diet. On the contrary, the choline-deficient ethionine-supplemented model showed a limited stem/progenitor cell distribution of up to 2.45% of the hepatocytes. A comparable setup was performed by Rodrigo-Torres and colleagues,[44] which showed similar outcomes. Only mice fed with the choline-deficient ethionine-supplemented-diet had a contribution of stem/progenitor cells up to 1.86% of the total hepatocytes after recovery. Thereby, Malato and colleagues[42] minimized the importance of HPCs in traditional liver homeostasis.

Taking into account all these findings, one could debate the relevance of the HPCs in liver regeneration.[45] However, not one of these studies were able to mimic complete senescence of all the hepatocytes as is present in advanced human liver diseases. The importance of senescence was illustrated by a study of our group. We showed that the proliferative capacity of the hepatocytes needed to be decreased and a threshold of a least 50% loss of hepatocytes was required before a significant proliferation of HPCs was observed.[46] The classic model for an entire senescence state is the use of 2-acetylaminofluorene in rats. This carcinogenic substance is a substrate for cytochrome P-450 and is known for its direct interaction with DNA to produce DNA adducts in hepatocytes. 2-Acetylaminofluorene is used to induce a complete blockage of the proliferative capacity of hepatocytes after a partial HPx. Making use of this rat model in practice, several studies implied a differentiation of oval cells toward hepatocytes.[47–52] Additionally, an attractive zebrafish model of Choi and colleagues[53] revealed the regenerative capacity of BECs toward hepatocytes after depletion of the hepatocytes due to usage of metronidazole, causing severe liver damage. Furthermore, supporting evidence is found in the histologic study of cirrhotic human livers. Small regenerative nodules, also known as buds, are seen in these injured livers and are composed of hepatocytes with only a few ductules.[54] Three-dimensional reconstruction showed that intraseptal hepatocytes were derived from the CK19-positive ductular reaction. This strongly suggests the active participation of HPCs and confirms their location in the smaller branches of the biliary tract, more accurately the canals of Hering.[55] A recent study of Stueck and Wanless[56] stressed the importance of these buds as a mechanism for regeneration in cirrhotic livers and also underlined the stem/progenitor-like characteristics of these cells. Regarding the emphasis toward the senescence of hepatocytes, Lu and colleagues[57] demonstrated what happens if the proliferative capacity of hepatocytes is exhausted. Their mouse model had an inducible deletion of Mdm2, an E3 ubiquitin ligase involved in the degradation of p53, present in almost all hepatocytes. Subsequent apoptosis, necrosis, and particularly the senescence was observed by the expression of p21. After this induced injury, they recognized a significant contribution of HPCs to the renewal of hepatocytes and BECs. Taking into account all this evidence, it seems that there is a role for the HPC in the regeneration of human liver diseases.

However, the previously mentioned studies do not exclude that subpopulations of hepatocytes are capable of self-renewal during mild liver injuries. A recent study by Wang and colleagues[58] identified such a particular, unique niche of hepatocytes next to the central vein. These pericentral hepatocytes were followed by using the Wnt-responsive gene Axin2 in mice models over a 1-year period. They observed a significant homeostatic renewal of descendants of these Axin2+ cells toward the periportal area. They demonstrated that the secretion of Wnt signals of central vein endothelial cells contributed to the proliferation of this niche (**Fig. 2**). However, Font-Burgada and colleagues[59] showed that another niche of periportal Sox9+ hepatocytes was able to undergo an extensive proliferation by replenishing the liver mass in chronic liver injuries. One can conclude that liver restore is the result of hepatocyte and HPC regeneration and that the contribution of each compartment depends on the setting.

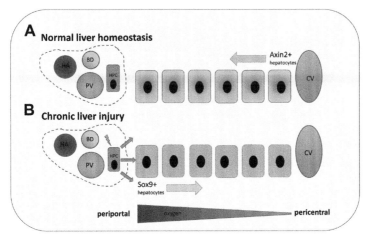

Fig. 2. Schematic illustration of normal liver homeostasis and a chronically injured liver model. (*A*) Self-renewing Axin2+ hepatocytes are located near the central vein and show the continuous renewal of hepatocytes under normal conditions. The participation of these cells when an injury is present is still unclear. (*B*) In contrast, HPCs are known for their supporting role in chronic liver injury when all other parenchymal cells become senescent. The Sox9+ hepatocytes, which are located in the periportal area, contribute to the parenchymal regeneration until the senescent state of the hepatocytes is reached. BD, bile duct; CV, central vein; HA, hepatic artery; PV, portal vein.

THE HEPATIC PROGENITOR CELL NICHE

It is clear that the regeneration of the liver and the cells involved are part of a complex mechanism that is not controlled by only one determinant, but by multiple overlapping and balanced pathways (discussed later). Because of the complex functionality, one can hypothesize that the HPC has many interactions with the nearby environment. This is called the "HPC niche" and contains macrophages (Kupffer cells or stellate macrophages), hepatic stellate cells (HSCs), liver sinusoidal endothelial cells (LSECs), and the extracellular matrix (ECM) itself (**Fig. 3**).

Hepatic macrophages have been an exciting target because of their critical role in the maintenance and stimulation of the hepatic progenitor niche, which marks them as a possible therapeutic target in human liver diseases.[60] Macrophages are well known for their function as phagocytes, but they also actively participate in the inflammatory response. This is illustrated by their involvement in the recruitment of monocytes, leading to several hepatic diseases that are followed by regeneration of the parenchymal compartment through proliferation of the HPCs.[61] The tumor necrosis factor–like weak inducer of apoptosis (TWEAK) is an important regulator of HPCs' activation and proliferation, secreted by the surrounding macrophages and other inflammatory cells.[62–64] The expression of its receptor, fibroblast growth factor–inducible 14 (Fn14), is significantly increased after HPx compared with healthy liver models.[65] This TWEAK/Fn14 cascade has been shown to be a necessity for the regeneration of liver tissue.[66] Another intriguing characteristic of TWEAK was seen in a study using anti-TWEAK antibodies, which was followed by an augmentation of the fibrotic liver regeneration.[67] The macrophages are involved in differentiation of HPCs toward the hepatic lineage after stimulation of the canonical Wnt3a/β-catenin pathway.[33]

HSCs are also known as Ito cells and are mesenchymal cells located in the perisinusoidal space of the liver (space of Disse). Histologically they are characterized by the

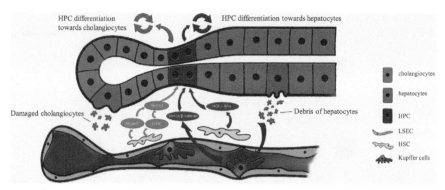

Fig. 3. Illustration of the HPC niche and its histologic position. In a healthy liver the niche is located near the periportal area and within the smaller branches of the bile duct, also known as the canals of Hering. The niche harbors the Kupffer cells (hepatic macrophages), hepatic stellate cells, and liver sinusoidal endothelial cells, which are necessary for the regeneration process of injured liver. When a mild liver injury occurs, the parenchymal compartment is capable of self-renewal without a significant interference of HPCs. After several years of liver injury, the regenerative capacity of the hepatocytes becomes exhausted, and the HPCs start to provide a dominant supportive role. Differentiation of the HPC toward the hepatic lineage has especially been linked to the Wnt3a/β-catenin and HGF/c-Met pathways that are initiated by Kupffer cells and HSCs. Note the stimulatory effect of hepatic debris on the macrophages, which stimulates these Kupffer cells to initiate the Wnt3a/β-catenin pathway. Regeneration toward the biliary component is mainly influenced by Notch1, which is stimulated by secretion of Jagged1 and epidermal growth factor receptor. For the sake of simplicity, the Angpt2 and the fibroblast growth factor 7 pathways are not shown. EGFR, epidermal growth factor receptor; HGF, hepatocyte growth factor.

presence of lipid droplets that are filled with stored retinoids.[68] Another interesting function of the HSC is their dominant role in liver fibrosis. On liver injury, these cells differentiate into myofibroblasts and are responsible for the highest production of collagen toward the ECM.[69,70] This makes them an excellent target for new insights in liver fibrosis and future therapies. Furthermore, there seems to be a strong association between the hepatocyte growth factor (HGF) together with its c-Met receptor and the proliferative capabilities of the HPCs. This significant relationship was detected by Ishikawa and colleagues.[71] After losing the HGF/c-Met signal transduction system with its downstream components, the expansion and differentiation of the HPCs was damaged on liver injury. Although HGF/c-Met was shown to be a strong inducer of differentiation of HPCs toward the hepatocytes, another critical component, epidermal growth factor receptor, seems to trigger the HPCs differentiation toward the cholangiocyte lineage by stimulation of the Notch1 pathway.[71,72] Fibroblast growth factor 7 is suggested as another component of the HSC that is linked to HPC proliferation and the corresponding regeneration.[73] One later study demonstrated that the expression of fibroblast growth factor 7 led to the expression of HPC-like cells and increased hepatic dysfunction.[74] Meanwhile, the differentiation of HPCs toward cholangiocytes is promoted through secretion of Jagged1 by HSCs, which induces stimulation of the Notch signaling cascade.[33,75–77]

The third cell of the liver progenitor niche is the LSEC, which forms the endothelium barrier between the blood and the hepatocytes. The endothelium is in the presence of specialized fenestrae and in the absence of a basal lamina underneath.[78] A recent study of Ding and colleagues[79] revealed that some liver injuries induce an upregulation of CXCR7 and CXCR4. Depending on the type of injury (acute vs chronic), these receptors trigger a cascade of proregenerative or profibrotic factors. The orchestrating function of the LSEC is also underlined by new insights into the role of the angiogenic molecule angiopoietin-2 (Angpt2). By regulation of Angpt2, the LSEC was capable of controlling the hepatocytes and its own proliferation.[80]

Not only do particular cell types seem to be able to influence the behavior of the HPCs, but also the ECM has an impact on the expansion and differentiation of the HPC.[81] The ECM is a sophisticated complex with a wide variety of functions ranging from structural support to regulation of intercellular communication.[82] Several studies showed the importance of laminin and collagens in the proximity of the HPC niche in distinct liver injury models.[81,83,84] Other recent studies have illustrated the complexity and influence of the ECM on the environment of the HPC niche. A recent result by Kaylan and colleagues[85] showed interactions between Notch ligands, transforming growth factor-β, and ECM proteins in the bipotential differentiation of HPCs. Other results demonstrated the cooperation of integrin $\alpha v \beta 6$ and connective tissue growth factor for the clonogenic potential and differentiation of the HPCs.[86,87] These promising results toward potential targets merit further investigation.

HEPATIC PROGENITOR CELL AND CANCER

Hepatocellular carcinoma (HCC) is a complication in chronic viral hepatitis, nonalcoholic fatty liver diseases, and alcoholic liver disease, whereas cholangiocellular carcinomas are seen in the setting of chronic biliary diseases.[88] A common end point of all these diseases is the inability of the parenchymal compartment to repair the injured cells. The senescence of hepatocytes triggers the activation and proliferation of the HPC niche, suggesting that HCC may derive from an HPC origin.[28,89,90] This hypothesis supports differentiation of the HPC during cancer progression, thereby taking into account the existence of a subpopulation of cancer with histopathologic features of hepatocellular and biliary differentiation, the so-called hepatocholangiocarcinoma or mixed tumor.[91,92] Although the underlying mechanism remains elusive, HCCs with high expression of progenitor cell biomarkers have shown to have a poor prognosis.[93] One study by Villanueva and coworkers[94] demonstrated that the Notch signaling pathway is strongly correlated with the promotion of HCCs. Next to this HPC-related marker, CK19 has been reported as a prognostic marker in human HCCs.[95,96] Another hypothesis in the carcinogenesis of HCC implies the dedifferentiation of the hepatocyte itself toward an HPC-like state. This presumed plasticity of the hepatocyte by inducing dedifferentiation has been illustrated by Chen and colleagues.[97] In view of the prognostic importance and different reaction to treatment, a relevant histologic-based classification of primary liver cancers is necessary.

SUMMARY

The HPC has been under investigation for many years. Because of its complex involvement in regeneration and differentiation, it has not been possible to select one specific biomarker for the identification of the HPC. However, discrepancies between studies are explained because of variations between diverse animal models, type of induced liver damage, different tracing systems, and various selection criteria for the HPC. It seems clear that the HPC has a limited role in the regeneration of hepatocytes or cholangiocytes when these compartments are not too injured, such as after partial HPx. HPC regeneration becomes important when other mechanisms fail. This is the case in most chronic human liver diseases and in submassive acute liver injury. Additionally, we emphasize the role of the HPC niche, because these interactions are of irrefutable importance and harbor interesting possibilities for future treatment strategies.

REFERENCES

1. Michalopoulos GK. Principles of liver regeneration and growth homeostasis. Compr Physiol 2013;3(1):485–513.
2. Strong RW, Lynch SV, Ong TH, et al. Successful liver transplantation from a living donor to her son. N Engl J Med 1990;322(21):1505–7.
3. Hashikura Y, Makuuchi M, Kawasaki S, et al. Successful living-related partial liver transplantation to an adult patient. Lancet 1994;343(8907):1233–4.
4. Johnson RJ, Bradbury LL, Martin K, et al. Organ donation and transplantation in the UK-the last decade: a report from the UK national transplant registry. Transplantation 2014;97(Suppl 1):S1–27.
5. Shiota G, Itaba N. Progress in stem cell-based therapy for liver disease. Hepatol Res 2016;47(2):127–41.
6. Fagoonee S, Famulari ES, Silengo L, et al. Prospects for adult stem cells in the treatment of liver diseases. Stem Cells Dev 2016;25(20):1471–82.
7. Duncan AW, Dorrell C, Grompe M. Stem cells and liver regeneration. Gastroenterology 2009;137(2):466–81.
8. Lunz JG 3rd, Contrucci S, Ruppert K, et al. Replicative senescence of biliary epithelial cells precedes bile duct loss in chronic liver allograft rejection: increased expression of p21(WAF1/Cip1) as a disease marker and the influence of immunosuppressive drugs. Am J Pathol 2001;158(4):1379–90.
9. Zhu C, Ikemoto T, Utsunomiya T, et al. Senescence-related genes possibly responsible for poor liver regeneration after hepatectomy in elderly patients. J Gastroenterol Hepatol 2014;29(5):1102–8.
10. Gutierrez-Reyes G, del Carmen Garcia de Leon M, Varela-Fascinetto G, et al. Cellular senescence in livers from children with end stage liver disease. PLoS One 2010;5(4):e10231.
11. Libbrecht L, Roskams T. Hepatic progenitor cells in human liver diseases. Semin Cell Dev Biol 2002;13(6):389–96.
12. Tan J, Hytiroglou P, Wieczorek R, et al. Immunohistochemical evidence for hepatic progenitor cells in liver diseases. Liver 2002;22(5):365–73.
13. Theise ND, Saxena R, Portmann BC, et al. The canals of Hering and hepatic stem cells in humans. Hepatology 1999;30(6):1425–33.
14. Roskams TA, Theise ND, Balabaud C, et al. Nomenclature of the finer branches of the biliary tree: canals, ductules, and ductular reactions in human livers. Hepatology 2004;39(6):1739–45.
15. Ziol M, Nault JC, Aout M, et al. Intermediate hepatobiliary cells predict an increased risk of hepatocarcinogenesis in patients with hepatitis C virus-related cirrhosis. Gastroenterology 2010;139(1):335–343 e332.
16. Parent R, Marion MJ, Furio L, et al. Origin and characterization of a human bipotent liver progenitor cell line. Gastroenterology 2004;126(4):1147–56.
17. Strick-Marchand H, Morosan S, Charneau P, et al. Bipotential mouse embryonic liver stem cell lines contribute to liver regeneration and differentiate as bile ducts and hepatocytes. Proc Natl Acad Sci U S A 2004;101(22):8360–5.
18. Shinozuka H, Lombardi B, Sell S, et al. Early histological and functional alterations of ethionine liver carcinogenesis in rats fed a choline-deficient diet. Cancer Res 1978;38(4):1092–8.
19. Yovchev MI, Grozdanov PN, Joseph B, et al. Novel hepatic progenitor cell surface markers in the adult rat liver. Hepatology 2007;45(1):139–49.
20. Roskams T, Desmet V. Ductular reaction and its diagnostic significance. Semin Diagn Pathol 1998;15(4):259–69.

21. Zhou H, Rogler LE, Teperman L, et al. Identification of hepatocytic and bile ductular cell lineages and candidate stem cells in bipolar ductular reactions in cirrhotic human liver. Hepatology 2007;45(3):716–24.

22. Williams MJ, Clouston AD, Forbes SJ. Links between hepatic fibrosis, ductular reaction, and progenitor cell expansion. Gastroenterology 2014;146(2):349–56.

23. Gouw AS, Clouston AD, Theise ND. Ductular reactions in human liver: diversity at the interface. Hepatology 2011;54(5):1853–63.

24. Yoon SM, Gerasimidou D, Kuwahara R, et al. Epithelial cell adhesion molecule (EpCAM) marks hepatocytes newly derived from stem/progenitor cells in humans. Hepatology 2011;53(3):964–73.

25. Spee B, Carpino G, Schotanus BA, et al. Characterisation of the liver progenitor cell niche in liver diseases: potential involvement of Wnt and Notch signalling. Gut 2010;59(2):247–57.

26. Gadd VL, Skoien R, Powell EE, et al. The portal inflammatory infiltrate and ductular reaction in human nonalcoholic fatty liver disease. Hepatology 2014;59(4): 1393–405.

27. Carpino G, Nobili V, Renzi A, et al. Macrophage activation in pediatric nonalcoholic fatty liver disease (NAFLD) correlates with hepatic progenitor cell response via Wnt3a pathway. PLoS One 2016;11(6):e0157246.

28. Clouston AD, Powell EE, Walsh MJ, et al. Fibrosis correlates with a ductular reaction in hepatitis C: roles of impaired replication, progenitor cells and steatosis. Hepatology 2005;41(4):809–18.

29. Yovchev MI, Grozdanov PN, Zhou H, et al. Identification of adult hepatic progenitor cells capable of repopulating injured rat liver. Hepatology 2008;47(2):636–47.

30. Dorrell C, Erker L, Schug J, et al. Prospective isolation of a bipotential clonogenic liver progenitor cell in adult mice. Genes Dev 2011;25(11):1193–203.

31. Libbrecht L, Desmet V, Van Damme B, et al. The immunohistochemical phenotype of dysplastic foci in human liver: correlation with putative progenitor cells. J Hepatol 2000;33(1):76–84.

32. Roskams TA, Libbrecht L, Desmet VJ. Progenitor cells in diseased human liver. Semin Liver Dis 2003;23(4):385–96.

33. Boulter L, Govaere O, Bird TG, et al. Macrophage-derived Wnt opposes Notch signaling to specify hepatic progenitor cell fate in chronic liver disease. Nat Med 2012;18(4):572–9.

34. Boulter L, Lu WY, Forbes SJ. Differentiation of progenitors in the liver: a matter of local choice. J Clin Invest 2013;123(5):1867–73.

35. Weinstein GD, McCullough JL, Ross P. Cell proliferation in normal epidermis. J Invest Dermatol 1984;82(6):623–8.

36. Umar S. Intestinal stem cells. Curr Gastroenterol Rep 2010;12(5):340–8.

37. Magami Y, Azuma T, Inokuchi H, et al. Cell proliferation and renewal of normal hepatocytes and bile duct cells in adult mouse liver. Liver 2002;22(5):419–25.

38. Furuyama K, Kawaguchi Y, Akiyama H, et al. Continuous cell supply from a Sox9-expressing progenitor zone in adult liver, exocrine pancreas and intestine. Nat Genet 2011;43(1):34–41.

39. Zajicek G, Oren R, Weinreb M Jr. The streaming liver. Liver 1985;5(6):293–300.

40. Español-Suñer R, Carpentier R, Van Hul N, et al. Liver progenitor cells yield functional hepatocytes in response to chronic liver injury in mice. Gastroenterology 2012;143(6):1564–75.e1567.

41. Carpentier R, Suner RE, van Hul N, et al. Embryonic ductal plate cells give rise to cholangiocytes, periportal hepatocytes, and adult liver progenitor cells. Gastroenterology 2011;141(4):1432–8.e1-4.

42. Malato Y, Naqvi S, Schurmann N, et al. Fate tracing of mature hepatocytes in mouse liver homeostasis and regeneration. J Clin Invest 2011;121(12):4850–60.

43. Schaub JR, Malato Y, Gormond C, et al. Evidence against a stem cell origin of new hepatocytes in a common mouse model of chronic liver injury. Cell Rep 2014;8(4):933–9.

44. Rodrigo-Torres D, Affo S, Coll M, et al. The biliary epithelium gives rise to liver progenitor cells. Hepatology 2014;60(4):1367–77.

45. Reid LM. Paradoxes in studies of liver regeneration: relevance of the parable of the blind men and the elephant. Hepatology 2015;62(2):330–3.

46. Katoonizadeh A, Nevens F, Verslype C, et al. Liver regeneration in acute severe liver impairment: a clinicopathological correlation study. Liver Int 2006;26(10): 1225–33.

47. Sarraf C, Lalani EN, Golding M, et al. Cell behavior in the acetylaminofluorene-treated regenerating rat liver. Light and electron microscopic observations. Am J Pathol 1994;145(5):1114–26.

48. Evarts RP, Nagy P, Marsden E, et al. A precursor-product relationship exists between oval cells and hepatocytes in rat liver. Carcinogenesis 1987;8(11): 1737–40.

49. Alison MR, Golding M, Sarraf CE, et al. Liver damage in the rat induces hepatocyte stem cells from biliary epithelial cells. Gastroenterology 1996;110(4): 1182–90.

50. Evarts RP, Nagy P, Nakatsukasa H, et al. In vivo differentiation of rat liver oval cells into hepatocytes. Cancer Res 1989;49(6):1541–7.

51. Paku S, Nagy P, Kopper L, et al. 2-acetylaminofluorene dose-dependent differentiation of rat oval cells into hepatocytes: confocal and electron microscopic studies. Hepatology 2004;39(5):1353–61.

52. Golding M, Sarraf CE, Lalani EN, et al. Oval cell differentiation into hepatocytes in the acetylaminofluorene-treated regenerating rat liver. Hepatology 1995; 22(4 Pt 1):1243–53.

53. Choi TY, Ninov N, Stainier DY, et al. Extensive conversion of hepatic biliary epithelial cells to hepatocytes after near total loss of hepatocytes in zebrafish. Gastroenterology 2014;146(3):776–88.

54. Wanless IR, Nakashima E, Sherman M. Regression of human cirrhosis. Morphologic features and the genesis of incomplete septal cirrhosis. Arch Pathol Lab Med 2000;124(11):1599–607.

55. Falkowski O, An HJ, Ianus IA, et al. Regeneration of hepatocyte 'buds' in cirrhosis from intrabiliary stem cells. J Hepatol 2003;39(3):357–64.

56. Stueck AE, Wanless IR. Hepatocyte buds derived from progenitor cells repopulate regions of parenchymal extinction in human cirrhosis. Hepatology 2015; 61(5):1696–707.

57. Lu W, Bird T, Boulter L, et al. Hepatic progenitor cells of biliary origin with liver repopulation capacity. Nature Cell Biology 2015;17(8):971–83.

58. Wang B, Zhao L, Fish M, et al. Self-renewing diploid Axin2(+) cells fuel homeostatic renewal of the liver. Nature 2015;524(7564):180–5.

59. Font-Burgada J, Shalapour S, Ramaswamy S, et al. Hybrid periportal hepatocytes regenerate the injured liver without giving rise to cancer. Cell 2015; 162(4):766–79.

60. Ju C, Tacke F. Hepatic macrophages in homeostasis and liver diseases: from pathogenesis to novel therapeutic strategies. Cell Mol Immunol 2016;13(3): 316–27.

61. Elsegood CL, Chan CW, Degli-Esposti MA, et al. Kupffer cell-monocyte communication is essential for initiating murine liver progenitor cell-mediated liver regeneration. Hepatology 2015;62(4):1272–84.

62. Jakubowski A, Ambrose C, Parr M, et al. TWEAK induces liver progenitor cell proliferation. J Clin Invest 2005;115(9):2330–40.

63. Bird TG, Lu WY, Boulter L, et al. Bone marrow injection stimulates hepatic ductular reactions in the absence of injury via macrophage-mediated TWEAK signaling. Proc Natl Acad Sci U S A 2013;110(16):6542–7.

64. Tirnitz-Parker JE, Viebahn CS, Jakubowski A, et al. Tumor necrosis factor-like weak inducer of apoptosis is a mitogen for liver progenitor cells. Hepatology 2010;52(1):291–302.

65. Ochoa B, Syn WK, Delgado I, et al. Hedgehog signaling is critical for normal liver regeneration after partial hepatectomy in mice. Hepatology 2010;51(5):1712–23.

66. Karaca G, Swiderska-Syn M, Xie G, et al. TWEAK/Fn14 signaling is required for liver regeneration after partial hepatectomy in mice. PLoS One 2014;9(1):e83987.

67. Kuramitsu K, Sverdlov DY, Liu SB, et al. Failure of fibrotic liver regeneration in mice is linked to a severe fibrogenic response driven by hepatic progenitor cell activation. Am J Pathol 2013;183(1):182–94.

68. Hautekeete ML, Geerts A. The hepatic stellate (Ito) cell: its role in human liver disease. Virchows Arch 1997;430(3):195–207.

69. Friedman SL, Roll FJ, Boyles J, et al. Hepatic lipocytes: the principal collagen-producing cells of normal rat liver. Proc Natl Acad Sci U S A 1985;82(24):8681–5.

70. Mederacke I, Hsu CC, Troeger JS, et al. Fate tracing reveals hepatic stellate cells as dominant contributors to liver fibrosis independent of its aetiology. Nat Commun 2013;4:2823.

71. Ishikawa T, Factor VM, Marquardt JU, et al. Hepatocyte growth factor/c-met signaling is required for stem-cell-mediated liver regeneration in mice. Hepatology 2012;55(4):1215–26.

72. Kitade M, Factor VM, Andersen JB, et al. Specific fate decisions in adult hepatic progenitor cells driven by MET and EGFR signaling. Genes Dev 2013;27(15):1706–17.

73. Tsai SM, Wang WP. Expression and function of fibroblast growth factor (FGF) 7 during liver regeneration. Cell Physiol Biochem 2011;27(6):641–52.

74. Takase HM, Itoh T, Ino S, et al. FGF7 is a functional niche signal required for stimulation of adult liver progenitor cells that support liver regeneration. Genes Dev 2013;27(2):169–81.

75. Carpino G, Renzi A, Franchitto A, et al. Stem/progenitor cell niches involved in hepatic and biliary regeneration. Stem Cells Int 2016;2016:3658013.

76. Kitade M, Kaji K, Yoshiji H. The relationship between hepatic progenitor cell-mediated liver regeneration and non-parenchymal cells. Hepatol Res 2016;46(12):1187–93.

77. Yin C, Evason KJ, Asahina K, et al. Hepatic stellate cells in liver development, regeneration, and cancer. J Clin Invest 2013;123(5):1902–10.

78. Poisson J, Lemoinne S, Boulanger C, et al. Liver sinusoidal endothelial cells: physiology and role in liver diseases. J Hepatol 2016;66(1):212–27.

79. Ding BS, Cao Z, Lis R, et al. Divergent angiocrine signals from vascular niche balance liver regeneration and fibrosis. Nature 2014;505(7481):97–102.

80. Hu J, Srivastava K, Wieland M, et al. Endothelial cell-derived angiopoietin-2 controls liver regeneration as a spatiotemporal rheostat. Science 2014;343(6169):416–9.

81. Van Hul NK, Abarca-Quinones J, Sempoux C, et al. Relation between liver progenitor cell expansion and extracellular matrix deposition in a CDE-induced murine model of chronic liver injury. Hepatology 2009;49(5):1625–35.

82. Bedossa P, Paradis V. Liver extracellular matrix in health and disease. J Pathol 2003;200(4):504–15.

83. Zhang W, Chen XP, Zhang WG, et al. Hepatic non-parenchymal cells and extracellular matrix participate in oval cell-mediated liver regeneration. World J Gastroenterol 2009;15(5):552–60.

84. Lorenzini S, Bird TG, Boulter L, et al. Characterisation of a stereotypical cellular and extracellular adult liver progenitor cell niche in rodents and diseased human liver. Gut 2010;59(5):645–54.

85. Kaylan KB, Ermilova V, Yada RC, Underhill GH. Combinatorial microenvironmental regulation of liver progenitor differentiation by Notch ligands, TGFbeta, and extracellular matrix. Sci Rep 2016;6:23490.

86. Pi L, Robinson PM, Jorgensen M, et al. Connective tissue growth factor and integrin alphavbeta6: a new pair of regulators critical for ductular reaction and biliary fibrosis in mice. Hepatology 2015;61(2):678–91.

87. Peng ZW, Ikenaga N, Liu SB, et al. Integrin alphavbeta6 critically regulates hepatic progenitor cell function and promotes ductular reaction, fibrosis, and tumorigenesis. Hepatology 2016;63(1):217–32.

88. Waller LP, Deshpande V, Pyrsopoulos N. Hepatocellular carcinoma: a comprehensive review. World J Hepatol 2015;7(26):2648–63.

89. Richardson MM, Jonsson JR, Powell EE, et al. Progressive fibrosis in nonalcoholic steatohepatitis: association with altered regeneration and a ductular reaction. Gastroenterology 2007;133(1):80–90.

90. Roskams T. Liver stem cells and their implication in hepatocellular and cholangiocarcinoma. Oncogene 2006;25(27):3818–22.

91. Komuta M, Govaere O, Vandecaveye V, et al. Histological diversity in cholangiocellular carcinoma reflects the different cholangiocyte phenotypes. Hepatology 2012;55(6):1876–88.

92. Akiba J, Nakashima O, Hattori S, et al. Clinicopathologic analysis of combined hepatocellular-cholangiocarcinoma according to the latest WHO classification. Am J Surg Pathol 2013;37(4):496–505.

93. Yang XR, Xu Y, Yu B, et al. High expression levels of putative hepatic stem/progenitor cell biomarkers related to tumour angiogenesis and poor prognosis of hepatocellular carcinoma. Gut 2010;59(7):953–62.

94. Villanueva A, Alsinet C, Yanger K, et al. Notch signaling is activated in human hepatocellular carcinoma and induces tumor formation in mice. Gastroenterology 2012;143(6):1660–9.e1667.

95. Govaere O, Komuta M, Berkers J, et al. Keratin 19: a key role player in the invasion of human hepatocellular carcinomas. Gut 2014;63(4):674–85.

96. Kim H, Choi GH, Na DC, et al. Human hepatocellular carcinomas with "Stemness"-related marker expression: keratin 19 expression and a poor prognosis. Hepatology 2011;54(5):1707–17.

97. Chen Y, Wong PP, Sjeklocha L, et al. Mature hepatocytes exhibit unexpected plasticity by direct dedifferentiation into liver progenitor cells in culture. Hepatology 2012;55(2):563–74.

Heart Disease and the Liver
Pathologic Evaluation

Anne Knoll Koehne de Gonzalez, MD, Jay H. Lefkowitch, MD*

KEYWORDS

- Liver • Congestive hepatopathy • Cardiac cirrhosis • Fontan
- Acute cardiogenic liver injury

KEY POINTS

- Congestive hepatopathy is progressive liver dysfunction resulting from chronic heart failure.
- MELD-XI scores and liver histology may be used in conjunction to risk-stratify patients for cardiac transplantation.
- After surgical repair of congenital cardiac abnormalities, sequelae of congestive hepatopathy include an increased risk for hepatocellular carcinoma.
- Cardiac medications, including amiodarone and calcium-channel blockers, have been implicated in progressive liver dysfunction.

HISTORICAL PERSPECTIVE

The structural and functional changes that develop in the liver in patients with cardiac disease have intrigued clinicians and pathologists for at least 2 centuries. The microscopic description of the "nutmeg," congested liver in heart failure (**Fig. 1**) is attributed to Kiernan in 1833.[1] Once Kiernan's "lobule" had become firmly entrenched in the conceptual microanatomy of the liver, by the early twentieth century more complete morphologic studies of centrilobular congestion began to emerge,[2] and in 1901, Mallory[3] (of Mallory-Denk body fame) described the features of centrilobular necrosis in autopsy specimens (see **Fig. 1**C). By the 1950s, during the formative years of modern hepatology, the liver in cardiac disease was addressed in publications by 2 of the giants in the field, Dame Professor Sheila Sherlock (The Royal Free Hospital, London, UK) and Professor Hans Popper (The Mount Sinai Medical Center, New York City) (**Fig. 2**),.[4,5] Wallach and Popper[5] examined centrilobular necrosis in individuals with cardiac disease, whereas Sherlock's seminal paper was a correlative study of

Disclosure Statement: The authors have nothing to disclose.
Department of Pathology and Cell Biology, Columbia University, 630 West 168th Street, PH 15 West, Rm 1574, New York, NY 10032-3725, USA
* Corresponding author.
E-mail address: jhl3@cumc.columbia.edu

Gastroenterol Clin N Am 46 (2017) 421–435
http://dx.doi.org/10.1016/j.gtc.2017.01.012
0889-8553/17/© 2017 Elsevier Inc. All rights reserved.

gastro.theclinics.com

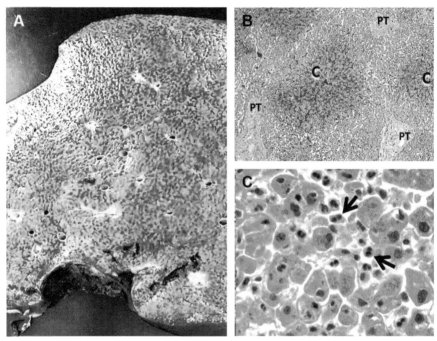

Fig. 1. (*A*) Postmortem example of the classical "nutmeg" liver with centrilobular conges-tion in CH. (*B*) Centrilobular regions (C) show congestion. The liver parenchyma around the portal tracts (PT) is spared (hematoxylin-eosin, original magnification ×25). (*C*) Many cases of CH at postmortem show evidence of associated acute left ventricular dysfunction and centrilobular coagulative necrosis, as seen here. If the patient was sustained for several days with pressor agents, there may also be a neutrophil infiltrate (*arrows*) near the hepa-tocytes with coagulative necrosis (hematoxylin-eosin, original magnification ×400).

serum liver tests, cardiac catheterization results, and hepatic abnormality in a cohort of individuals with cardiac disease of multifactorial cause. Sherlock's clinical cases reflected the general state of medicine in that period: cases of rheumatic heart dis-ease were abundant, and there was a comparatively high number of cases of constrictive pericarditis. Hypertensive heart disease and atherosclerotic cardiovas-cular disease were, as today, also represented in the heart failure study subjects. The hepatic lesions shown in photomicrographs in Professor Sherlock's study remain, even now, some 65 years after publication, representative of the histologic spectrum of "congestive hepatopathy," (**Box 1**) including centrilobular congestion and sinusoidal dilatation, atrophy of liver-cell plates and fibrosis involving centrilobu-lar regions and, later, even portal tracts (**Figs. 3–5**). "Reversed lobulation" was also described in her treatise, the process whereby relatively uninvolved portal tracts come to lie at the centers of hepatic parenchymal units circumscribed peripherally by fibrosis linking central veins. As with other publications of that period and later, the term "cardiac cirrhosis" was often used (while, in fact, a true cirrhosis was not pre-sent morphologically), chiefly because the criteria for cirrhosis were less stringent than those of today. In many instances, the term "cardiac cirrhosis" was used to describe combinations of central-to-central or central-to-portal bridging fibrosis with nodularity due to periportal regenerative hyperplasia or in cases of perivenular fibrosis (cardiac *sclerosis*) with frank nodular regenerative hyperplasia (NRH)[6]

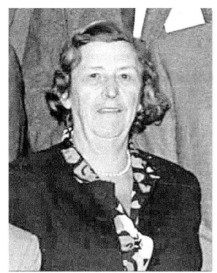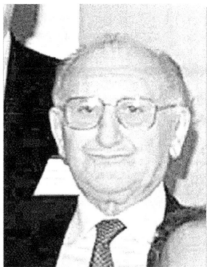

Fig. 2. These giants of hepatology, Professor Dame Sheila Sherlock (*left*) and Professor Hans Popper (*right*), of London, UK and New York City, respectively, contributed seminal papers on cardiac hepatopathy in the 1950s. Photographs taken in 1988 at a postgraduate conference on liver pathology at Columbia University Medical Center, New York, New York. (*Courtesy of* Charles Manley, New York, NY.)

(**Fig. 6**). Today, because of the increased prevalence of patients with ischemic and other forms of late stage cardiomyopathy, many await cardiac transplantation, and clinical concerns are directed to the state of hepatic fibrosis in the event that combined heart-liver transplantation may be required.[7]

Box 1
Hepatic morphology in cardiac hepatopathy

Major lesions
   Centrilobular congestion
   Centrilobular sinusoidal dilatation
   Hepatocyte atrophy
   Perivenular/perisinusoidal fibrosis ("cardiac sclerosis")
   Periportal fibrosis
   Bridging fibrosis (central-central; central-portal)
   Periportal nodularity (regenerative hyperplasia)
   Cirrhosis

Nodular lesions
   Nodular regenerative hyperplasia
   Focal nodular hyperplasia-like
   Hepatocellular adenoma-like
   Hepatocellular carcinoma
   Combined hepatocellular-cholangiocarcinoma

Other
   Steatosis; steatohepatitis
   Glycogen nuclei
   Extramedullary hematopoiesis (especially megakaryocytosis)
   Centrilobular cholestasis (typically minimal/mild)

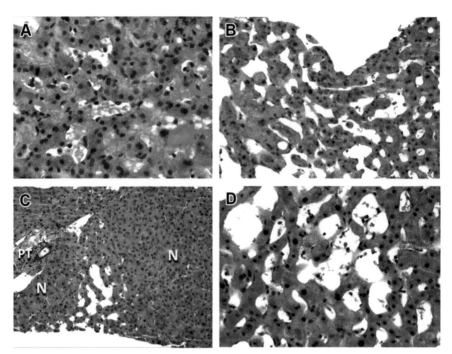

Fig. 3. Major histopathologic lesions in CH include centrilobular sinusoidal congestion (*A*), centrilobular sinusoidal dilatation (*B*), variable degrees of periportal hepatocyte regenerative hyperplasia, rendering nodularity (*C*), and atrophy of centrilobular liver-cell plates (*D*). (*A–D*, hematoxylin-eosin, original magnification ×200). N, nodule.

PATHOLOGIC HEPATIC ABNORMALITIES IN HEART FAILURE

Heart failure occurs when clinical symptoms result from an increase in the work performed by the heart in order to maintain circulation throughout the body. This may occur acutely, as cardiogenic shock, with damage due to sudden lack of perfusion, such as in cases of myocardial infarction, acute decompensation of chronic heart failure, infection/sepsis, or pulmonary embolism. The preferred term for damage to the liver arising in these cases of left-sided or forward failure is acute cardiogenic liver injury (ACLI),[8–10] sometimes referred to as "ischemic hepatitis" or "hypoxic hepatitis."[11,12] In ACLI, the pattern of injury seen in the liver is due to sudden lack of perfusion. Without sufficient oxygen, hepatocytes surrounding the central regions (acinar zone 3), which have the lowest baseline oxygen perfusion, are most affected and show features of coagulative necrosis of centrilobular hepatocytes (see **Fig. 1**). Intrasinusoidal hemorrhage may develop in tandem due to ischemic damage if the endothelium. Early (ie, <24 hours' duration) ischemic centrilobular coagulative necrosis is usually not accompanied by significant inflammation.[4,13] However, if the patient received pressor support, several days after the acute cardiac insult there may be an influx of neutrophils into the affected centrilobular regions[14] (see **Fig. 1**C).

Heart failure may also be chronic; there may be no acute insult, but a slow accumulation of damage. In the liver, these changes are associated with hepatic venous congestion, often called "congestive hepatopathy" (CH), resulting from increased central venous pressure due to prolonged right heart failure (sometimes referred to as "backward failure"), which can be seen in congestive heart failure, congenital heart

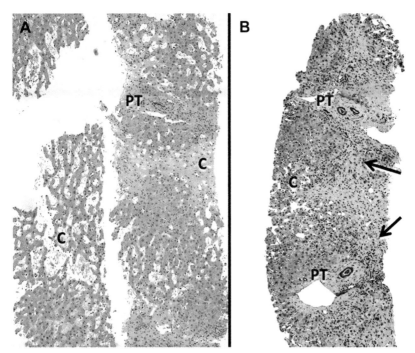

Fig. 4. Long-term CH results in progressive fibrosis emanating from centrilobular regions, with bridging fibrosis linking to other central veins (C) or to portal tracts (PT). (*A*) Needle liver biopsy from patient with chronic cardiac disease shows cardiac sclerosis involving centrilobular region in the core at right (C); note that the fibrosis may be heterogeneous, as in the nonfibrotic centrilobular region (C) seen in the core at left. (*B*) Needle liver biopsy with more advanced fibrosis, in this field bridging from the central vein (C) to adjacent portal tracts (PT). (*A, B,* hematoxylin-eosin, original magnification ×100).

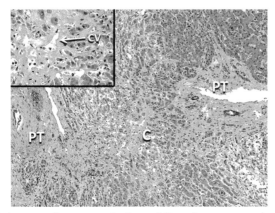

Fig. 5. The liver in longstanding congestive heart failure shows progressive fibrosis involving centrilobular regions (C), perisinusoidal spaces, and portal tracts (PT). Inset: Perivenular fibrosis extends outward into perisinusoidal spaces of Disse. (hematoxylin-eosin, original magnification ×25; inset, original magnification ×200). CV, central vein.

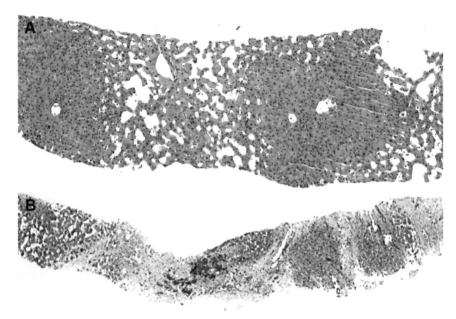

Fig. 6. Architectural changes in cardiac hepatopathy may include NRH (*A*) to cirrhosis with severe bridging fibrosis and regional nodularity (*B*). In the example of NRH shown in (*A*), note the centrilobular sinusoidal dilatation and liver-cell plate atrophy, with no obvious fibrosis. The nodules at left and right typically emerge from regenerative hyperplasia of periportal liver parenchyma. (*A*: hematoxylin-eosin, original magnification ×100; *B*: Masson trichrome, original magnification ×25).

disease, and cor pulmonale, among others. The histologic features of chronic cardiac failure can be summarized by the term "chronic venous outflow obstruction" (or "chronic HVOO"). The histopathology of chronic HVOO includes centrilobular congestion and sinusoidal dilatation, atrophy of centrilobular hepatocyte plates (cords), and variable degrees of perivenular, perisinusoidal, and bridging fibrosis accompanied by regenerative hyperplasia emerging from periportal regions[4,13,14] (see **Fig. 5**). Fibrosis surrounding centrilobular veins and within perisinusoidal spaces is referred to as "cardiac sclerosis" (**Fig. 7**); this term should not be equated with "cardiac cirrhosis," which is a relatively uncommon phenomenon in comparison to cardiac sclerosis. The microscopic distribution of these changes, particularly centrilobular fibrosis, is notable for its heterogeneity, as demonstrated in explant livers from Budd-Chiari patients.[15–17] Late in progressive CH associated with extensive centrilobular fibrosis, portal tracts may demonstrate ductular reaction as well as periportal fibrosis, which may be mistaken for the changes of biliary tract obstruction[18] (**Fig. 8**). Immunohistochemical staining for cytokeratin 7 is useful diagnostically for demonstrating this ductular reaction and its microanatomic relationship to centrilobular regions. The CK7 immunostain may also demonstrate cytoplasmic positivity of centrilobular hepatocytes (see **Fig. 6**C), presumed to be an adaptive "metaplastic" response.[19]

Nevertheless, acute and chronic heart failure are not mutually exclusive, and acute ischemic damage to the liver may be compounded by pre-existing changes of CH due to chronic heart failure. Indeed, some investigators[10,20–24] suggest that little liver damage accrues from an acute ischemic insult unless there is pre-existing cardiac disease with increased central venous pressure.

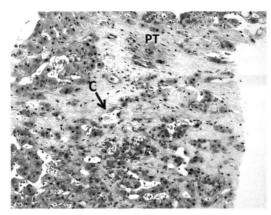

Fig. 7. Cardiac sclerosis. This term refers to the localization of fibrosis surrounding central veins (C) and extending into perisinusoidal spaces in individuals with chronic cardiac disease. Note that the fibrosis is both perisinusoidal, surrounding atrophic liver-cell plates, and "replacing" (see region above the central vein) where hepatocyte dropout previously occurred. In the case depicted here, fibrosis has linked to a nearby portal tract (PT). (Masson trichrome, original magnification ×200).

CLINICAL LIVER ABNORMALITIES IN HEART FAILURE

Laboratory abnormalities in liver tests in ACLI reflect the changes caused by acute ischemic necrosis of hepatocytes, that is, increases in transaminases (aspartate and alanine aminotransferases: AST and ALT) and lactate dehydrogenase (LDH), with elevations up to 10 to 20 times the upper limit of normal or greater.[8–10,25] These elevations generally peak at 1 to 3 days after the acute insult, returning to the normal range in 7 to 10 days if cardiac function resolves. It should be noted that the ALT:LDH ratio is nearly always less than 1.5 in ACLI, whereas with other causes of acute hepatitis, it is generally higher.[9,26,27] There may be an associated jaundice, with concomitant increase in serum bilirubin, with accompanying lesser elevations of alkaline phosphatase and gamma-glutamyl transpeptidase (GGT); derangements in coagulation factors may also be seen.[8–10,20,28]

In ACLI, a retrospective analysis of the SURVIVE (The Survival of Patients With Acute Heart Failure in Need of Intravenous Inotropic Support) trial, a multicenter trial comparing levosimendan and dobutamine in acutely decompensated heart failure patients, found that abnormal transaminases were correlated with greater 31-day and 180 day mortality, whereas elevations in alkaline phosphatase were correlated with greater 180-day mortality (but not 31-day mortality); serum bilirubin was not measured in this trial.[29] Similar results were seen in the RELAX-AHF (Relaxin in Acute Heart Failure) trial, where it was found that an increase of 20% or greater in ALT correlated with increased all-cause 180-day mortality.[30]

In chronic CH at physical examination, the liver may be enlarged and firm, reflecting congestion, and may also be tender. Jaundice is uncommon but may be seen. An increase in laboratory values associated with cholestasis is often seen, including increased alkaline phosphatase and GGT, with or without a mild increase in total bilirubin.[8,9,31,32] Interestingly, an assessment of liver function tests in heart failure patients in the CHARM (Candesartan in Heart Failure: Assessment of Reduction in Mortality and Morbidity) program found that bilirubin increases were significantly correlated with volume overload and were not seen in euvolemic heart failure patients.[10,33] The

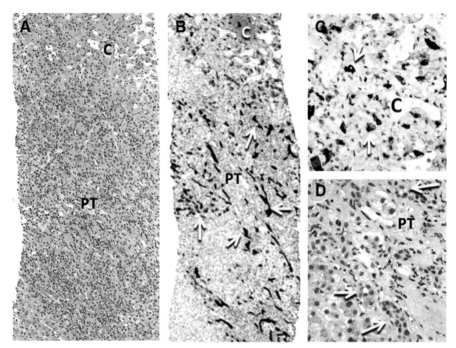

Fig. 8. Features of biliary obstruction in CH. Certain cases of CH may be associated with a sufficiently vigorous periportal ductular reaction (from activated hepatic progenitor cells) as to be mistaken for biliary tract obstruction. (*A*) At low power, the predominant feature appears to be the numerous bile ductular structures emerging from the periportal region near the portal tract (PT) and migrating toward the central vein (C) (hematoxylin-eosin, original magnification ×100). (*B*) Immunostain for cytokeratin 7 demonstrates numerous bile ductular structures (*arrows*) emanating from near the portal tract (PT) (Specific immunoperoxidase for cytokeratin 7, original magnification ×100). C, central vein. (*C*) Cytokeratin 7 also demonstrates many centrilobular hepatocytes with positive cytoplasm (*arrows*) (Specific immunoperoxidase for cytokeratin 7, original magnification ×200). (*D*) Higher magnification demonstrates the periportal ductular reaction (*arrows*) surrounding the portal tract (PT) (hematoxylin-eosin, original magnification ×200).

mechanism behind the increase in "cholestatic" laboratory measurements (alkaline phosphatase, GGT, and bilirubin) is thought to be due to the increased pressure in the centrally congested sinusoids compressing the bile canaliculi and small ductules, and preventing normal bile flow toward the portal region.[29] Modest elevations of transaminases (up to 2–3 times the upper limit of normal) may also be seen.[8,13] As a result of decreased hepatic synthetic function, serum albumin may be mildly decreased, while prothrombin time may be mildly increased[25]; however, because a large proportion of patients with chronic heart failure are undergoing anticoagulant therapy, laboratory measurements of these parameters may not be helpful.

Analysis of chronic heart failure patients in the CHARM program found that increased bilirubin was the strongest predictor for all-cause mortality,[33] as did a retrospective data analysis of the placebo arm of patients in the EVEREST (Efficacy of Vasopressin Antagonism in Heart Failure Outcome Study With Tolvaptan) trial, which showed increased mortality in patients with increased bilirubin and/or decreased albumin measurements.[31] At least 4 other studies have shown that GGT and bilirubin are prognostic factors in predicting mortality in patients with chronic heart failure.[32,34–36]

Bilirubin is therefore logically an important feature in the model for end-stage liver dysfunction (MELD) score, a composite measure of liver function, currently used in waitlist stratification for liver transplantation. The MELD score is based on laboratory measurements of total bilirubin, creatinine, and international normalized ratio (INR). MELD scoring has now been shown to be a useful predictor of postoperative mortality in cirrhotic patients[37] as well as heart transplant recipients.[38] However, as mentioned above, heart failure patients are often anticoagulated; in these cases, the artificial increase in the INR measurement renders the traditional MELD score less useful. Therefore, a modified MELD score, the MELD-XI (eXcluding INR), has been validated as highly correlated with MELD's predictive prognostic utility in a heart failure cohort requiring ventricular assist devices (VADs).[39] MELD-XI has now been shown to be useful at predicting mortality in heart failure patients[40,41] as well as postoperative mortality after the Fontan procedure,[42] and orthotopic heart transplantation in pediatric[43] and adult patients.[36,44]

HISTOPATHOLOGIC SCORING SYSTEMS FOR THE LIVER IN INDIVIDUALS WITH HEART FAILURE

The definitive treatment of heart failure is cardiac transplantation; when organs are not available, or in cases where recovery is possible, VAD support may be used as a temporizing measure. As the studies mentioned above show, liver dysfunction is implicated in mortality in patients with heart failure, including those treated with VADs and transplant. Historically, it has been thought that the early changes of CH might be reversible with treatment of the underlying cardiac dysfunction, while more advanced fibrosis was a relative contraindication to transplantation,[45] making a scoring system evaluating the extent of both liver dysfunction and fibrosis desirable.

However, biopsy is generally needed to assess liver fibrosis; a study by Gelow and colleagues[46] demonstrated that although liver test abnormalities were associated with hepatic fibrosis, the severity of the abnormality did not predict the extent of the fibrosis, and imaging was also insufficient to predict the extent of fibrosis.

Louie and colleagues[15] analyzed a series of liver biopsy (precardiac transplant) and explant specimens (combined heart-liver transplants), along with outcome data for these patients. In the biopsy cohort, pretransplant MELD scores were not found to be significantly associated with the presence of fibrosis.

In another series of liver biopsies in 42 patients with heart failure, Dai and colleagues[16] showed a correlation between the histologic features of centrilobular fibrosis, hepatocyte atrophy, and sinusoidal dilatation, and right atrial pressure, and were able to correlate the fibrosis score with the severity of right atrial and ventricular dilatation.

Farr and colleagues[47] have now proposed a scoring system that incorporates both a standard histologic fibrosis score (0–4) on biopsy and an MELD-XI score [(fibrosis + 1) $\times$ MELD-XI] for outcome prediction in patients with suspected liver dysfunction undergoing workup for heart transplant. A liver risk score of 45 or greater was significantly associated with a greater risk of death at 1 year after transplant.[47]

It must also be noted that several recent papers have questioned the degree to which hepatic fibrosis is irreversible. Normalization of liver test abnormalities has been reported after cardiac transplant.[38,48] Furthermore, Crespo-Leiro and colleagues[49] report a case of apparent regression of cirrhosis following cardiac transplant, and there have been reports of regression of fibrosis due to noncardiac causes following treatment.[50,51]

CONGENITAL HEART DISEASE, THE FONTAN PROCEDURE, AND THE LIVER

The impact of congenital heart disease on hepatic morphology is dependent on the relative severity of left- versus right-sided cardiac impairment and associated respective hypoxic liver injury (centrilobular necrosis) versus CH (centrilobular congestion, hepatocyte atrophy, perisinusoidal fibrosis) as well as the time frame (acute vs chronic cardiac decompensation)[52]. Several primary liver diseases are linked to congenital heart disease, including Alagille syndrome (syndromic paucity of intrahepatic bile ducts), which has associations with pulmonic stenosis and tetralogy of Fallot,[53] and extrahepatic biliary atresia, which is associated with multiorgan congenital anomalies, including a/polysplenia and congenital heart disease (pulmonic stenosis, ventricular septal defect, atrial septal defect, and others).[54] Congenital heart diseases with univentricular physiology and right ventricular functional overload (eg, hypoplastic left heart syndrome [HLHS], tricuspid atresia [TA]) are more likely to cause morphologic changes of HVOO, such as centrilobular sinusoidal congestion and dilatation, hepatocellular atrophy, and eventually, fibrosis.

The Fontan procedure (including the original atriopulmonary connection and variants such as total cavopulmonary connection) was developed some 40 years ago as a palliative procedure for single ventricle physiology as seen in TA and HLHS. The altered pulmonary and hepatic vascular pressures and morbidity and mortality of the Fontan procedure have been addressed in many publications.[41,55–57] High central venous pressure, low cardiac output (due to diminished cardiac preload and elevated systemic artery resistance), and mild but significant hypoxia are recognized complications post-Fontan, with ramifications for individuals who underwent the procedure and have now reached young adulthood. Hepatic fibrosis, cirrhosis, and mass lesions are important long-term complications that are now recognized in these patients. Hepatic fibrosis increases over time following Fontan surgery, and the liver stiffness can be evaluated by elastography.[58,59]

A recent study of 74 needle liver biopsies from subjects who had undergone Fontan procedure comprehensively examined the degree and location of fibrosis and other histologic lesions as well as the quantitative percentage of collagen deposition by Sirius red staining and image analysis.[60] The investigators showed centrilobular fibrosis in 100% and some degree of portal fibrosis in 93%. The investigators founds that few clinical or laboratory data could be correlated with the histologic data, although high-grade fibrosis was associated with prolonged prothrombin time/INR, and elevated serum alkaline phosphatase was associated with advanced portal fibrosis (METAVIR 3–4).

From the standpoint of hepatic abnormality and potential sequelae, Fontan patients resemble those with chronic HVOO, such as seen in Budd-Chiari syndrome. Hepatic masses, including hepatocellular adenomas, focal nodular hyperplasia-like masses, and hepatocellular carcinomas, may arise in this setting and are concerning for the long-term follow-up of Fontan patients.[55,61–66] In the histologic evaluation of these masses, particularly in differentiating adenomas from focal nodular hyperplasia (FNH)-like lesions, immunohistochemical stains play an important role.[66]

CARDIAC MEDICATIONS, NONALCOHOLIC FATTY LIVER DISEASE, AND LIVER DISEASE IN THE CARDIAC PATIENT

Drug-induced liver injury due to medications used in the treatment of heart disease is an uncommon complication and usually can be readily distinguished histologically from the typical changes of "cardiac hepatopathy." Calcium channel blocking agents nifedipine and diltiazem have been reported as causes of elevations of serum aminotransferases and bilirubin and features of idiopathic/idiosyncratic hepatocellular

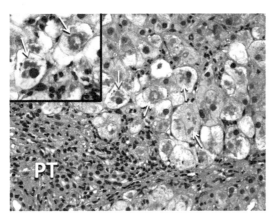

Fig. 9. Amiodarone hepatotoxicity. Amiodarone liver injury causes steatohepatitis (with or without steatosis) with a periportal predilection (in contrast to classical alcoholic or nonalcoholic steatohepatitis, which shows preferential centrilobular involvement). In this example, the portal tract shows chronic inflammation, and periportal hepatocytes are ballooned and contain numerous Mallory-Denk bodies (*arrows*). Inset: higher magnification of the intra-hepatocellular Mallory-Denk bodies (*arrows*). (hematoxylin-eosin, original magnification ×200; inset, original magnification ×400).

and/or cholestatic injury. In addition, histologic features resembling alcoholic steatohepatitis have also been described for both agents,[67,68] including the presence of Mallory-Denk bodies. Diltiazem has also resulted in hepatitis with granulomas.[69] Amiodarone may result in 2 hepatic lesions: phospholipidosis (aggregates of phospholipids within sinusoidal Kupffer cells) and Mallory-Denk bodies, with or without fat.[70,71] The periportal location of Mallory-Denk bodies is diagnostically important (**Fig. 9**) for distinction from changes of typical nonalcoholic fatty liver disease (NAFLD), which are centrilobular.

Many individuals with atherosclerotic cardiovascular disease and chronic cardiac ischemia have common risk factors that are also associated with NAFLD, namely, obesity, diabetes, insulin resistance, hypertension, metabolic syndrome, and dyslipidemia.[72] Histopathologic examination for macrovesicular steatosis and/or steatohepatitis in centrilobular regions should therefore be included in the routine evaluation of liver specimens in subjects with cardiac disease. The primary involvement of centrilobular regions (acinar zone 3) in both CH and NAFLD may represent an etiopathogenetic challenge for the pathologist, particularly when centrilobular and perisinusoidal fibrosis are present, but steatosis is minimal or absent (as may be seen in late NAFLD with progressive fibrosis). In most cases of active steatohepatitis, however, there are sufficiently distinctive hepatocyte ballooning and associated inflammation to distinguish it from the typical fibrosing and congestive changes of cardiac disease.

SUMMARY

The effects of cardiac disease on the liver have been investigated for several centuries and the clinical as well as pathologic hallmarks of acute and chronic cardiac decompensation are now well described. The landmark hepatic lesions in CH were comprehensively described in 1951 by Sherlock. The histologic distinctions between ACLI with centrilobular coagulative necrosis versus chronic congestive heart failure (with centrilobular congestion, sinusoidal dilatation, and perivenular fibrosis) remain important parameters for correlating clinical findings, serum liver tests, and abnormal hepatic and cardiac physiology in a given patient. This review also discusses several potential scoring systems for hepatic fibrosis in the setting of cardiac disease, a topic of concern for patients who are under consideration for either a heart or a combined heart-liver transplant.

REFERENCES

1. Kiernan F. The Anatomy and Physiology of the Liver. Paper presented at: Philosophical Transactions of the Royal Society of London. London, January 1, 1833.
2. Lambert RA, Allison BR. Types of lesion in chronic passive congestion of the liver. Bull Johns Hopkins Hosp 1916;27:350–6.
3. Mallory FB. Necroses of the liver. J Med Res 1901;6(1):264–80, 267.
4. Sherlock S. The liver in heart failure; relation of anatomical, functional, and circulatory changes. Br Heart J 1951;13(3):273–93.
5. Wallach HF, Popper H. Central necrosis of the liver. AMA Arch Pathol 1950;49(1): 33–42, illust.
6. Reshamwala PA, Kleiner DE, Heller T. Nodular regenerative hyperplasia: not all nodules are created equal. Hepatology 2006;44(1):7–14.
7. Reich HJ, Awad M, Ruzza A, et al. Combined heart and liver transplantation: the Cedars-Sinai experience. Transplant Proc 2015;47(9):2722–6.
8. Cagli K, Basar FN, Tok D, et al. How to interpret liver function tests in heart failure patients? Turkish J Gastroenterol 2015;26(3):197–203.
9. Alvarez AM, Mukherjee D. Liver abnormalities in cardiac diseases and heart failure. Int J Angiol 2011;20(3):135–42.
10. Samsky MD, Patel CB, DeWald TA, et al. Cardiohepatic interactions in heart failure: an overview and clinical implications. J Am Coll Cardiol 2013;61(24): 2397–405.
11. Tapper EB, Sengupta N, Bonder A. The incidence and outcomes of ischemic hepatitis: a systematic review with meta-analysis. Am J Med 2015;128(12): 1314–21.
12. Waseem N, Chen PH. Hypoxic hepatitis: a review and clinical update. J Clin Transl Hepatol 2016;4(3):263–8.
13. Giallourakis CC, Rosenberg PM, Friedman LS. The liver in heart failure. Clin Liver Dis 2002;6(4):947–67, viii-ix.
14. Lefkowitch JH, Mendez L. Morphologic features of hepatic injury in cardiac disease and shock. J Hepatol 1986;2(3):313–27.
15. Louie CY, Pham MX, Daugherty TJ, et al. The liver in heart failure: a biopsy and explant series of the histopathologic and laboratory findings with a particular focus on pre-cardiac transplant evaluation. Mod Pathol 2015;28(7):932–43.
16. Dai DF, Swanson PE, Krieger EV, et al. Congestive hepatic fibrosis score: a novel histologic assessment of clinical severity. Mod Pathol 2014;27(12):1552–8.
17. Cazals-Hatem D, Vilgrain V, Genin P, et al. Arterial and portal circulation and parenchymal changes in Budd-Chiari syndrome: a study in 17 explanted livers. Hepatology 2003;37(3):510–9.
18. Kakar S, Batts KP, Poterucha JJ, et al. Histologic changes mimicking biliary disease in liver biopsies with venous outflow impairment. Mod Pathol 2004;17(7): 874–8.
19. Pai RK, Hart JA. Aberrant expression of cytokeratin 7 in perivenular hepatocytes correlates with a cholestatic chemistry profile in patients with heart failure. Mod Pathol 2010;23(12):1650–6.
20. Henrion J. Hypoxic hepatitis. Liver Int 2012;32(7):1039–52.

21. Henrion J, Descamps O, Luwaert R, et al. Hypoxic hepatitis in patients with cardiac failure: incidence in a coronary care unit and measurement of hepatic blood flow. J Hepatol 1994;21(5):696–703.
22. Henrion J, Schapira M, Luwaert R, et al. Hypoxic hepatitis: clinical and hemodynamic study in 142 consecutive cases. Medicine 2003;82(6):392–406.
23. Seeto RK, Fenn B, Rockey DC. Ischemic hepatitis: clinical presentation and pathogenesis. Am J Med 2000;109(2):109–13.
24. Fuhrmann V, Kneidinger N, Herkner H, et al. Hypoxic hepatitis: underlying conditions and risk factors for mortality in critically ill patients. Intensive Care Med 2009;35(8):1397–405.
25. Myers RP, Cerini R, Sayegh R, et al. Cardiac hepatopathy: clinical, hemodynamic, and histologic characteristics and correlations. Hepatology 2003;37(2):393–400.
26. Gitlin N, Serio KM. Ischemic hepatitis: widening horizons. Am J Gastroenterol 1992;87(7):831–6.
27. Cassidy WM, Reynolds TB. Serum lactic dehydrogenase in the differential diagnosis of acute hepatocellular injury. J Clin Gastroenterol 1994;19(2):118–21.
28. Naschitz JE, Yeshurun D, Shahar J. Cardiogenic hepatorenal syndrome. Angiology 1990;41(11):893–900.
29. Nikolaou M, Parissis J, Yilmaz MB, et al. Liver function abnormalities, clinical profile, and outcome in acute decompensated heart failure. Eur Heart J 2013;34(10):742–9.
30. Metra M, Cotter G, Davison BA, et al. Effect of serelaxin on cardiac, renal, and hepatic biomarkers in the Relaxin in Acute Heart Failure (RELAX-AHF) development program: correlation with outcomes. J Am Coll Cardiol 2013;61(2):196–206.
31. Ambrosy AP, Vaduganathan M, Huffman MD, et al. Clinical course and predictive value of liver function tests in patients hospitalized for worsening heart failure with reduced ejection fraction: an analysis of the EVEREST trial. Eur J Heart Fail 2012;14(3):302–11.
32. Poelzl G, Eberl C, Achrainer H, et al. Prevalence and prognostic significance of elevated gamma-glutamyltransferase in chronic heart failure. Circ Heart Fail 2009;2(4):294–302.
33. Allen LA, Felker GM, Pocock S, et al. Liver function abnormalities and outcome in patients with chronic heart failure: data from the Candesartan in Heart Failure: assessment of Reduction in Mortality and Morbidity (CHARM) program. Eur J Heart Fail 2009;11(2):170–7.
34. Poelzl G, Ess M, Mussner-Seeber C, et al. Liver dysfunction in chronic heart failure: prevalence, characteristics and prognostic significance. Eur J Clin Invest 2012;42(2):153–63.
35. Ruttmann E, Brant LJ, Concin H, et al. Gamma-glutamyltransferase as a risk factor for cardiovascular disease mortality: an epidemiological investigation in a cohort of 163,944 Austrian adults. Circulation 2005;112(14):2130–7.
36. Szygula-Jurkiewicz B, Zakliczynski M, Andrejczuk M, et al. The model for end-stage liver disease (MELD) can predict outcomes in ambulatory patients with advanced heart failure who have been referred for cardiac transplantation evaluation. Kardiochir Torakochirurgia Pol 2014;11(2):178–81.
37. Teh SH, Nagorney DM, Stevens SR, et al. Risk factors for mortality after surgery in patients with cirrhosis. Gastroenterology 2007;132(4):1261–9.
38. Chokshi A, Cheema FH, Schaefle KJ, et al. Hepatic dysfunction and survival after orthotopic heart transplantation: application of the MELD scoring system for outcome prediction. J Heart Lung Transplant 2012;31(6):591–600.

39. Yang JA, Kato TS, Shulman BP, et al. Liver dysfunction as a predictor of outcomes in patients with advanced heart failure requiring ventricular assist device support: use of the model of end-stage liver disease (MELD) and MELD eXcluding INR (MELD-XI) scoring system. J Heart Lung Transplant 2012;31(6):601–10.

40. Kim MS, Kato TS, Farr M, et al. Hepatic dysfunction in ambulatory patients with heart failure: application of the MELD scoring system for outcome prediction. J Am Coll Cardiol 2013;61(22):2253–61.

41. Abe S, Yoshihisa A, Takiguchi M, et al. Liver dysfunction assessed by model for end-stage liver disease excluding INR (MELD-XI) scoring system predicts adverse prognosis in heart failure. PLoS One 2014;9(6):e100618.

42. Assenza GE, Graham DA, Landzberg MJ, et al. MELD-XI score and cardiac mortality or transplantation in patients after Fontan surgery. Heart 2013;99(7):491–6.

43. Grimm JC, Magruder JT, Do N, et al. Modified model for end-stage liver disease eXcluding INR (MELD-XI) score predicts early death after pediatric heart transplantation. Ann Thorac Surg 2016;101(2):730–5.

44. Deo SV, Al-Kindi SG, Altarabsheh SE, et al. Model for end-stage liver disease excluding international normalized ratio (MELD-XI) score predicts heart transplant outcomes: evidence from the registry of the United Network for organ sharing. J Heart Lung Transplant 2016;35(2):222–7.

45. Hsu RB, Chang CI, Lin FY, et al. Heart transplantation in patients with liver cirrhosis. Eur J Cardiothorac Surg 2008;34(2):307–12.

46. Gelow JM, Desai AS, Hochberg CP, et al. Clinical predictors of hepatic fibrosis in chronic advanced heart failure. Circ Heart Fail 2010;3(1):59–64.

47. Farr M, Mitchell J, Lippel M, et al. Combination of liver biopsy with MELD-XI scores for post-transplant outcome prediction in patients with advanced heart failure and suspected liver dysfunction. J Heart Lung Transplant 2015;34(7):873–82.

48. Dichtl W, Vogel W, Dunst KM, et al. Cardiac hepatopathy before and after heart transplantation. Transpl Int 2005;18(6):697–702.

49. Crespo-Leiro MG, Robles O, Paniagua MJ, et al. Reversal of cardiac cirrhosis following orthotopic heart transplantation. Am J Transplant 2008;8(6):1336–9.

50. Wanless IR, Nakashima E, Sherman M. Regression of human cirrhosis. Morphologic features and the genesis of incomplete septal cirrhosis. Arch Pathol Lab Med 2000;124(11):1599–607.

51. Serpaggi J, Carnot F, Nalpas B, et al. Direct and indirect evidence for the reversibility of cirrhosis. Hum Pathol 2006;37(12):1519–26.

52. Moller S, Bernardi M. Interactions of the heart and the liver. Eur Heart J 2013;34(36):2804–11.

53. Hartley JL, Gissen P, Kelly DA. Alagille syndrome and other hereditary causes of cholestasis. Clin Liver Dis 2013;17(2):279–300.

54. Guttman OR, Roberts EA, Schreiber RA, et al. Biliary atresia with associated structural malformations in Canadian infants. Liver Int 2011;31(10):1485–93.

55. Ohuchi H. Adult patients with Fontan circulation: what we know and how to manage adults with Fontan circulation? J Cardiol 2016;68(3):181–9.

56. Pundi K, Pundi KN, Kamath PS, et al. Liver disease in patients after the Fontan operation. Am J Cardiol 2016;117(3):456–60.

57. Wu FM, Ukomadu C, Odze RD, et al. Liver disease in the patient with Fontan circulation. Congenit Heart Dis 2011;6(3):190–201.

58. DiPaola FW, Schumacher KR, Goldberg CS, et al. Effect of Fontan operation on liver stiffness in children with single ventricle physiology. Eur Radiol 2016. [Epub ahead of print].

59. Poterucha JT, Venkatesh SK, Novak JL, et al. Liver nodules after the Fontan operation: role of magnetic resonance elastography. Tex Heart Inst J 2015;42(4): 389–92.

60. Surrey LF, Russo P, Rychik J, et al. Prevalence and characterization of fibrosis in surveillance liver biopsies of patients with Fontan circulation. Hum Pathol 2016; 57:106–15.

61. Ghaferi AA, Hutchins GM. Progression of liver pathology in patients undergoing the Fontan procedure: chronic passive congestion, cardiac cirrhosis, hepatic adenoma, and hepatocellular carcinoma. J Thorac Cardiovasc Surg 2005;129(6): 1348–52.

62. Asrani SK, Warnes CA, Kamath PS. Hepatocellular carcinoma after the Fontan procedure. N Engl J Med 2013;368(18):1756–7.

63. Elder RW, Parekh S, Book WM. More on hepatocellular carcinoma after the Fontan procedure. N Engl J Med 2013;369(5):490.

64. Josephus Jitta D, Wagenaar LJ, Mulder BJ, et al. Three cases of hepatocellular carcinoma in Fontan patients: review of the literature and suggestions for hepatic screening. Int J Cardiol 2016;206:21–6.

65. Bryant T, Ahmad Z, Millward-Sadler H, et al. Arterialised hepatic nodules in the Fontan circulation: hepatico-cardiac interactions. Int J Cardiol 2011;151(3): 268–72.

66. Sempoux C, Paradis V, Komuta M, et al. Hepatocellular nodules expressing markers of hepatocellular adenomas in Budd-Chiari syndrome and other rare hepatic vascular disorders. J Hepatol 2015;63(5):1173–80.

67. Babany G, Uzzan F, Larrey D, et al. Alcoholic-like liver lesions induced by nifedipine. J Hepatol 1989;9(2):252–5.

68. Beaugrand M, Poupon R, Levy VG, et al. Hepatic lesions due to perhexiline maleate. Gastroenterol Clin Biol 1978;2:579–88.

69. Toft E, Vyberg M, Therkelsen K. Diltiazem-induced granulomatous hepatitis. Histopathology 1991;18(5):474–5.

70. Lewis JH, Ranard RC, Caruso A, et al. Amiodarone hepatotoxicity: prevalence and clinicopathologic correlations among 104 patients. Hepatology 1989;9(5): 679–85.

71. Lewis JH, Mullick F, Ishak KG, et al. Histopathologic analysis of suspected amiodarone hepatotoxicity. Hum Pathol 1990;21(1):59–67.

72. Targher G, Arcaro G. Non-alcoholic fatty liver disease and increased risk of cardiovascular disease. Atherosclerosis 2007;191(2):235–40.

Index

Note: Page numbers of article titles are in **boldface** type.

A

Abacavir. *See* Antiretroviral therapy.
ABCC2 gene, 240
N-Acetylglutamate synthase deficiency, 247
Adenomas, hepatocellular, **253–272**
Adenomatosis, 266
Adrenoleukodystrophy, 247
Aglycogenosis, 241
AIH. *See* Autoimmune hepatitis.
Alagille syndrome, 236, 430
Alanine transaminase, in NAFLD, 218
ALDOB gene, 244
Aldolase A deficiency, 243
ALK gene, 211
Alkaline phosphatase, in AIH overlap syndromes, 348
Alpha-1-antitrypsin deficiency, 237
Alpha-fetoprotein, in HCC, 313
Amino acid metabolic disorders, 244–245
Amprenavir. *See* Antiretroviral therapy.
Amyloid A, in HCAs, 259
Andersen disease, 242
Antibody-mediated rejection, after liver transplantation, **297–309**
Antimitochondrial antibodies, in AIH overlap syndromes, 348, 351–352
Antioxidants, for NAFLD, 226
Antiretroviral therapy, liver pathology in, 332–338
Arginase-1, in HCC, 312, 314–316
Arginase deficiency, 247
Arginosuccinate lyase deficiency, 247
ART. *See* Antiretroviral therapy.
Atazanavir. *See* Antiretroviral therapy.
ATP7B gene, 248
Autochthonous hepatitis E, 400–401, 403
Autoimmune hepatitis, 290
    overlap syndromes, **345–364**
        clinical indications of, 348–349
        diagnosis of, 349–353
        phenotypes of, 346–348
        treatment of, 353–358
Azathioprine, for AIH overlap syndromes, 355–358

Gastroenterol Clin N Am 46 (2017) 437–447
http://dx.doi.org/10.1016/S0889-8553(17)30038-9
0889-8553/17

Printed and bound by CPI Group (UK) Ltd, Croydon, CR0 4YY

07/10/2024

01040504-0009